Neurons, Networks, and Motor Behavior

edited by Paul S. G. Stein,
Sten Grillner, Allen I. Selverston,
and Douglas G. Stuart

Neurons, Networks, and Motor Behavior

A Bradford Book
The MIT Press
Cambridge, Massachusetts
London, England

© 1997 Massachusetts Institute of Technology
All rights reserved. No part of this book may be reproduced in any form by any electronic or mechanical means (including photocopying, recording, or information storage and retrieval) without permission in writing from the publisher.

This book was set in Palatino on the Monotype "Prism Plus" PostScript Imagesetter by Asco Trade Typesetting Ltd., Hong Kong and was printed and bound in the United States of America.

Library of Congress Cataloging-in-Publication Data

Neurons, networks, and motor behavior / edited by Paul S. G. Stein ... [et al.].
    p.   cm. — (Computational neuroscience)
Includes index.
ISBN 0-262-19390-6 (alk. paper)
  1. Sensorimotor cortex. 2. Locomotion. 3. Neural networks (Neurobiology) 4. Neuromuscular transmission. 5. Muscles—Innervation. I. Stein, Paul S. G. II. Series.
QP383.15.N48   1997
612.8'252—dc21   97-1551
                                                                          CIP

Contents

Series Foreword

Computational neuroscience is an approach to understanding the information content of neural signals by modeling the nervous system at many different structural scales, including the biophysical, the circuit, and the systems levels. Computer simulations of neurons and neural networks are complementary to traditional techniques in neuroscience. This book series welcomes contributions that link theoretical studies with experimental approaches to understanding information processing in the nervous system. Areas and topics of particular interest include biophysical mechanisms for computation in neurons, computer simulations of neural circuits, models of learning, representation of sensory information in neural networks, systems models of sensory-motor integration, and computational analysis of problems in biological sensing, motor control, and perception.

Terrence J. Sejnowski
Tomaso A. Poggio

Preface

The twenty-five chapters of *Neurons, Networks, and Motor Behavior* focus on cellular, network, and behavioral levels of organization. For the cellular level, the volume describes the computational characteristics of individual neurons and how those characteristics can be modified by neuromodulators. For the network and the behavioral levels, it discusses how network structure is dynamically modulated to produce adaptive behavior. Recent advances in our understanding of the complex coordination of motor output generated during a variety of motor behaviors have relied on detailed knowledge of the characteristics of the neurons and networks that generate those motor behaviors. An emerging principle of organization is that the nervous system is remarkably efficient in the construction of neural networks. New results point to remarkable multitasking by the networks of neurons that generate motor behavior.

This 1997 volume is the third in a once-a-decade series that began with the 1976 volume *Neural Control of Locomotion*, edited by Richard M. Herman, Sten Grillner, Paul S. G. Stein, and Douglas G. Stuart. The second volume of the series, *Neurobiology of Vertebrate Locomotion*, edited by Sten Grillner, Paul S. G. Stein, Douglas G. Stuart, Hans Forssberg, and Richard M. Herman, was published in 1986. Each volume marks, for its decade, a mid-decade understanding of specific research in neural control of motor behavior. The 1986 volume focuses on a comparative approach toward vertebrate motor systems; the 1976 and 1997 volumes take a broader perspective, with comparative emphases on both invertebrate and vertebrate systems. The three volumes share common concepts: neuronal networks generate motor behavior, and comparisons of model systems distributed throughout the animal kingdom provide insights into general principles of motor control.

All three volumes recognize that understanding the neural control of movement requires a multilevel approach. The multilevel approach emphasizes the importance of both analysis and synthesis. Reductionist analysis reveals properties of components of the system: specific motor patterns generated by networks, neurons, and neuromolecules (channels, receptors, transmitters, and modulators). Synthesis uses a systems approach regarding the levels of networks and behavior: motor patterns generate movements that are modulated by movement-related sensory feedback. Such a multilevel approach has been supported elsewhere: Bunge (1989) stressed the importance of multilevel approaches in neuroscience; Stein (1995) applied Bunge's perspectives to neural control of movement; and Getting (1989) emphasized the utilization of reductionist results in the construction of synthetic mathematical models of neuronal networks that generate motor patterns.

Many of the chapter authors in the three volumes were speakers at the corresponding once-a-decade international conferences organized by the volumes' editors. Herman chaired the 1975 Valley Forge conference; Grillner, the 1985 Stockholm conference; and Stein, the 1995 Tucson conference. The 1975 and 1985 chairs also served as local coordinators of those conferences; Stuart served as local coordinator of the 1995 conference. Abstracts of the 1995 conference were published as part of the *Proceedings of the International Symposium on Neurons, Networks, and Motor Behavior* (Stein et al., 1995). The World Wide Web site http://www.physiol.arizona.edu/CELL/Department/Conferences.html currently provides access to an electronic version of the proceedings. Important financial support for the 1995 conference was provided by several institutes of the National Institutes of Health (NINDS, NIMH, NIDCD, NICHD, NIA, and NCRR), the Office of Naval Research, the National Science Foundation, the University of Arizona, and the International Science Foundation. Their support led to the success of the 1995 conference (Katz, 1996) and played a critical role in the writing of chapters that appear in the present volume.

At each of the three conferences, there was an exciting sense that new understanding had just been or was about to be reached, and each conference served as a catalyst for the emerging ideas of its decade. Prior to the 1975 conference, researchers of vertebrate systems tended to view only vertebrate research as relevant, whereas researchers of invertebrate systems tended to focus only on other invertebrate research. The 1975 conference and its accompanying 1976 volume revealed common neuron, network, and behavior organizational principles for both vertebrates and invertebrates. That discovery led to a change in the way many investigators and university training programs approached the neural control of movement. The 1985 conference and its accompanying 1986 volume offered further support for the view that the nervous systems of lower vertebrates share important common features with the nervous systems of mammals. Incorporating these previous insights,

the 1995 conference and this volume add the emerging concept of the current decade: the modulatory abilities of the neurons that make up a neuronal network confer abilities onto the modulated network that allow it to generate an array of motor patterns responsible for a set of motor behaviors.

A historical theme common to the three volumes and the three conferences is the important role of the Moscow School of Motor Control in the investigation of the neural control of motor behavior. A seminal contribution by this school was the 1965 demonstration in a mesencephalic cat that locomotion could be elicited by electrical stimulation of a site in the midbrain (Shik, Severin, and Orlovsky, 1965; see also Arshavsky, Gelfand, and Orlovsky, 1986). Several members of the Moscow School (Gurfinkel, Shik, Orlovsky, and Kashin) were invited to the 1975 Valley Forge meeting, but the political climate of the day prevented their attendance. Herman expressed the disappointment over that missed opportunity in his preface to the 1976 volume. Invited to the 1985 Stockholm meeting, the Members of the Moscow School were again unable to attend, but they were successful in providing manuscripts that were published in the 1986 volume. Grillner ended the preface of the 1986 volume with the note that "the Soviet authors in this volume were unfortunately unable to attend, despite their great contributions to the field." In the 1995 meeting, we were very pleased to have members of that important group present: Arshavsky, Feldman, and Orlovsky—contributing authors to the 1986 volume—as well as Deliagina and Panchin.

The present volume departs from the previous volumes in one organizational feature. For many of the chapters in the 1976 and the 1986 volumes, only the senior author of the chapter was a conference speaker. For the 1995 Tucson conference, however, two or three speakers were invited to collaborate on some of the chapters. Some of those invitations were accepted, resulting in such jointly authored chapters. Other invitations were declined, so some chapters were singly authored by an individual speaker or, in some cases, co-authored with the speaker's collaborators. Whether authored individually or collaboratively, the twenty-five chapters here are the product of many spirited dialogues between the volume editors and authors.

References

Arshavsky YI, Gelfand IM, Orlovsky GN (1986) *Cerebellum and Rhythmical Movements.* Berlin: Springer.

Bunge M (1989) From neuron to mind. *News Physiol Sci* 4:206–209.

Getting PA (1989) Emerging principles governing the operation of neural networks. *Annu Rev Neurosci* 12:185–204.

Grillner S, Stein PSG, Stuart DG, Forssberg H, Herman RM, eds. (1986) *Neurobiology of Vertebrate Locomotion*. Hampshire, England: Macmillan.

Herman RM, Grillner S, Stein PSG, Stuart DG, eds. (1976) *Neural Control of Locomotion*. New York: Plenum.

Katz PS (1996) Neurons, networks, and motor behavior meeting review. *Neuron* 16:245–253.

Shik ML, Severin FV, Orlovsky GN (1966) Control of walking and running by means of electrical stimulation of the midbrain. *Biophysics* 11:756–765.

Stein PSG (1995) A multiple-level approach to motor pattern generation. In: *Neural Control of Movement* (Ferrell WR, Proske U, eds.), 159–165. New York: Plenum.

Stein PSG, Grillner S, Selverston AI, Stuart DG, eds. (1995) *Proceedings of the International Symposium on Neurons, Networks, and Motor Behavior*. Tucson: University of Arizona.

Part I

Selection and Initiation of Motor Patterns

Selection and Initiation of Motor Behavior

Sten Grillner,
Apostolos P. Georgopoulos,
and Larry M. Jordan

Abstract

Successful locomotion in vertebrates requires not only generation of the appropriate propulsive synergy (flying, swimming, or walking), but also goal-directed steering and control of body orientation. In most vertebrates, a correct positioning of each foot is also required during selected phases of the movement. This review focuses on the role of the forebrain and brainstem control in the initiation of locomotion. It considers the basal ganglia, hypothalamus, the mesencephalic locomotor region, including the cuneiform and pedunculopontine regions, as well as the medullary reticular areas. The various corticospinal systems are also reviewed because they most likely contribute to accurate foot placement during locomotion over a complex terrain.

In the absence of their forebrain, mammals like decerebrate cats and rats can be made to walk, trot, and gallop by activation of different locomotor regions in the brainstem. Corresponding findings have been made in all classes of vertebrates. The movements are well coordinated and accompanied by a largely appropriate equilibrium control. In character, however, the movements are robotlike—neither goal directed nor adapted to the environment. The latter qualities are added by neural structures in the forebrain. However, even in advanced mammals like the cat, goal-directed locomotion is retained after an ablation of the entire cerebral cortex that leaves the rest of the forebrain intact (including the basal ganglia and hypothalamus). Kittens, decorticated during their first few weeks of life (Bjursten et al., 1976), can be kept alive for years. The casual observer finds it difficult to distinguish their movements from those of cats with intact nervous systems. They exhibit periods of rest (and possibly sleep), become active, search for food, and are able to remember the location of food. Complex patterns of behavior, such as searching for and finding water or food, or attacking other individuals, require a sequential recruitment of the motor programs coordinating locomotion in combination with other motor patterns. Such patterns of behavior can be so activated without the participation of the cerebral cortex. The neuronal substrate contained in a forebrain devoid of the cerebral cortex is thus able to produce surprisingly complex, goal-directed patterns of behavior.

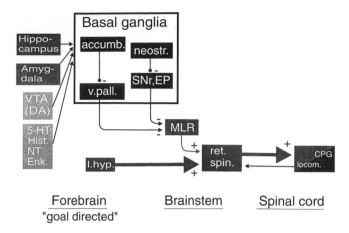

Forebrain
"goal directed"   **Brainstem**   **Spinal cord**

Figure 1.1

Forebrain and brainstem structures important for initiation of the basic locomotor synergy in mammals. The basal ganglia are included within the box (accumb, n. accumbens; v.pall., ventral pallidum; neostr., neostriatum; SNr,EP, substantia nigra pars reticulata, n. entopeduncularis). The inputs to accumb are indicated to the left, including modulation by dopamine (DA) from the ventral tegmental area (VTA) and also by 5-HT, histamine (Hist.), neurotensin (NT), and enkephalin (Enk.). The descending control from the MLR activates reticulospinal neurons (ret. spin.), which in turn activate the spinal central pattern generator (CPG). The reticulospinal neurons can also be activated by a direct projection from the lateral hypothalamus (l. hyp.).

Stimulation of different areas in the basal forebrain, such as the lateral hypothalamus, can evoke different types of goal-directed behavior (Hess, 1949) related to fluid and food intake, attack/escape behavior, or sexual behavior and drive. An important component of these different patterns of behavior is the locomotion that brings the animal to or away from a particular location. Locomotion itself is dependent on several different control systems (see Grillner, 1981, 1985; Mori, 1987; Shik and Orlovsky, 1976), including those that: (1) produce the actual propulsive moments (walking, flying, or swimming); (2) maintain body orientation (balance) during locomotion; (3) ensure that each foot is placed appropriately during each step (visuomotor coordination); and (4) plan the overall locomotor episode to bring the animal from one point to another through what often can be a complex terrain.

One brainstem locomotor area from which locomotion can be activated is termed the mesencephalic locomotor region (MLR), which appears to be present in all classes of vertebrates and is located at the mesopontine border lateral to the aqueduct. When stimulated, it produces the motor synergies underlying flying in birds (Steeves et al., 1987); walking in tetrapods (Shik et al., 1966; Eidelberg et al., 1981; also see review in Jordan, 1991); and swimming in fish and cyclostomes (McClellan

and Grillner, 1984; Kashin and Feldman, 1974). Moreover, a simple continuous stimulation of this region can elicit locomotion involving the coordinated activation of hundreds of different muscles throughout the body. The more intense the stimulation, the faster the animal will locomote. The MLR projects to reticulospinal neurons in the lower brainstem, which in turn form the major locomotor pathway to the spinal cord. There is, in addition, a direct projection from the lateral hypothalamus to the reticulospinal locomotor activating system (Sinnamon and Stopford, 1987). This area appears to correspond to the area designated by Orlovsky (1970) as the subthalamic locomotor area. The axonal bundles from this area course through the ventral mesencephalon and appear to be distinctly different from the MLR system (figure 1.1). Thus, these two areas appear to have the independent capacity to elicit and control locomotor activity. They are referred to in this chapter as the MLR and the diencephalic locomotor region, respectively. An important consideration is obviously how the neurons in these areas are controlled and modulated by other regions of the central nervous system (CNS).

The Basal Ganglia and Locomotor Control in Mammals

If the caudate nucleus of the basal ganglia is removed selectively on both sides (in cat; Villablanca et al., 1976), a remarkable syndrome develops referred to as the "compulsory approaching syndrome." The cat will faithfully follow any moving object that catches its attention, seemingly unable to terminate the behavior (cf., also "obstinate progression"; Bailey and Davis, 1942). Although the exact limits of the lesions may be unclear, these results imply that the basal ganglia are involved in locomotor control. Mogenson and collaborators have shown that the older parts of the basal ganglia, n. accumbens and the ventral pallidum, take part in locomotor control (see figure 1.1). Administration of dopamine agonists or excitatory amino acids in n. accumbens elicits increased levels of locomotor activity (in rats, for example). These effects are obviated by local blockage of the MLR with lidocaine (see Mogenson, 1991; Slawinska and Kasicki, 1995), thereby suggesting that accumbens exerts its action via the MLR. Similarly, locomotor effects can also be elicited by activation of the excitatory input to n. accumbens from the hippocampus or amygdala, or by the dopaminergic input from the ventral tegmental area. Clearly, this part of the basal ganglia is involved in the control of locomotion.

The output from accumbens is made up of GABAergic, medium spiny neurons that project to the ventral pallidum. Neurons in the latter area project, in turn, to several areas including the MLR, as shown by both anatomical and electrophysiological criteria (Swanson and Mogenson, 1981). Part of these ventral pallidal projections are inhibitory (GABAergic), whereas other neurons or axons in this area appear to be excitatory, as shown in stimulation experiments (Mogenson, 1991).

The MLR appears to be under tonic inhibitory control under resting conditions because a local injection of bicuculline (a GABA$_A$ receptor antagonist) into this structure will cause a release of locomotor activity (Garcia-Rill et al., 1990). The dorsal pallidal output to the thalamus and superior colliculus provides a powerful tonic inhibition (a resting rate of output cell discharge near 90 Hz) and a release of different motor programs (such as specific saccades) through disinhibition (Hikosaka, 1991). As an analogy, the accumbens–ventral pallidum–MLR projection might release locomotion by a disinhibition of the MLR (see figure 1.1). If so, striatal GABAergic neurons, which are silent at rest, would become activated and thereby inhibit GABAergic ventral pallidal neurons, resulting in a disinhibition of MLR neurons. Although this scenario appears to be a likely possibility, it needs further investigation. For example, there is need to demonstrate that ventral pallidal neurons that project to the MLR have a high resting rate of discharge (in analogy to dorsal pallidal neurons) and that they become inhibited during initiation of locomotion. Injection of different GABA antagonists and uptake blockers into these relatively undefined areas have, however, produced conflicting results. There *may* be a neuronal link with double inhibition between n. accumbens and the MLR. This suggestion is compelling, but in need of further investigation.

The above-mentioned forebrain areas involve components of the dopaminergic "reward system" (ventral tegmental area), and they are implicated in diverse patterns of behavior (some involving the hippocampus and amygdala). Possibly these circuits are used to initiate locomotion in the context of different types of behavior, such as foraging and allied tasks (Kasicki et al., 1991; Sinnamon, 1993). The more recently evolved parts of the basal ganglia, such as the neostriatum–dorsal pallidum (globus pallidus–substantia nigra reticulata), may also play a role in locomotor control and perhaps in other behavioral contexts. The dorsal pallidum also projects to the MLR (Garcia-Rill and Skinner, 1986; Garcia-Rill, 1986). It seems likely that there are subcompartments in both neostriatum–dorsal pallidum and accumbens–

ventral pallidum that are involved in the locomotor control.

The Lamprey Locomotor Control System

The lamprey system is much like the mammalian system (Grillner et al., 1995); it is a reticulospinal system that activates spinal pattern generators. The reticulospinal system can be activated from two areas corresponding to the MLR (McClellan and Grillner, 1984; Sirota et al., 1995) and the diencephalic locomotor region (El Manira et al., 1995). The input to the lamprey MLR is not yet known. The diencephalic locomotor region consists of cells projecting from the ventral thalamus area to neurons in the middle and posterior reticular nuclei of the rhombencephalon (MRRN, PRRN). They provide monosynaptic glutamatergic excitation to reticular neurons. When the diencephalic locomotor region is stimulated, fictive locomotor activity can be recorded in the spinal cord (El Manira et al., 1995, Pombal et al., 1995).

Cells in the diencephalic locomotor region receive a GABAergic projection from the ventral pallidum, which in turn receives input from GABAergic striatal neurons as deduced from immunohistochemical and tracing data (Pombal et al., 1995). Thus, evidence suggests that the lamprey CNS and the mammalian CNS utilize a similar locomotor circuit: a double inhibitory circuit. The input to the striatum is from the dorsal thalamus and selected telencephalic structures. In addition, there are a number of modulatory inputs, including dopamine, serotonin, histamine, neurotensin, and enkephalins (Pombal et al., 1995). Such organization of input is identical to that of mammals (see Graybiel, 1995), thereby providing evidence for an ancient organization of the vertebrate basal ganglia (the lamprey line of evolution became separate from the line leading up to mammals 450 million years ago).

Midbrain Locomotor Regions

Although the MLR is now well established as a functional region of the brain stem involved in the initiation of locomotion, the nature of the MLR activity in behaving animals is still an open issue. Two nuclei in the midbrain that have been implicated as the major components of the MLR are the *nucleus cuneiformis* and the *pedunculopontine nucleus*. The MLR area also includes other cell groups, but most recent studies have focused on one or the other of these two nuclei.

Shik and others (1967) first showed that stimulation of the mesencephalon could produce locomotion in decerebrate cats. Nucleus cuneiformis was regarded as the effective site. Work with intact cats revealed that electrical stimulation of an area corresponding to the nucleus cuneiformis produced a significant increase in the speed of locomotion (Sterman and Fairchild, 1966; Mori et al., 1989). Stimulus sites were located "within and around the nucleus cuneiformis, possibly including a part of the pedunculopontine nucleus" (Mori et al., 1989, p. 71). A great many studies have been conducted involving histological verification of sites with electrical stimulation and injection of neuroactive substances effective in eliciting locomotion in cats, rats, and guinea pigs. Such sites were invariably located in and around the nucleus cuneiformis (Amemiya and Yamaguchi, 1984; Brudzynski et al., 1986; Milner and Mogenson, 1988; Coles et al., 1989; Depoortere et al., 1990a, 1990b; Garcia-Rill et al., 1985; Garcia-Rill et al., 1983a, 1983b; Marlinsky and Voitenko, 1991; Mitchell et al., 1988a, 1988b; Mori et al., 1983; Mori et al., 1989; Shefchyk et al., 1984; Shefchyk and Jordan, 1985; Shimamura et al., 1984; Shimamura et al., 1987; Shimamura et al., 1990; Sirota and Shik, 1973; Steeves and Jordan, 1984). The MLR has also been localized in a few submammalian species, including the carp (Kashin and Feldman, 1974), lamprey (McClellan and Grillner, 1984), and stingray (Bernau et al., 1991). According to Bernau and coworkers, "the stingray MLR is associated with the caudal portion of the cuneiform nucleus."

The pedunculopontine nucleus was first implicated in the initiation of locomotion on the basis of its connections with limbic structures and the basal ganglia (Armstrong, 1986; Garcia-Rill, 1991; Skinner and Garcia-Rill, 1990; Skinner and Garcia-Rill, 1993; Mogenson et al., 1993; Reese et al., 1995a, 1995b; Inglis and Winn, 1995). Among researchers there is considerable confusion concerning the role of the pedunculopontine nucleus in the initiation of locomotion. It consists of both cholinergic and noncholinergic cells, with borders now considered to be defined by the presence of cholinergic neurons (Inglis and Winn, 1995; Reese et al., 1995a, 1995b). (Previous studies considered its borders to be somewhat broader; see Swanson et al., 1984.) Mogenson and coworkers (Brudzynski and Mogenson, 1985; Milner and Mogenson, 1988; Brudzynski et al., 1993) have ascribed the effects of stimulation, drug injection, and lesions to actions on the pedunculopontine nucleus, but their results may have involved other structures, including the nucleus cuneiformis. The pedunculopontine nucleus and nucleus cuneiformis are in such close proximity that any

effects produced by electrical stimulation or drug injections cannot always be attributed clearly to one or the other. Garcia-Rill and Skinner (1987a, 1987b; Garcia-Rill et al., 1990) have used markers for cholinergic neurons to show convincingly that locomotion can be induced by electrical or chemical stimulation within the pedunculopontine nucleus.

Lesions within the MLR region must be rather large to eliminate locomotion evoked by stimulation of more rostral structures. Such large lesions are effective if they involve the nucleus cuneiformis as well as more ventral areas of the midbrain, including the pedunculopontine nucleus (Jordan, 1986). A recent case report shows that similar lesions in humans can prevent standing and stepping movements (Masdeu et al., 1994). In this instance, a hemorrhage at the pontomesencephalic junction—including the nucleus cuneiformis, pedunculopontine nucleus, and other nearby areas—was detected using magnetic resonance imaging. When limited to the pedunculopontine nucleus or the nucleus cuneiformis, smaller lesions in experimental animals may not result in a locomotor deficit (Shik et al., 1968; Sinnamon and Stopford, 1987). On the other hand, it is possible to reduce locomotor activity by procaine injections into the MLR (Brudzynski and Mogenson, 1985) or by excitotoxic lesions and cobalt injections into the MLR (Brudzynski et al., 1993). There is controversy, however, regarding whether the neurons affected by such lesions are located in the pedunculopontine nucleus or the nucleus cuneiformis (Inglis and Winn, 1995). Lesions of the pedunculopontine nucleus do not appear to produce deficits in spontaneous or drug-induced locomotion (Steckler et al., 1994; Inglis and Winn, 1995). Procaine injection into the pedunculopontine nucleus, however, appears to block locomotion elicited by stimulation of the lateral hypothalamus (Levy and Sinnamon, 1990).

Only brief episodes of chemically induced locomotion were produced with injection sites in the pedunculopontine nucleus in rats and cats (Garcia-Rill et al., 1990), but sustained locomotion occurred with sites in the nucleus cuneiformis (Garcia-Rill et al., 1985). Effective sites for chemically evoked locomotion in freely moving rats appear to be located predominantly in the nucleus cuneiformis and not in the pedunculopontine nucleus, as currently defined (Milner and Mogenson, 1988). The activity-dependent expression of c-fos following treadmill locomotion in rats is detectable in nucleus cuneiformis and not in the pedunculopontine nucleus area as defined by NADPH-diaphorase staining (Shojania et al., 1992; Livingston et al., submitted). Similarly, labeling with 2-deoxyglucose (Shimamura et al., 1987; Jordan, 1986) revealed increased activity only in the nucleus cuneiformis as a result of MLR-evoked locomotion. Stimulation of the periaqueductal gray (Sandner and Di Scala, 1992) or of the medial hypothalamus (Leite-Silveira et al., 1995)—which produce flight or escape responses and defensive or aversive behavior with concomitant locomotor activity in freely moving animals—results in c-*fos* labeling in the nucleus cuneiformis. The pedunculopontine nucleus is labeled with c-*fos*, however, during REM sleep (Shiromani et al., 1992, 1995).

The suggestion that stimulation of the nucleus cuneiformis is associated with aversive or escape reactions has considerable support. In freely moving cats or rats such stimulation produces—in addition to locomotor activity—behavior suggesting that the animal is attempting to avoid a noxious stimulus and escape (Sirota and Shik, 1973; Mori et al., 1989; Depoortere et al., 1990a, 1990b). Injections of glutamate into the nucleus cuneiformis of freely moving rats results in freezing, darting, and fast running (Mitchell et al., 1988a, 1988b).

There is evidence that the pedunculopontine nucleus is associated with startle responses (Ebert and Ostwald, 1991). When GABA antagonists were injected into this structure, a "slight jump preceded each bout of locomotion" (Garcia-Rill et al., 1990). These authors also described "audiogenic stepping," induced when GABA antagonists were injected into a locomotor site in the inferior colliculus. Stimulation of the cochlear nuclei can elicit locomotion (Beresovskii and Bayev, 1988), and auditory-evoked potentials have been detected in the pedunculopontine nucleus (Reese et al., 1995a, 1995b), which appears to express c-*fos* in response to startle-eliciting acoustic stimuli (Reese et al., 1992). The cholinergic cells in the pedunculopontine nucleus appear to project to the pontine reticular nucleus, an obligatory relay station in the primary startle pathway (Koch et al., 1993). Perhaps the pedunculopontine nucleus is important for locomotor activity resulting from startle-eliciting stimuli.

Three types of locomotor systems that function in different behavioral or motivational contexts have been proposed (Sinnamon, 1993): an *appetitive* system, a *primary defensive* system, and an *exploratory* system—all eventually converging on lower brainstem locomotor areas. According to this view, the preoptic and perifornical/lateral hypothalamic locomotor regions and their connections make up the appetitive system, with a direct projection to the brain stem. The primary defensive system consists of the medial hypothalamic and perifornical regions, plus their connections with the central gray and the MLR. The exploratory system is said to involve the subpallidal area, including hippocampal projections to n. accumbens, as well as accumbens projections to the subpallidum, the zona incerta, and the pedunculopontine nucleus. If such separate channels exist at the diencephalic and mesencephalic levels, with the primary defensive system somewhat distinct from the overlapping appetitive and exploratory systems, then the pedunculopontine nucleus and the nucleus cuneiformis may be involved in locomotor activity related to different behavioral goals. Thus, the nucleus cuneiformis might be more related to the medial hypothalamus and associated structures, with a role in escape, flight, aversion, and defensive behavior. The pedunculopontine nucleus might be more related to subpallidal systems or exploratory locomotion. The MLR may, therefore, include subcomponents involved in locomotion produced in different behavioral contexts. If this is correct, then the results of lesions studies involving the MLR should be interpreted on the basis of their behavioral contexts.

Pontomedullary Locomotor Areas

In all species examined, the pathways for initiation of locomotion that descend to the spinal cord are considered to arise from reticulospinal cells. This view was originally expressed by Orlovsky (1970) and has been extensively reviewed (Grillner, 1981; Armstrong, 1986; McClellan, 1986; Arshavsky et al., 1988; Jordan, 1991; Skinner and Garcia-Rill, 1993; Rossignol, 1996). Considerable evidence indicates the involvement of a lateral *pontomedullary locomotor strip* and a more medial *medullary reticular formation* (Garcia-Rill and Skinner, 1987a, 1987b) in the initiation of locomotion.

The medial reticular formation (Skinner and Garcia-Rill, 1993) is the source of the reticulospinal cells that supply a "locomotor command" to spinal locomotor systems (figure 1.1). Locomotor defects result from lesions in the reticulospinal areas that receive input from the MLR (Zemlan et al., 1983). Reversible cooling (Shefchyk et al., 1984), GABA injections (Garcia-Rill and Skinner, 1987a, 1987b), and procaine injections (Marlinsky and Voitenko, 1991) into the medial reticular formation block locomotion induced by MLR stimulation and pontomedullary, locomotor-strip stimulation (Noga et al., 1991). Activation of neurons in the medial reticular formation with cholinergic agonists, substance P, and excitatory amino acids (Garcia-Rill and Skinner, 1987a, 1987b; Sholomenko et al., 1991; Noga et al., 1988; Kinjo et al., 1990) produces locomotion in mammals and birds.

Precise anatomical identification of the reticulospinal cells that form the descending locomotor command pathway has not yet been accomplished for any species. It is presumed that glutamatergic cells predominate in this pathway because initiation of locomotion from the brain stem can be blocked by antagonists of excitatory amino acids (Fenaux et al., 1991; Douglas et al., 1993; Hagevik and McClellan, 1994). The pharmacology of the descending control of locomotion has been reviewed recently (Jordan et al., 1992; Rossignol and Dubuc, 1994). For example, excitatory amino acids can elicit a locomotor rhythm when applied directly to the isolated spinal cord. In the lamprey, reticulospinal monosynaptic excitation of all types of neurons recognized as having a role in the central pattern generator (CPG) for swimming is mediated by excitatory amino acids (Ohta and Grillner, 1989). The same reticulospinal nerves provide monosynaptic excitatory postsynaptic potentials (EPSPs) to the inhibitory and excitatory interneurons responsible for the CPG operation.

Other descending pathways are also likely to be sufficient, however, including pathways that contain 5-hydroxytryptamine (5-HT or serotonin) and norepinephrine. The raphe-spinal system deserves special attention because 5-HT promotes the development of plateau potentials in spinal cord neurons (Kiehn, 1991). This system is effective for induction of locomotor activity in the isolated neonatal rat spinal cord (Cazalets et al., 1992; Cowley and Schmidt, 1994) and it is necessary for the initiation of oscillatory membrane behavior in *Rana temporaria* embryos (Sillar and Simmers, 1994). Application of 5-HT antagonists blocks pharmacologically induced locomotor rhythms in the isolated neonatal rat spinal cord (MacLean and Schmidt, 1995). 5-HT cells in the caudal raphe nuclei increase their firing rate during treadmill locomotion in freely moving cats (Jacobs and Fornal, 1993; Veasey and Fornal, 1995), and 5-HT levels increase in the spinal cord during locomotion (Gerin et al., 1995).

Cortical Contribution to Locomotor Movements

Thus far we have focused on forebrain and brainstem control of the basic propulsive locomotor synergy, but what specific adaptations are necessary for accurate foot placement during each step (see Armstrong, 1986)? This action requires elaborate visuomotor processing, and it appears to depend on intact corticospinal projections. Liddell and Phillips (1944) showed that a transection of the pyramidal tract in cats resulted in an inability to

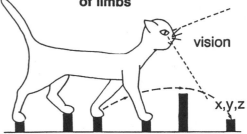

Locomotion with accurate positioning of limbs

vision

x,y,z

Accurate positioning of limbs without locomotion

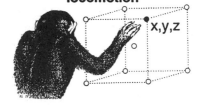

x,y,z

Figure 1.2
Precision movements during locomotion and reaching. During ordinary locomotion in a complex terrain, the limbs need to be placed with great accuracy (see drawing of a cat), which requires integration between general locomotor commands as well as corticospinal visuomotor coordination, leading to an accurate placement of the foot in each step. This aspect of visuomotor coordination has been shown to depend on a corticospinal contribution in the cat (see text), and presumably applies to other mammals. Arboreal primates move from branch to branch, and very accurate reaching and grasping are required in practically each step cycle. Positioning the limb accurately in relation to the environment, as the body is continuously moving, is in fact a more difficult task than a normal reaching situation. In this case, the body is kept semi-stationary while the arm and hand reach out to different points in the surrounding space. It is therefore likely that the neuronal systems used for accurate positioning of the limb during locomotion involve overlapping circuits to those used during reaching, as exemplified in the drawing of a monkey in the lower part of the illustration (A. P. Georgopoulos, S. Grillner, and G. N. Orlovsky, unpublished).

locomote on a ladder (which requires precise foot placement), but it had no effect on overground locomotion on a flat floor. The pyramidal tract includes projections from different precentral motor areas that are important in the control of a variety of motor patterns including reaching, grasping, and fine motor skills (Georgopoulos, 1991, 1995). Some types of locomotion (figure 1.2) over complicated terrain require adaptations for each foot placement, which, in their complexity, resemble reaching and grasping (Georgopoulos and Grillner, 1989). This analogy is the basis for the following review of cortical motor systems.

Precentral Motor Areas

The precentral motor areas comprise the motor cortex and several premotor areas anterior to it. These include,

Grillner, Georgopoulos, and Jordan

from lateral to medial, the inferior premotor area, the arcuate premotor area, the dorsal premotor area, the supplementary and presupplementary motor areas, and the cingulate premotor area. The precentral motor areas have been investigated intensely for the past fifteen years, using both morphological and physiological methods. Here, we focus on new developments, especially those concerning the connectivity patterns and functional cell properties of these areas.

All premotor areas are interconnected with the motor cortex. In addition, precentral motor areas are interconnected with parietal areas of the ipsilateral hemisphere and with areas of the contralateral hemisphere. Recent studies (Johnson et al., 1996) have shown an orderly arrangement in the connectivity patterns such that frontal areas, from anterior to posterior (e.g., the dorsal premotor cortex to the motor cortex), connect with parietal areas, from posterior to anterior (e.g., medial intraparietal area, area 5), respectively. This pattern of anatomical connectivity is reflected in the discharge characteristics of cells in these areas (Kalaska et al., 1983; Johnson et al., 1996), suggesting that these interconnected areas process similar information with respect to arm movements (leg movements have not yet been studied).

C3/C4 System

Precentral motor areas can influence spinal interneuronal systems by influencing neuronal activity in the C3/C4 propriospinal system (Lundberg, 1979). This system is made up of interneurons that are intercalated between descending supraspinal systems and spinal segments innervating proximal muscles. Lesion studies in the cat (Alstermark et al., 1981) have provided evidence of a role for this system in reaching, and a general scheme has been proposed for the use of the C3/C4 system by descending precentral motor commands (Georgopoulos, 1988).

Thalamic Connections

Single thalamocortical axons in the cat terminate in the motor cortex in a multifocal pattern (Shinoda et al., 1992). Terminal plexuses are about 0.5 mm in diameter, separated by terminal-free gaps and distributed mainly in the rostrocaudal direction for a distance of up to 6 mm. A similar pattern has been observed for projections from postcentral to precentral areas in the monkey (DeFelipe et al., 1986). Conversely, there is substantial convergence of these projections as well, such that several nuclei converge on a small cortical area (Darian-Smith et al., 1990).

The information conveyed to a small area in the motor cortex, therefore, comes from diverse sources, underscoring the highly integrative nature of motor cortical processing.

Another issue concerns the differential projections of the basal ganglia and cerebellum to various precentral motor areas. Motor and premotor areas receive partially overlapping input from the thalamus, and the bulk of the projections from thalamic nuclei receiving projections from the globus pallidus are directed to premotor areas (Shindo et al., 1995). Cerebellar influences to the motor cortex are also well established (Shinoda et al., 1992).

Corticospinal Projections

Pyramidal tract axons diverge and terminate along several spinal segments (Shinoda et al., 1981). Conversely, there is substantial convergence onto single motoneurons from a wide area of the motor cortex (Porter and Lemon, 1993). Thus, divergence and convergence are hallmarks of corticospinal projections. All precentral motor areas project to the spinal cord; some projections from premotor areas are as dense as those from the motor cortex (Dum and Strick, 1991). These findings have invalidated the earlier belief that premotor areas exert their influence on the spinal cord only by way of the motor cortex. It now seems that the precentral motor areas form a parallel system within which each premotor area, like the motor cortex, possesses a direct communication line with spinal structures.

Cortico-Brainstem Connections

There are extensive connections between all precentral motor areas and various brainstem structures, including the red nucleus, the reticular formation, and the pontine nuclei (Kuypers, 1981). The functional role of these connections is only partially understood but easy to infer when the recipient nuclei is considered to be a "relay" station (e.g., precerebellar nuclei). In most cases, this role still needs to be elucidated, as it does, for example, in the case of corticorubral and corticoreticular projection (Armstrong, 1986).

Microstimulation

Electrical microstimulation has been used to investigate the somatotopic organization of the motor cortex and to determine which motor variables are represented (Porter and Lemon, 1993). Microstimulation of a number of precentral motor areas can elicit motor responses. The result is in accord with the existence of direct projections from these areas to the spinal cord. Microstimulation in the motor cortex results in activation of a number of muscles, and particular muscles can be activated from various locations. Interestingly, the motor cortex has "silent" zones in which microstimulation does not elicit motor responses (Waters et al., 1990). These zones are found between the hand and face representations. Neuroanatomical studies (Huntley and Jones, 1991) have documented a separation between the two representations and have also demonstrated extensive local connectivity *within* the forelimb and face representations but a lack of connectivity *between* these two representations.

Postspike Facilitation

The technique of spike-triggered averaging has been applied to motor cortical discharge in an attempt to determine the patterns of possible facilitation of motor cortical spike trains on electromyographic (EMG) activity (Porter and Lemon, 1993). The main finding was that postspike facilitation can be produced in a number of muscles of the contralateral forearm, hand, and fingers. Recently, postspike facilitation was observed in extensive groups of muscles spanning two or more joints (McKieman et al., 1994). This suggests that monosynaptic connections extend to large groups of muscles spanning several joints and that this pattern may be the substrate for integrated muscle synergies during reaching.

Combined Behavioral-Neurophysiological Studies

Recordings of single-cell activity in behaving monkeys, and to a lesser extent in cats, have provided important insights into the differential role of various precentral areas in motor control. It is important to realize that the behavioral task used in a particular experiment is crucial for interpreting the results. All tasks involve the generation of arm or hand movements under various conditions, which may relate to (1) the kind of motor output itself (e.g., making a movement or exerting an isometric force); (2) the functional aspects of the same kind of motor output (e.g., static vs. dynamic isometric force; precision vs. power grip); (3) the conditional requirements in the generation of movement (e.g., imposed delays to withhold the movement until a go signal is given); (4) more complex manipulations (e.g., memorized delays), or (5) imposed transformations of an intended movement (e.g., moving at an angle from a stimulus direction).

Static Force

In the original and later work of Evarts, and in subsequent work by others (reviewed in Porter and Lemon, 1993), the force exerted by the animal was restricted to one joint and to the activation of reciprocal groups of muscles. In these experiments, the steady-state activity of a number of motor cortical cells varied with the level of force exerted. The neural relations to static force were extended to the direction of multijoint, two-dimensional (Kalaska et al., 1989), and three-dimensional (Taira et al., 1996) static forces. Cellular activity in the motor cortex varies with and is broadly tuned to the direction of force.

Precision Grip

The original use of precision grip as an experimental tool (Smith et al., 1975) was in accord with the idea that the motor cortex may be particularly involved in the control of precise forces. A precision grip involves the simultaneous activation of a large number of muscles (Smith, 1981; Maier et al., 1990) and, at the same time, an accurate control of force levels as an output motor parameter. Earlier results on the relations between motorcortical cell activity and isometric force in a single joint were interpreted in a simple fashion (Fromm, 1983). For precision grip, however, these relations cannot be interpreted as easily. The desired force levels can be attained by various combinations of muscle activations, and the amount of activation of a particular muscle does not vary in a simple fashion with the amount of force exerted (Maier et al., 1990, 1993). The activity of motor cortical cells is *not* solely or exclusively determined by the motor output; rather, it reflects other processes pertaining to specific aspects of task performance.

The dynamic relations of cellular activity in the motor cortex to the direction of 2-D isometric force pulses were investigated, using an experimental arrangement that dissociated the dynamic and static components of the force exerted (Georgopoulos et al., 1992). Monkeys produced pure force pulses on an isometric handle in the presence of a constant bias force so that the net force (i.e., the vector sum of the monkey's force and the bias force) was in a visually specified direction. The net force developed over time had to stay in the specified direction and to increase in magnitude in order to exceed a required intensity threshold. Now consider the case in which the directions of the net and bias forces differ by being, for example, orthogonal. Under these conditions, the animal's force has to change continuously in direction and magnitude such that, at any moment during force development, the vector sum of this force and the bias force is in the visually specified direction. This experimental arrangement effectively dissociated the animal's force vector, the direction of which changed continuously in a trial, from the net force vector, whose direction remained invariant. Eight net-force directions and eight bias-force directions were employed. Recordings of neuronal activity in the motor cortex revealed that the activity of single cells was directionally tuned in the absence of bias force and that this tuning remained invariant when the same net forces were produced in the presence of different directions of bias force. These results demonstrated that cell activity does not relate to the direction of the animal's force. Because the net force is equivalent to the dynamic component of the force exerted by the animal, after a static component vector (equal and opposite to the bias force) is subtracted, *these findings suggest that the motor cortex provides the dynamic force signal during force development; other, possibly subcortical, structures might provide the static compensatory signal.* This latter signal could be furnished by antigravity neural systems, given that most static loads encountered are gravitational in nature. According to this general view, the force exerted by the subject consists of dynamic and static components, each of which is controlled by different neural systems. These signals presumably converge in the spinal cord to provide an ongoing integrated signal to the motoneuronal pools.

Locomotion

Single-cell activity in the motor cortex of the locomoting cat is modulated periodically during the stance and swing phases of locomotion (Armstrong and Drew, 1984; Drew, 1993; Beloozerova and Sirota, 1993). However, the amplitude of this periodic modulation was hardly influenced when cats had to locomote uphill, even when the EMG activity increased by approximately 50% (Armstrong and Drew, 1984). This finding led Armstrong and Drew (1984) to question the "central dogma" (p. 492) of that time—namely, that motor cortical activity reflects the magnitude of force exerted or the intensity of activation of target muscles. Instead, the periodicity in cell activity changed with the speed of locomotion, and phase shifts were also observed (Armstrong and Drew, 1984). This finding is in accord with previous findings that motor cortical activity reflects temporal and directional factors probably associated with the selection of muscles to be activated rather than with the intensity of muscle activation.

A clue as to the important determinants of motor cortical activation was obtained by studies involving the locomoting cat in which the cat had to overcome an obstacle (Drew, 1993) or walk in situations that demanded greater precision, such as on the flat rungs of a horizontal ladder (Beloozerova and Sirota, 1993). Such maneuvers produced marked changes in single-cell activity. These observations suggest that the motor cortex is involved when the motor output has to be reorganized into a new pattern, according to the demands of the particular situation. Such reorganization is usually encountered during visuomotor control of the locomoting limbs (Georgopoulos and Grillner, 1989). The role of the motor cortex has thus been shifted from that of a simple *producer* of motor output to a *specifier* of new motor patterns to be produced as a particular condition may demand (Drew, 1993).

Reaching

Reaching is a complex motor pattern involving the concomitant activation of several joints and a larger number of muscles, and yet it is performed gracefully and almost effortlessly. Changes in cell activity were analyzed with respect to a parameter of the reaching movement that captured in a global fashion most of the changes in muscles and joints—namely, its direction in space. A surprisingly orderly relation between the frequency of cell discharge and the direction of reaching was revealed (Georgopoulos et al., 1993). Motor cortical cells are directionally tuned such that their activity varies in a sinusoidal manner with the direction of the movement in space. The tuning curve is broad and covers the entire directional continuum. This means that there is a particular movement direction for which cell activity will be the highest (the "preferred direction" of the cell). Preferred directions differ among cells and are distributed throughout the directional continuum.

Neuronal Population Coding

These findings of cell activity during reaching indicate that the neuronal ensemble engaged with reaching movements consists of directionally tuned cells with diverse directional preferences. The broad tuning of individual cells indicates that a cell will be engaged with movements in many directions. Conversely, many cells will be engaged with movements in a particular direction. Therefore, a unique encoding of the direction of movement may reside within the whole ensemble. This information was extracted by the population vector analysis (Georgopoulos et al., 1983; see also Sparks et al., chapter 2, this volume), which considers a given cell as a vector pointing in its preferred direction and with length proportional to the intensity of the cell activation. The population vector is the vector sum of the cell vectors and points in the direction of the movement. It is a robust predictor of direction under different postures (Caminiti et al., 1991; Georgopoulos, 1995) and different muscle patterns (Georgopoulos et al., 1992), as well as in various motor areas (Georgopoulos, 1991). In addition, it provides an accurate, time-varying directional signal that can be used to monitor the directional tendency of the neuronal ensemble during the generation, transformation, and selection of motor commands (Georgopoulos et al., 1993).

Finger Movements

The question of coding for and selecting from combinations of finger movements is a basic issue in motor behavior and in motor cortical physiology. Behaviorally, this is an important issue because, during natural manipulation of objects, the fingers are used in groups rather than as isolated entities. Although the ability to move single fingers is, by itself, one of the hallmarks of primate motor behavior, the use of fingers in combinations during object manipulation is the more behaviorally meaningful motor action. In fact, such combinations are being reconfigured dynamically as one manipulates an object in different ways (Schieber and Hibbard, 1993). In their study, Schieber and Hibbard discovered that movements of a particular finger were represented multiply in the motor cortex of the monkey. Conversely, single cells were related to movement of more than one finger. Moreover, neuronal populations active in movements of different fingers overlapped extensively. The authors concluded that "control of any finger movement ... appears to utilize a population of neurons distributed throughout the M1 hand area rather than a somatotopically segregated population" (Schieber and Hibbard, 1993, p. 489). They also remarked (p. 491) on the similarity of this distributed coding of finger movements to the distributed coding of movement direction in reaching, as suggested by Georgopoulos and others (1993).

Instructed Delay Tasks

In an instructed delay task, a sensory stimulus is delivered and a motor response is required *after a period of time*. This task has been used as a probe to identify changes in cell activity during a period in which the information about the upcoming movement has to be retained in the absence of an immediate motor output. Changes in cell activity during an instructed delay period have been observed in practically all precentral motor areas, although they tend to be more common in premotor areas (Tanji and Evarts, 1976; for review, see Wise, 1985; Georgopoulos, 1991; Tanji, 1994). Moreover, the neuronal population vector pointed in the direction of the instructed movement during the delay period (Georgopoulos et al., 1989).

Memorized Delay Tasks

The typical memorized delay task is like the instructed delay task except that the instructing signal is turned off during the delay period. Thus, there is a time period during which information about the upcoming movement has to be kept in memory and used to generate the movement after the go stimulus is given. Several studies have documented changes in cell activity during the memorized delay in motor (Hocherman and Wise, 1991; Smyrnis et al., 1992; Ashe et al., 1993), dorsal premotor (Hocherman and Wise, 1991), and supplementary motor areas (see Tanji, 1994). As in the instructed delay task, the neuronal population vector pointed in the direction of the memorized movement during the memory delay period (Smyrnis et al., 1992).

A study conducted by Alexander and Crutcher (1990a, 1990b) is remarkable because it showed that the direction of movement was dissociated from the pattern of muscle activity within a memorized delay task. The question asked was: Do changes in cell activity during the memorized delay period reflect the muscle pattern or the direction of movement? Three motor areas were studied: the motor cortex, the supplementary motor area, and the putamen. The effect of the intended direction of movement on neural activity was dissociated from the effect of muscle pattern, which was dictated by the applied loads. It was found that (1) many cells in the motor cortex (37%, n = 202), the supplementary motor area (55%, n = 222), and the putamen (33%, n = 317) showed changes in activity during the preparatory period; (2) these changes were selective in anticipation of elbow movements in a particular direction (87% in the motor cortex, 86% in the supplementary motor area, and 78% in the putamen); and (3) these changes were independent of the loading conditions (83% in the motor cortex, 80% in the supplementary motor area, and 84% in the putamen). Alexander and Crutcher concluded, "The near absence of preparatory 'loading effects' in all three motor areas suggests that directional preparatory activity, at least in these structures, may not play a significant role in coding for either the dynamics or the muscle activation patterns of preplanned movements. Instead, such activity may be coding for the intended direction of movement at a more abstract level of processing (e.g., trajectory and/or kinematics), independent of the forces that the movement will require" (1990a, p. 133).

A study done by Ashe and colleagues (1993) investigated the representation of *memorized trajectories* in the motor cortex. For that purpose, a trajectory with an orthogonal directional bend was used. This task was unique in several respects. First, monkeys had to generate from memory a complex movement trajectory involving a change in direction. Second, the movement was truly internally generated: there was no "go" signal to trigger it. And third, the monkeys were never given a visual signal, either during the recordings or during training, to indicate the endpoint of the movement; therefore, the movement was internally planned. A substantial percentage (62.8%) of cells changed activity during a waiting period preceding the beginning of movement. An interesting observation was that a few cells changed activity *exclusively during the execution of the memorized movement*; these cells were completely inactive during performance of similar movements in the visually guided control task. These findings suggest that *performance of a movement trajectory from memory may involve a specific set of cells*, in addition to the cells activated during both visually guided and memorized movements.

Movement Sequences

When a movement is a simple key press, the complexity of neural responses is more evident in the supplementary motor area than in the motor cortex (Tanji and Kurata, 1985). It seems that the motor cortex is more involved in planning or preparing the motor command when the upcoming movement possesses spatial characteristics (e.g., direction) specified by visuospatial information. Conversely, evidence for a more specific role of the supplementary motor area to memorized sequences of movements was provided recently (Tanji and Shima, 1994).

Transformation of Motor Commands: Mental Rotation of an Intended Movement Direction

The mental rotation task required monkeys to move a handle orthogonally and counterclockwise from a reference direction defined by a visual stimulus in one plane. Because the reference direction changed from trial to trial, the task required that, in a given trial, the direction of movement be specified according to this reference direction (Lurito et al., 1991). When the time-varying neuronal population vector was calculated during the reaction time, it was found that it rotated from the stim-

ulus direction to the movement direction through the counterclockwise angle. It is remarkable that the population vector rotated at all *and* that it rotated through the smaller, 90° counterclockwise angle. The results showed that the cognitive process in this task truly involved rotation of an analog signal. The rotation process, "sweeping" through the directionally tuned ensemble, provided for the first time a direct visualization of a dynamic cognitive process. Interestingly, the rotation rates observed in the neurophysiological studies were very similar to those obtained in psychological studies on human subjects (Georgopoulos and Massey, 1987).

Selection of Motor Commands Based on Context-Recall

The studies done by Lurito and others exemplified the *spatial rule* operating in the mental rotation task, which required the production of a movement at an angle from a stimulus direction. In a different study, Pellizzer and others (1995) sought, instead, to determine the neural correlates of a cognitive process, the rule of which was based not on a spatial constraint, but on the *serial position* of stimuli in a sequence. Given an arbitrary sequence of stimuli on a circle, one of which was identified as the test stimulus, the motor response had to be toward the stimulus that followed the test stimulus in the sequence. When the test stimulus was the first in the sequence, cell activity continued to reflect the direction of the second stimulus, which in this case was the appropriate motor response. However, when the test stimulus was the second in the sequence, neural activity switched abruptly—within approximately 100–150 ms after the "go" signal—to reflect the pattern associated with the direction of the third stimulus, which was now the appropriate motor response. These findings identify the neural correlates of a switching process that is different from a mental rotation task, as described in the previous paragraph. Thus, it seems that the time taken to derive the motor direction in a mental rotation task reflects a transformation, whereas the time taken in a context-recall task reflects a selection process.

Complex Visuomotor Interactions: Inferior Premotor Cortex

The inferior premotor cortex (lateral to the arcuate sulcus) stands apart from other areas by virtue of the presence of complex relations of its cells to visual and motor events. With respect to motor functions, some neurons are activated with proximal arm movements, such as reaching to a goal or bringing the hand to the mouth

(Gentilucci et al., 1988); other neurons with hand movements such as grasping, holding, and tearing (di Pellegrino et al., 1992); and still other neurons with combined reaching-and-grasping actions (Rizzolatti et al., 1990). These functional properties resemble those described in previous studies for area 7 of the posterior parietal cortex (Hyvärinen and Poramen, 1974; Mountcastle et al., 1975). With respect to visual responses, receptive fields are spatially, not retinotopically, organized (Fogassi et al., 1992), and they move with the arm (Graziano et al., 1994).

In summary, visuomotor interaction is clearly an important element in the adaptation of the locomotor movements to the environment, as it is for all reaching, grasping, or pointing movements. During the last decade, the knowledge regarding the neural basis of reaching in three dimensions has markedly expanded. A number of modules in the motor and premotor cortici are involved. Although we know a substantial amount about neuronal processing and population coding in cortex, we are nonetheless left with meager information on cortical level interaction, on the integration between cortical and subcortical motor centers, and on the different mechanisms of spinal-level action. Supraspinal control involves not only the monosynaptic effects on different combinations of target motor neurons, but also effects exerted on different types of interneurons and on spinal neural networks of different types.

Concluding Remarks

In addition to basic propulsive locomotor movements, behaviorally relevant movements require most tetrapods and bipeds to place each foot accurately in each step. In most instances, this accuracy requires a very precise visuomotor coordination, in which the animal strives to modify the limb trajectory in each step, so that the foot lands on an appropriate spot on the ground. In addition, some animals use the foot (with footpads), the fingers, or both to secure attachment to the target structure, a behavior most pronounced in species with arboreal locomotion, such as many primates. They move in the trees or branches and swing themselves between branches, requiring a precise "reaching out" toward the target, as well as a powerful and well-timed grasp. Most likely, not only are many of the cortical systems we have discussed utilized to achieve isolated precise reaching, grasping, and manipulatory movements, but also are used during locomotion (Georgopoulos and Grillner, 1989).

In the first part of this review we dealt with the forebrain and lower brainstem circuitry that initiates and controls the basic locomotor synergy. We considered the role of the basal ganglia in relation to the limbic system and to the lateral and medial hypothalamus. Most of the effects we discussed appear to be channeled via the MLR to the medullary reticulospinal locomotor command. We also evaluated the possibility that the cuneiform nucleus of the MLR is particularly involved in escape reactions, whereas the pedunculopontine part of the MLR might be involved during exploratory behavior and startle reactions involving locomotor activation. During locomotion, which is a part of overall foraging behavior, direct projections from the lateral hypothalamus to the medulla may also be involved. Thus, for the animal in its natural environment, the underlying type of motivation may determine which parts of the forebrain circuitry will be used to initiate a locomotor episode. The different systems will converge, in turn, on the lower brainstem and spinal cord circuitry that generates the basic locomotor synergy. This synergy requires cycle-to-cycle modifications, including visuomotor coordination that involves the motor cortex.

Acknowledgments

Sten Grillner supported by the Swedish Medical Research Council (project 3026) and Science Research Council; Apostolos Georgopoulos by USPHS grant MS-17413, U.S. Department of Veterans Affairs, and American Legion Brain Sciences Chair; Larry Jordan by Medical Research Council of Canada, Networks of Centres of Excellence (Canada), and International Human Frontier Science Program Organization.

References

Alexander GE, Crutcher MD (1990a) Preparation for movement: Neural representation of intended direction in three motor areas of the monkey. *J Neurophysiol* 64:133–150.

Alexander GE, Crutcher MD (1990b) Neural representations of the target (goal) of visually guided arm movements in three motor areas of the monkey. *J Neurophysiol* 64:164–178.

Alstermark B, Lundberg A, Norrsell U, Sybirska E (1981) Integration in descending motor pathways controlling the forelimb in the cat. 9. Differential behavioral defects after spinal cord lesions interrupting defined pathways from higher centres to motorneurones. *Exp Brain Res* 42:299–318.

Amemiya M, Yamaguchi T (1984) Fictive locomotion of the forelimb evoked by stimulation of the mesencephalic locomotor region in the decerebrate cat. *Neurosci Lett* 50:91–96.

Armstrong DM (1986) Supraspinal contributions to the initiation and control of locomotion in the cat. *Prog Neurobiol* 26:273–361.

Armstrong DM, Drew T (1984) Discharges of pyramidal tract and other motor cortical neurones during locomotion in the cat. *J Physiol (London)* 346:471–495.

Arshavsky YI, Deliagina TG, Gelfand IM, Orlovsky GN, Panchin YV, Pavlova GA (1988) Stance and motion: Facts and concepts. In: *Neuronal Mechanisms Controlling Rhythmic Movements in Gastropod Molluscs* (Gurfinkel VS, Ioffe ME, Massion J, Roll JP, eds.), 107–121. New York: Plenum.

Ashe J, Taira M, Smyrnis N, Pellizzer G, Georgakopoulos T, Lurito JT, Georgopoulos AP (1993) Motor cortical activity preceding a memorized movement trajectory with an orthogonal bend. *Exp Brain Res* 95:118–130.

Bailey P, Davis EW (1942) The syndrome of obstinate progression in the cat. *Proc Soc Exp Biol Med* 51:307.

Beloozerova IN, Sirota MG (1993) The role of motor cortex in the control of accuracy of locomotor movements in the cat. *J Physiol (London)* 461:1–25.

Beresovskii VK, Bayev KV (1988) New locomotor regions of the brainstem revealed by means of electrical stimulation. *Neuroscience* 26:863–869.

Bernau NA, Puzdrowski RL, Leonard RB (1991) Identification of the midbrain locomotor region and its relation to descending locomotor pathways in the Atlantic stingray, *Dasyatis-Sabina*. *Brain Res* 557:83–94.

Bjursten L-M, Norrsell K, Norrsell U (1976) Behavioral repertory of cats without cerebral cortex from infancy. *Exp Brain Res* 25:115–130.

Brudzynski SM, Houghton PE, Brownlee RD, Mogenson GJ (1986) Involvement of neuronal cell bodies of the mesencephalic locomotor region in the initiation of locomotor activity of freely behaving rats. *Brain Res Bull* 16:377–381.

Brudzynski SM, Mogenson GJ (1985) Association of the mesencephalic locomotor region with locomotor activity induced by injections of amphetamine into the nucleus accumbens. *Brain Res* 334:77–84.

Brudzynski SM, Wu M, Mogenson GJ (1993) Decreases in rat locomotor activity as a result of changes in synaptic transmission to neurons within the mesencephalic locomotor region. *Can J Physiol Pharmacol* 71:394–406.

Caminiti R, Johnson PB, Galli C, Ferraina S, Burnod Y, Urbano A (1991) Making arm movements within different parts of space: The premotor and motor cortical representation of a coordinate system for reaching at visual targets. *J Neurosci* 11:1182–1197.

Cazalets JR, Sqalli-Houssaini Y, Clarac F (1992) Activation of the central pattern generators for locomotion by serotonin and excitatory amino acids in neonatal rat. *J Physiol* 455:187–204.

Coles SK, Iles JF, Nicolopoulos-Stournaras S (1989) The mesencephalic centre controlling locomotion in the rat. *Neuroscience* 28:149–157.

Cowley KC, Schmidt BJ (1994) A comparison of motor patterns induced by N-methyl-D-aspartate, acetylcholine and serotonin in the in-vitro neonatal rat spinal-cord. *Neurosci Lett* 171:147–150.

Darian-Smith C, Darian-Smith I, Cheema SS (1990) Thalamic projections to sensorimotor cortex in the macaque monkey: Use of multiple retrograde fluorescent tracers. *J Comp Neurol* 299:17–46.

DeFelipe J, Conley M, Jones EG (1986) Long-range focal collaterization of axons arising from corticocortical cells in monkey sensory-motor cortex. *J Neurosci* 6:3749–3766.

Depoortere R, Di Scala G, Sandner G (1990a) Treadmill locomotion and aversive effects induced by electrical stimulation of the mesencephalic locomotor region in the rat. *Brain Res Bull* 25:723–727.

Depoortere R, Sandner G, Di Scala G (1990b) Aversion induced by electrical stimulation of the mesencephalic locomotor region in the intact and freely moving rat. *Physiol Behav* 47:561–567.

Di Pellegrino G, Fadiga L, Fogassi L, Gallese V, Rizzolatti G (1992) Understanding motor events: A neurophysiological study. *Exp Brain Res* 91:176–180.

Douglas JR, Noga BR, Dai X, Jordan LM (1993) The effects of intrathecal administration of excitatory amino-acid agonists and antagonists on the initiation of locomotion in the adult cat. *J Neurosci* 13:990–1000.

Drew T (1993) Motor cortical activity during voluntary gait modifications in the cat. I. Cells related to the forelimbs. *J Neurophysiol* 70:179–199.

Dum RP, Strick PL (1991) The origin of corticospinal projections from the premotor areas in the frontal lobe. *J Neurosci* 11:667–689.

Ebert U, Ostwald J (1991) The mesencephalic locomotor region is activated during the auditory startle response of the unrestrained rat. *Brain Res* 565:209–217.

Eidelberg E, Walden JG, Nguyen LH (1981) Locomotor control in macaque monkeys. *Brain* 104:647–663.

El Manira A, Pombal MA, Grillner S (1995) Diencephalic control of reticulospinal neurons involved in the initiation of locomotion in the lamprey. *Fourth IBRO Cong Neurosci Abstr* 57.

Fenaux F, Corio M, Palisses R, Viala D (1991) Effects of an NMDA-receptor antagonist, MK-801, on central locomotor programming in the rabbit. *Exp Brain Res* 86:393–401.

Fogassi L, Gallese V, di Pellegrino G, Fadiga L, Gentilucci M, Luppino G, Matelli M, Pedotti A, Rizzolatti G (1992) Space coding by premotor cortex. *Exp Brain Res* 89:686–690.

Fromm C (1983) Changes of steady state activity in motor cortex consistent with the length-tension relation of the muscle. *Pflügers Arch* 398:318–323.

Garcia-Rill E (1986) The basal ganglia and the locomotor regions. *Brain Res Rev* 11:47–63.

Garcia-Rill E (1991) The pedunculopontine nucleus. *Prog Neurobiol* 36:363–389.

Garcia-Rill E, Kinjo N, Atsuta Y, Ishikawa Y, Webber M, Skinner RD (1990) Posterior midbrain-induced locomotion. *Brain Res Bull* 24:499–508.

Garcia-Rill E, Skinner RD (1986) The basal ganglia and the mesencephalic locomotor region. In: *Neurobiology of Vertebrate Locomotion* (Grillner S, Stein PSG, Stuart D, Forssberg H, Herman R, eds.), 77–104. London: Macmillan.

Garcia-Rill E, Skinner RD (1987a) The mesencephalic locomotor region. I. Activation of a medullary projection site. *Brain Res* 411:1–12.

Garcia-Rill E, Skinner RD (1987b) The mesencephalic locomotor region. II. Projections to reticulospinal neurons. *Brain Res* 411:13–20.

Garcia-Rill E, Skinner RD, Fitzgerald JA (1985) Chemical activation of the mesencephalic locomotor region. *Brain Res* 330:43–54.

Garcia-Rill E, Skinner RD, Gilmore SA, Owings R (1983a) Connections of the mesencephalic locomotor region (MLR). II. Afferents and efferents. *Brain Res Bull* 10:63–71.

Garcia-Rill E, Skinner RD, Jackson MB, Smith MM (1983b) Connections of the mesencephalic locomotor region (MLR). I. Substantia nigra afferents. *Brain Res Bull* 10:57–62.

Gentilucci M, Fogassi L, Luppino G, Matelli M, Camarda R, Rizzolatti G (1988) Functional organization of inferior area 6 in the macaque monkey. I. Somatotopy and control of proximal movements. *Exp Brain Res* 71:475–490.

Georgopoulos AP (1988) Neural integration of movement: Role of motor cortex in reaching. *FASEB J* 2:2849–2857.

Georgopoulos AP (1991) Higher order motor control. *Ann Rev Neurosci* 14:361–377.

Georgopoulos AP (1995) Current issues in directional motor control. *Trends Neurosci* 18:506–510.

Georgopoulos AP, Ashe J, Smyrnis N, Taira M (1992) Motor cortex and the coding of force. *Science* 256:1692–1695.

Georgopoulos AP, Caminiti R, Kalaska JF, Massey JT (1983) Spatial coding of movement: A hypothesis concerning the coding of movement direction by motor cortical populations. *Exp Brain Res Suppl* 7:327–336.

Georgopoulos AP, Crutcher MD, Schwartz AB (1989) Cognitive spatial motor processes. 3. Motor cortical prediction of movement direction during an instructed delay period. *Exp Brain Res* 75:183–194.

Georgopoulos AP, Grillner S (1989) Visuomotor coordination in reaching and locomotion. *Science* 245:1209–1210.

Georgopoulos AP, Massey JT (1987) Cognitive spatial-motor processes. 1. The making of movements at various angles from a stimulus direction. *Exp Brain Res* 65:361–370.

Georgopoulos AP, Taira M, Lukashin AV (1993) Cognitive neurophysiology of the motor cortex. *Science* 260:47–52.

Gerin C, Becquet D, Privat A (1995) Direct evidence for the link between monoaminergic descending pathways and motor activity. I. A study with microdialysis probes implanted in the ventral funiculus of the spinal cord. *Brain Res* 704:191–201.

Graziano MSA, Yap GS, Gross CG (1994) Coding of visual space by premotor neurons. *Science* 266:1054–1057.

Graybiel AM (1995) The basal ganglia (review). *Trends Neurosci* 18:60–62.

Grillner S (1981) Control of locomotion in bipeds, tetrapods, and fish. In: *Handbook of Physiology, sect. 1. The Nervous System II. Motor Control* (Brooks VB, ed.), 1179–1236. Bethesda Md.: American Physiol Soc, Waverly.

Grillner S (1985) Neurobiological bases of rhythmic motor acts in vertebrates. *Science* 228:143–149.

Grillner S, Deliagina T, Ekeberg Ö, El Manira A, Hill RH, Lansner A, Orlovsky G, Wallén P (1995) Neural networks that coordinate locomotion and body orientation in lamprey. *Trends Neurosci* 18:270–279.

Hagevik A, McClellan AD (1994) Role of excitatory amino-acids in brain-stem activation of spinal locomotor networks in larval lamprey. *Brain Res* 636:147–152.

Hess WR (1949) Das zwischenhirn. Basel, Switzerland: Benno Schwabe.

Hikosaka O (1991) Basal ganglia: Possible role in motor coordination and learning. *Curr Opin Neurobiol* 1:638–643.

Hocherman S, Wise SP (1991) Effects of hand movement path on motor cortical activity in awake, behaving rhesus monkeys. *Exp Brain Res* 83:285–302.

Huntley GW, Jones EG (1991) Relationship of intrinsic connections to forelimb movement representations in monkey cortex: A correlative anatomic and physiological study. *J Neurophysiol* 66:390–413.

Hyvärinen J, Poramen A (1974) Function of the parietal associative area 7 as revealed from cellular discharges in alert monkeys. *Brain* 97:673–692.

Inglis WL, Winn P (1995) The pedunculopontine tegmental nucleus: Where the striatum meets the reticular formation. *Prog Neurobiol* 47:1–29.

Jacobs BL, Fornal CA (1993) 5-HT and motor control: A hypothesis. *Trends Neurosci* 16:346–352.

Johnson PB, Ferraina S, Bianchi L, Caminiti R (1996) Cortical networks for visual reaching: Physiological and anatomical organization of frontal and parietal lobe arm regions. *Cerebral Cortex* 6:102–119.

Jordan LM (1986) Initiation of locomotion from the mammalian brainstem. In: *Neurobiology of Vertebrate Locomotion* (Grillner S, Stein PSG, Stuart D, Forssberg H, Herman R, eds.), 21–37. London: Macmillan.

Jordan LM (1991) Brainstem and spinal cord mechanisms for the initiation of locomotion. In: *Neurobiological Basis of Human Locomotion* (Shimamura M, Grillner S, Edgerton VR, eds.), 3–20. Tokyo: Japan Scientific Societies.

Jordan LM, Brownstone RM, Noga BR (1992) Control of functional systems in the brainstem and spinal cord. *Curr Opin Neurobiol* 2:794–801.

Kalaska JF, Caminiti R, Georgopoulos AP (1983) Cortical mechanisms related to the direction of two-dimensional arm movements: Relations in parietal area 5 and comparison with motor cortex. *Exp Brain Res* 51:247–260.

Kalaska JF, Cohen DAD, Hyde ML, Prud'homme M (1989) A comparison of movement direction-related versus load direction-related activity in primate motor cortex, using a two-dimensional reaching task. *J Neurosci* 9:2080–2102.

Kashin SM, Feldman AG (1974) Locomotion of fish evoked by electrical stimulation of the brain. *Brain Res* 82:41–47.

Kasicki S, Korczynski R, Romaniuk JR, Slawinska U (1991) Two locomotor strips in the diencephalon of thalamic cats. *Acta Neurobiol Exp* 51:137–143.

Kiehn O (1991) Plateau potentials and active integration in the 'final common pathway' for motor behavior. *Trends Neurosci* 14:68–73.

Kinjo N, Atsuta Y, Webber M, Kyle R, Skinner RD, Garcia-Rill E (1990) Medioventral medulla-induced locomotion. *Brain Res Bull* 24:509–516.

Koch M, Kungel M, Herbert H (1993) Cholinergic neurons in the pedunculopontine tegmental nucleus are involved in the mediation of prepulse inhibition of the acoustic startle response in the rat. *Exp Brain Res* 97:71–82.

Kuypers HGJM (1981) Anatomy of the descending pathways. In: *Handbook of Physiology. The Nervous System II* (Brooks VB, ed.), 597–666. Bethesda, Md.: American Physiological Society.

Leite-Silveira MC, Sandner G, Di Scala G, Graeff FG (1995) C-*fos* immunoreactivity in the brain following electrical or chemical stimulation of the medial hypothalamus of freely moving rats. *Brain Res* 674:265–274.

Levy DI, Sinnamon HM (1990) Midbrain areas required for locomotion initiated by electrical stimulation of the lateral hypothalamus in the anesthetized rat. *Neuroscience* 39:665–674.

Liddell EGT, Phillips CG (1944) Pyramidal sections in the cat. *Brain* 67:1–9.

Livingston CA, Pylypas S, Shojania K, Sorensen C, Wang M, Nance DM, Jordan LM (submitted) Brainstem projections from mesencephalic locomotor regions (MLR) in the rat. I. Identification of the MLR by induction of c-*fos* in the nucleus cuneiformis following treadmill locomotion.

Lundberg A (1979) Integration in a propriospinal motor centre controlling the forelimb in the cat. In: *Integration in the Nervous System* (Asanuma H, Wilson VS, eds.), 47–69. Tokyo: Igaku-Shoin.

Lurito JT, Georgakopoulos T, Georgopoulos AP (1991) Cognitive spatial-motor processes. 7. The making of movements at an angle from a stimulus direction: Studies of motor cortical activity at the single cell and population levels. *Exp Brain Res* 87:562–580.

MacLean JN, Schmidt BJ (1995) TTX-resistant NMDA receptor-mediated voltage oscillations in mammalian lumbar motoneurons are modulated by serotonin. Proceedings of the International Symposium on Neurons, Networks, and Motor Behavior (Stein PSG, Grillner S, Selverston AI, Stuart DG, eds.), 59. Tucson: University of Arizona.

Maier MA, Hepp-Reymond M-C, Meyer M (1990) EMG coactivation patterns and isometric grip force in human. *European J Neurosci Suppl* 3:65.

Maier MA, Bennett KMB, Hepp-Reymond M-C, Lemon RN (1993) Contribution of the monkey corticomotoneuronal system to the control of force in precision grip. *J Neurophysiol* 69:772–785.

Marlinsky VV, Voitenko LP (1991) The effect of procaine injection into the medullary reticular formation on forelimb muscle activity evoked by mesencephalic locomotor region and vestibular stimulation in the decerebrated guinea-pig. *Neuroscience* 45:753–759.

Masdeu JC, Alampur U, Cavaliere R, Tavoulareas G (1994) Astasia and gait failure with damage of the pontomesencephalic locomotor region. *Ann Neurol* 35:619–621.

McClellan AD (1986) In vitro CNS preparations: Unique approaches to the study of command and pattern generation systems in motor control. *J Neurosci Meth* 17:209–210.

McClellan AD, Grillner S (1984) Activation of 'fictive swimming' by electrical microstimulation of brainstem locomotor regions in an in vitro preparation of the lamprey central nervous system. *Brain Res* 300:357–361.

McKieman BJ, Marcario JK, Karrer JH, Cheney PD (1994) Corticomotoneuronal (CM) postspike effects on shoulder, elbow, wrist, digit, and intrinsic hand muscles during a reaching task in the monkey. *Soc Neurosci Abst* 20:983.

Milner KL, Mogenson GJ (1988) Electrical and chemical activation of the mesencephalic and subthalamic locomotor regions in freely moving rats. *Brain Res* 452:273–285.

Mitchell IJ, Dean P, Redgrave P (1988a) The projection from superior colliculus to cuneiform area in the rat II. Defence-like responses to stimulation with glutamate in cuneiform nucleus and surrounding structures. *Exp Brain Res* 72:626–639.

Mitchell IJ, Redgrave P, Dean P (1988b) Plasticity of behavioral response to repeated injection of glutamate in cuneiform area of rat. *Brain Res* 460:394–397.

Mogenson GJ (1991) The role of mesolimbic dopamine projections to the ventral striatum in response initiation. In: *Neurobiological Basis of Human Locomotion* (Shimamura M, Grillner S, Edgerton VR, eds.), 33–44. Tokyo: Japan Scientific Societies.

Mogenson GJ, Brudzynski SM, Wu M, Yang CR, Yim CCY (1993) From motivation to action: A review of dopaminergic regulation of limbic–nucleus accumbens–ventral pallidum–pedunculopontine nucleus circuitries involved in limbic-motor integration. In: *Limbic Motor Circuits and Neuropsychiatry* (Kalivas PW, ed.), 193–236. Boca Raton, Fl.: CRC.

Mori S (1987) Integration of posture and locomotion in acute decerebrate cats in awake, freely moving cats. *Prog Neurobiol* 28:161–195.

Mori S, Kawahara K, Sakamoto T (1983) Supraspinal aspects of locomotion in the mesencephalic cat. In: *Neural Origin of Rhythmic Movements* (Roberts A, Roberts B, eds.), Symp. Soc. Exp. Biol. 37, 445–468. New York: Cambridge University Press.

Mori S, Sakamoto T, Ohta Y, Takakusaki KMK (1989) Site-specific postural and locomotor changes evoked in awake, freely moving intact cats by stimulating the brainstem. *Brain Res* 505:66–74.

Mountcastle VB, Lynch JC, Georgopoulos A, Sakata H, Acuna C (1975) Posterior parietal association cortex of the monkey: Command functions for operations within extrapersonal space. *J Neurophysiol* 38:871–908.

Noga BR, Kettler J, Jordan LM (1988) Locomotion produced in mesencephalic cats by injections of putative transmitter substances and antagonists into the medial reticular formation and the pontomedullary locomotor strip. *J Neurosci* 8:2074–2086.

Noga BR, Kriellaars DJ, Jordan LM (1991) The effect of selective brainstem or spinal cord lesions on treadmill locomotion evoked by stimulation of the mesencephalic or pontomedullary locomotor regions. *J Neurosci* 11:1691–1700.

Ohta Y, Grillner S (1989) Monosynaptic excitatory amino acid transmission from the posterior rhombencephalic reticular nucleus to spinal neurons involved in the control of locomotion in lamprey. *J Neurophysiol* 62:1079–1089.

Orlovsky GN (1970) Work of reticulospinal neurones during locomotion. *Biofizika* 15:728–737.

Pellizzer G, Sargent P, Georgopoulos AP (1995) Motor cortical activity in a context-recall task. *Science* 269:702–705.

Pombal MA, El Manira A, Orlovsky G, Grillner S (1995) Identification of the striatum and its inputs, and the role of the ventral thalamus in the control of reticulospinal neurons and locomotion in the lamprey. *Soc Neurosci Abstr* 21:142.

Porter R, Lemon R (1993) *Corticospinal Function and Voluntary Movement*. Oxford: Clarendon.

Reese NB, Garcia-Rill E, Skinner RD (1992) Auditory input to the pedunculopontine nucleus. *Soc Neurosci Abst* 18:139.11.

Reese NB, Garcia-Rill E, Skinner RD (1995a) Auditory input to the pedunculopontine nucleus: II. Unit responses. *Brain Res Bull* 37:265–273.

Reese NB, Garcia-Rill E, Skinner RD (1995b) The pedunculopontine nucleus—Auditory input, arousal, and pathophysiology. *Prog Neurobiol* 47:105–133.

Rizzolatti G, Gentilucci M, Camarda RM, Gallese V, Luppino G, Matelli M, Fogassi L (1990) Neurons related to reaching-grasping arm movements in the rostral part of area 6 (area 6a beta). *Exp Brain Res* 82:337–350.

Rossignol S (1996) Neural control of stereotypic limb movements. In: *Handbook of Physiology*, sec. 12 (Rowell LB, Shepherd JT, eds.), 173–216. New York: Oxford University Press.

Rossignol S, Dubuc R (1994) Spinal pattern generation. *Curr Opin Neurobiol* 4:894–902.

Sandner G, Di Scala GR (1992) C-*fos* immunoreactivity in the brain following unilateral electrical stimulation of the dorsal periaqueductal gray in freely moving rats. *Brain Res* 573:276–283.

Schieber MH, Hibbard LS (1993) How somatotopic is the motor cortex hand area? *Science* 261:489–492.

Shefchyk SJ, Jordan LM (1985) Excitatory and inhibitory postsynaptic potentials in alpha-motoneurons produced during fictive locomotion by stimulation of the mesencephalic locomotor region. *J Neurophysiol* 53:1345–1355.

Shefchyk SJ, Jell RM, Jordan LM (1984) Reversible cooling of the brainstem reveals areas required for mesencephalic locomotor region evoked treadmill locomotion. *Exp Brain Res* 56:257–262.

Shik ML, Orlovsky GN (1976) Neurophysiology of locomotor automatism. *Physiol Rev* 56:465–501.

Shik ML, Orlovsky GN, Severin FV (1968) Locomotion of the mesencephalic cat elicited by stimulating the pyramids. *Biofizika* 13:127–135.

Shik ML, Severin FV, Orlovsky GN (1966) Control of walking and running by means of electrical stimulation of the mid-brain. *Biophysics* 11:756–765.

Shik ML, Severin FV, Orlovsky GN (1967) Structures of the brain stem responsible for evoking locomotion. *Fiziol Zh (SSSR)* 53:1125–1132.

Shimamura M, Edgerton VR, Kogure I (1987) Application of autoradiographic analysis of 2-deoxyglucose in the study of locomotion. *J Neurosci Meth* 21:303–310.

Shimamura M, Kugure I, Fuwa T (1984) Role of joint afferents in relation to the initiation of forelimb stepping in thalamic cats. *Brain Res* 297:225–234.

Shimamura M, Tanaka I, Fuwa T (1990) Comparison between spinobulbo-spinal and propriospinal reflexes in thalamic cats during stepping. *Neurosci Res* 7:358–368.

Shindo K, Shima K, Tanji J (1995) Spatial distribution of thalamic projections to the supplementary motor area and the primary motor cortex: A retrograde multiple labeling study in the macaque monkey. *J Comp Neurol* 357:98–116.

Shinoda Y, Futami T, Kakei S (1992) Inputs from the cerebellar nuclei to the forelimb area of the motor cortex. *Exp Brain Res Suppl* 22:65–84.

Shinoda Y, Yokota JI, Futami T (1981) Divergent projections of individual corticospinal axons to motoneurons of multiple muscles in the monkey. *Neurosci Lett* 23:7–12.

Shiromani PJ, Kilduff TS, Bloom FE, McCarley RW (1992) Cholinergically induced REM-sleep triggers *fos*-like immunoreactivity in dorsolateral pontine regions associated with REM-sleep. *Brain Res* 580:351–357.

Shiromani PJ, Malik M, Winston S, McCarley RW (1995) Time-course of *fos*-like immunoreactivity associated with cholinergically induced REM-sleep. *J Neurosci* 15:3500–3508.

Shojania K, Livingston CA, Pylypas S, Jordan LM, Nance DM (1992) Descending projections of the mesencephalic locomotor region (MLR) based upon treadmill induced c-*fos* protein and anterograde tract tracing. *Soc Neurosci Abstr* 18:591.15.

Sholomenko GN, Funk GD, Steeves JD (1991) Avian locomotion activated by brainstem infusion of neurotransmitter agonists and antagonists. II. Gamma-aminobutyric acid. *Exp. Brain Res* 85:674–681.

Sillar KT, Simmers AJ (1994) 5HT induces NMDA receptor–mediated intrinsic oscillations in embryonic amphibian spinal neurons. *Proc Royal Soc London (B)* 255:139–145.

Sinnamon HM (1993) Preoptic and hypothalamic neurons and the initiation of locomotion in the anesthetized rat. *Prog Neurobiol* 41:323–344.

Sinnamon HM, Stopford CK (1987) Locomotion elicited by lateral hypothalamic stimulation in the anesthetized rat does not require the dorsal midbrain. *Brain Res* 402:78–86.

Sirota MG, Shik ML (1973) The cat locomotion on stimulation of the midbrain. *Fiziol Zh (SSSR)* 59:1314–1321.

Sirota M, Viana di Prisco G, Dubuc R (1995) Electrical microstimulation of a mesencephalic locomotor region elicits controlled swimming in semi-intact lampreys. *Soc Neurosci Abstr* 21(1):142.

Skinner RD, Garcia-Rill E (1990) Brainstem modulation of rhythmic functions and behaviors. In: *Brainstem Mechanisms and Behavior* (Klemm W, Vertes R, eds.), 465–496. New York: Wiley and Sons.

Skinner RD, Garcia-Rill E (1993) Mesolimbic interactions with mesopontine modulation of locomotion. In: *Limbic Motor Circuits and Neuropsychiatry* (Kalivas PW, ed.), 155–191. Boca Raton, Fl.: CRC.

Slawinska U, Kasicki S (1995) Theta-like rhythm in depth EEG activity of hypothalamic areas during spontaneous or electrically induced locomotion in the rat. *Brain Res* 678:117–126.

Smith AM (1981) The coactivation of antagonist muscles. *Can J Physiol Pharmacol* 59:733–747.

Smith AM, Hepp-Reymond M-C, Wyss UR (1975) Relation of activity in precentral cortical neurons to force and rate of force change during isometric contractions of finger muscles. *Exp Brain Res* 23:315–332.

Smyrnis N, Taira M, Ashe J, Georgopoulos AP (1992) Motor cortical activity in a memorized delay task. *Exp Brain Res* 92:139–151.

Grillner, Georgopoulos, and Jordan

Steckler T, Inglis W, Winn P, Sahgal A (1994) The pedunculopontine tegmental nucleus: A role in cognitive processes? *Brain Res Rev* 19:298–318.

Steeves JD, Jordan LM (1984) Autoradiographic demonstration of the projections from the mesencephalic locomotor region. *Brain Res* 307:263–276.

Steeves JD, Sholomenko GN, Webster DMS (1987) Stimulation of the pontomedullary reticular formation initiates locomotion in decerebrate birds. *Brain Res* 401:205–212.

Sterman MB, Fairchild MD (1966) Modification of locomotor performance by reticular formation and basal forebrain stimulation in the cat: Evidence for reciprocal systems. *Brain Res* 2:205–217.

Swanson LW, Mogenson GJ (1981) Neural mechanisms for the functional coupling of autonomic, endocrine, and somatomotor responses in adaptive behavior (review). *Brain Res* 228:1–34.

Swanson LW, Mogenson GJ, Gerfen CR, Robinson P (1984) Evidence for a projection from the lateral preoptic area and substantia innominata to the 'mesencephalic locomotor region' in the rat. *Brain Res* 295:161–178.

Taira M, Boline J, Smyrnis N, Georgopoulos AP, Ashe J (1996) On the relations between single cell activity in the motor cortex and the direction and magnitude of three-dimensional static isometric force. *Exp Brain Res* 109:367–376.

Tanji J (1994) The supplementary motor area in the cerebral cortex. *Neurosci Res* 19:251–268.

Tanji J, Evarts EV (1976) Anticipatory activity of motor cortex neurons in relation to direction of an intended movement. *J Neurophysiol* 39:1062–1068.

Tanji J, Kurata K (1985) Contrasting neuronal activity in supplementary and precentral motor cortex of monkeys. I. Responses to instructions determining motor responses to forthcoming signals of different modalities. *J Neurophysiol* 53:129–141.

Tanji J, Shima K (1994) Role for supplementary motor area cells in planning several movements ahead. *Nature* 371:413–416.

Veasey SC, Fornal CA (1995) Response of serotonergic caudal raphe neurons in relation to specific motor activities in freely moving cats. *J Neurosci* 15:5346–5359.

Villablanca JR, Marcus RJ, Olmstead CE (1976) Effects of caudate nuclei or frontal cortical ablations in cats. I. Neurology and gross behavior. *Exp Neurol* 52:389–420.

Waters RS, Samulack DD, Dykes RW, McKinley PA (1990) Topographic organization of baboon primary motor cortex: Face, hand, forelimb, and shoulder representation. *Somatosens Mot Res* 7:485–514.

Wise SP (1985) The primate premotor cortex: Past, present, and preparatory. *Annu Rev Neurosci* 8:1–19.

Zemlan FP, Kow L-M, Pfaff DW (1983) Effect of interruption of bulbospinal pathways on lordosis, posture, and locomotion. *Exp Neurol* 81:177–194.

2

The Role of Population Coding in the Control of Movement

David L. Sparks,
William B. Kristan, Jr.,
and Brian K. Shaw

Abstract

This chapter presents findings that stimulated the formulation of population-coding hypotheses of motor control, outlines the essential features of selected hypotheses, and describes the results of experiments designed to test predictions based on these hypotheses. The predictions of certain population-coding hypotheses have been confirmed in studies of the primate superior colliculus, and in invertebrate systems by selectively activating or inactivating specific subsets of neurons with known functional properties. In principle, testing predictions of other population-coding hypotheses should be straightforward; in practice, such tests are often difficult. We suggest that future research directions include finding how nervous systems select a particular behavioral response represented by a population code and how individual neurons in overlapping populations can help to mediate more than one behavior.

The question of how spatial and temporal patterns of neural activity in various regions of the nervous system are related to bodily movements has received much experimental and theoretical attention (for a recent review, see Fetz, 1992). In general, sensory neurons—both exteroceptors and proprioceptors—that provide signals for selecting and guiding movements are broadly tuned to the features of the stimuli that they encode, and central neurons discharging in association with movements are broadly tuned with respect to the parameters of the movements they produce (e.g., force, velocity, direction, amplitude). Fundamental questions emerge from these observations. How can coarsely tuned sensory neurons select and guide specific, spatially accurate actions? How can motor cells that discharge before and during a broad range of movements be responsible for initiating and executing accurate and precise movements? The broad tuning of sensory cells and neurons with motor-related activity means that large populations of cells respond to each stimulus and that large populations of cells are active before and during each movement. Moreover, different populations of "sensory" and "motor" cells in widely distributed areas of the nervous system are active simultaneously both before and during any movement. Therefore, the overriding concern is to explain how nervous systems extract the signals needed to select, initiate, guide, and control movements from the spatial and temporal profiles of large populations of widely distributed and coarsely tuned neurons.

In this chapter we present findings that stimulated the formulation of population-coding hypotheses, outline the essential features of selected hypotheses and models, and describe experiments designed to test the predictions of these models. In addition, many neurons identified for their role in one behavior also take part in one or more other behaviors. This observation raises issues about overlapping codes. For instance, can the same neuron be part of a population that codes for one behavior, and, in addition, participate in the network of neurons that generates the pattern for another behavior (Harris-Warrick et al., chapter 19, this volume)? What happens when the two behaviors are brought into conflict? Will the overlapping interneurons help to make the decision about which behavior is executed? This chapter is divided into separate sections on vertebrate and invertebrate studies to accommodate differences in individual authors' familiarity with the burgeoning literature on this subject and because different issues have been addressed more thoroughly in the different types of nervous systems. It should become apparent to the reader, however, that this artificial division does not represent fundamental differences in the way different nervous systems confront similar problems.

Population Codes for Movements in Vertebrates

In vertebrates, the issue of population coding has been addressed most vigorously in studies of the role of the superior colliculus (SC) in orienting movements of the eyes (e.g., McIlwain, 1975; Sparks et al., 1976 and 1990), as well as in experiments related to the role of the motor cortex in the planning and execution of reaching movements of the arm (e.g., Humphrey et al., 1970; Fetz, 1992; Georgopoulos et al., 1986, 1988, and 1992). This chapter focuses on studies of the primate SC. Population coding in the motor cortex is also considered elsewhere (Grillner et al., chapter 1, this volume).

Population Coding in the Superior Colliculus

Experimental Basis of the Population-Coding Hypotheses

The intermediate and deeper layers of the SC receive convergent auditory, visual, and somatosensory signals, and generate motor commands for orienting movements of the eyes and head. SC neurons related to saccadic eye movements have been studied most extensively in ani-

mals with their heads restrained. Under these conditions, many SC neurons discharge before saccadic eye movements. Each cell discharges before saccades that have a particular range of directions and amplitudes (termed the *movement field* of the cell). The topographical organization of movement fields within the SC forms a map of motor (saccadic) space (Wurtz and Goldberg, 1972; Robinson, 1972; Sparks et al., 1976; Sparks, 1978).

Because each neuron in the SC fires before a broad range of saccades, a large population of neurons is active before each saccade (Sparks et al., 1976; Sparks and Mays, 1980). How such broadly tuned activity precisely controls the direction and amplitude of a saccade might be accomplished in various ways. The movement might be based on a "winner-take-all" code in which the activity of the most intensely firing neurons within the population is selected at a subsequent stage of neural processing. Alternatively, the activity of each member of the population might contribute to the direction and amplitude of the movement. Various schemes by which this might be accomplished have been proposed (McIlwain, 1975; Sparks et al., 1976; van Gisbergen et al., 1987; van Opstal and van Gisbergen, 1989). The following two sections present the evidence for the most likely mechanism for generating saccades: vector averaging.

The Vector-Averaging Hypothesis: Description and Predictions

The vector-averaging hypothesis was first proposed by Sparks and colleagues (1976). This hypothesis assumes that the large population of collicular neurons active before a given saccade occupies a symmetrical area within the motor map on the SC (panel 1 of figure 2.1). Only the neurons in the center of the active population (marked A in the figure) discharge maximally before the programmed movement; however, for each subset of active neurons (marked B) discharging maximally before movements with a direction and amplitude other than the programmed movement, there will be a second subset of active neurons (marked C) discharging maximally before movements of other directions and amplitudes such that the average direction and amplitude will be the same as that coded by neurons in the center of the population. Thus, it is hypothesized that each member of the active population contributes to the ensuing saccade. Specifically, the direction and amplitude of each saccade is the average of the vectors that describe the movements coded by each of the active neurons. This hypothesis predicts that any perturbation in the spatial profile of collicular activity should produce an alteration in the

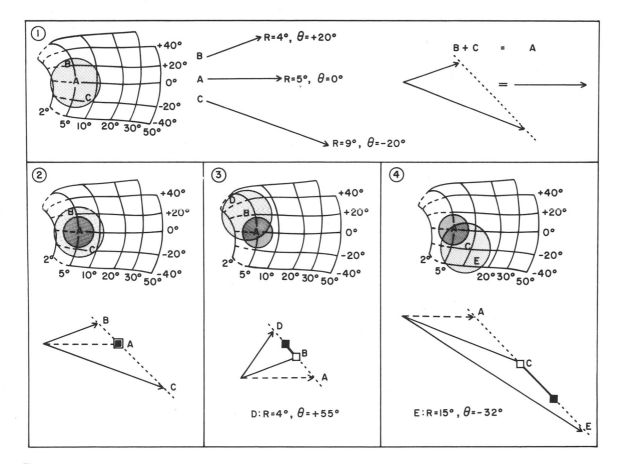

Figure 2.1

Using the vector-averaging hypothesis to predict the direction and amplitude of saccades. (Panel 1) Vector-averaging scheme of Sparks and colleagues (1976). On the left is the motor map of the left SC. The area within the circle represents the locus of neurons active before saccades to a target five degrees right of the fixation point. The locus is assumed to be symmetrical. Neurons at locations A, B, and C fire most vigorously for movements in the directions and with the amplitudes shown by the three vectors in the middle. As indicated on the right side of the panel, the weighted average of activity at points B and C yields approximately the same movement vector as does activity at A. (Panels 2–4) Predicted effect of deactivating a localized set of neurons in a specific region of the SC. The locus of deactivation (the darkly stippled circle) is the same in each panel, but the location of the active population (the lightly stippled area) is different, indicating saccades to three different targets (i.e., to a location corresponding to locus A in panel 2, to locus B in panel 3, and to locus C in panel 4). Beneath each map are the saccade vectors associated with neural activity at the center and the outside edges of each of the locations illustrated. The open square represents the vector of the intended saccade. The dashed line represents the vector of the movement tendency produced by the deactivated neurons. Because these neurons do not contribute to the saccade, the actual movement (indicated by the filled square) may be the same as (panel 2) or different from (panels 3 and 4) the intended movement. (Reprinted with permission from Lee et al., 1988).

direction and amplitude of the ensuing saccade. Specific predictions of the vector-averaging hypothesis regarding the effects of deactivating a portion of the SC are outlined in panels 2–4 of figure 2.1.

Panel 2 shows that deactivation restricted to the center of the activated population will have no effect upon saccade direction and amplitude. (A more recent version of this hypothesis [Sparks and Mays, 1990] assumes that the speed of the movement is related to the overall level of activity within the active population, so that the movement would be slower after deactivating the central region.) Panels 3 and 4 show that a systematic pattern of errors will be observed when the deactivated cells are on the periphery of the active population. Activation (instead of deactivation) by microstimulation, or by small injections of substances that produce local elevations in neuronal activity, is predicted to have effects upon direction, amplitude, speed, and latency that are opposite to those produced by deactivation of cellular activity. Experimental tests of these predictions are presented in the following section.

Evidence Related to the Predictions

Microstimulation experiments The vector-averaging hypothesis was based, in part, upon the finding of Robinson

(1972) that simultaneously stimulating two points in the SC evoked movements intermediate in amplitude and direction between movements produced by stimulating either site alone. This finding strongly suggested an averaging, rather than winner-take-all, strategy for combining activity throughout different regions of the SC. Sparks and Mays (1983) observed a similar interaction between visually guided saccades and stimulation-induced movements: the direction and amplitude of stimulation-evoked saccades were influenced toward the location of a visual target to which a saccade had not yet been directed. Such interactions were apparent even when the stimulation was at a sufficiently low frequency that it was subthreshold for producing any movement (Glimcher and Sparks, 1993). The subthreshold stimulation trains biased the direction and amplitude of spontaneous and visually guided eye movements in the direction and amplitude of movements induced by suprathreshold stimulation of the same collicular location. All of these data are consistent with the predictions of the vector-averaging hypothesis of Sparks et al. (1976).

Reversible inactivation or activation experiments Injection of substances that either depress or enhance activity in a localized collicular region perturb the spatial and temporal balance in the collicular motor map (Lee et al., 1988; Sparks et al., 1990). These experiments provide additional tests of predictions of the vector-averaging model. Following local deactivation of collicular neurons, the endpoints of visually guided saccades were biased away from the endpoint of the control stimulation-induced movement (figure 2.2A). The opposite perturbation—activating a small region by injecting bicuculline, which blocks input from inhibitory neurons—produced saccades to surrounding targets that displayed an "attraction" to the position commanded by the activated region (figure 2.2B). These results provide compelling support for the vector-averaging model. According to this model, saccadic accuracy results from the averaging of the movement tendencies produced by the entire active population rather than from the discharge of a small number of finely tuned cells. Small changes in the direction and amplitude of saccades are produced by slight shifts in the location of the large population of active cells.

Population Coding in Other Vertebrate Motor Systems

Recent experiments by Berkowitz and Stein (1994a, 1994b) suggest that the turtle nervous system may select the appropriate form of scratching, rostral or pocket, by

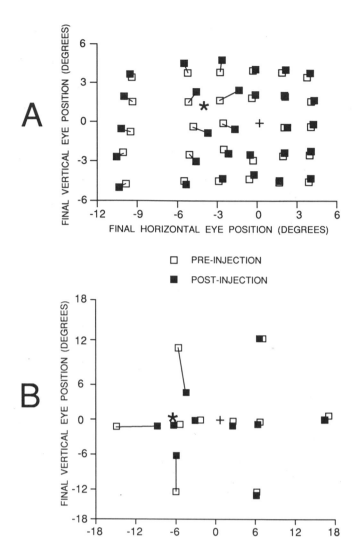

Figure 2.2
Modifications of saccades by injections that inactivate and activate small regions of the SC. Plots show the positions of the initial fixation (+) and the endpoint (*) of the best saccade. Each square represents the average endpoint of three to five visually guided saccades. Unfilled squares represent movements that occurred before the injections; filled squares represent postinjection trials for matching targets. Lines connecting the squares represent the average error introduced by modifying the spatial and temporal pattern of neuronal activity within the SC. (A) Effects of a single 200-nl injection of lidocaine. (B) Effects of a single 200-nl injection of bicuculline. (Modified from Sparks et al., 1990.)

activating populations of broadly tuned neurons, rather than highly specialized neurons (see also Stein and Smith, chapter 5, this volume). Testing whether a population-coding scheme controls turtle scratching is difficult, however, because the axons of propriospinal neurons maximally tuned for a particular form of scratching do not appear to be localized in particular regions of the spinal cord white matter (Berkowitz and Stein, 1994a). It may be impossible to use microstimulation or reversible activation/inactivation in this preparation to test the contributions of particular neuronal subsets. Berkowitz and Stein's studies do, however, raise an interesting issue about how nervous systems code for specific directions of movement (e.g., dorsal vs. ventral pocket scratching) as well as make choices between behaviors (e.g., rostral vs. pocket scratching). Within a scratch type, the same muscles are used in similar patterns. A population code similar to that described above for primate motor control could also be used for turtle pocket scratching—that is, a population of neurons could be activated in a slightly different pattern to produce a pocket scratch directed to a slightly different location. Berkowitz and Stein (1994b) have proposed an additional feature that may account for appropriate choice of scratch form: the knee extensor motoneuron pool may provide a possible integration site for the behavioral choice. The issue of behavioral choice will be considered further in the section on invertebrate motor control.

Georgopoulos and colleagues (1986) have described a possible population code in the monkey motor cortex that controls reaching movements of the arm. During an arm-reaching task, many broadly tuned cells discharge maximally in association with movements in a preferred direction, but less vigorously in association with movements in other directions. Georgopoulos and colleagues have shown that the sum of the activity of directionally tuned cells, weighted by their discharge rate, provides a population vector that points in the direction of the movement of the limb. Other studies suggest that the length of the vector is related to movement speed and that the population vector may also represent aspects of the intention to move (Georgopoulos et al., 1993). These findings have been interpreted as evidence that the direction of hand displacement by the arm, rather than muscle force or other movement parameters, is coded by populations of neurons in the motor cortex. This hypothesis is an extension of earlier work by Humphrey and colleagues (1970) showing that by optimally selecting weighting factors for each parameter, the output of neuron populations in the motor cortex can be made to match force trajectories and wrist displacements, as well as their temporal derivatives. Numerous experiments have extended the feasibility of the vector summation hypothesis of Georgopoulos and colleagues to a variety of conditions, including reaching movements in three-dimensional space (Georgopoulos et al., 1988; Schwartz et al., 1988) and drawing movements (Schwartz, 1994).

Repeated demonstrations of the feasibility of the population vector hypothesis of Georgopoulos and colleagues do not, however, constitute proof of the hypothesis. As others have emphasized, it is not so easy to decide which features of a movement are explicitly coded by the nervous system and which are consequences of the interaction of the output with the external world (Gottlieb, 1993; Kalaska and Crammond, 1992; Latash, 1993). Plausible arguments can be made that neurons in the motor cortex encode a variety of movement parameters—including force, rate of change of force, direction of movement, and muscle stiffness. Mussa-Ivaldi (1988) has shown that the solution of the matrix transform between the direction of endpoint handpath and shoulder muscle-state variables predicts that cells encoding information about shoulder muscle lengths and the rate of changes of muscle lengths would have directional tuning properties similar to cells in the motor cortex. This alternative interpretation of the data offered as support of the Georgopoulos hypothesis is also consistent with models of motor control in which the kinematic features of a movement, such as direction, are emergent properties of the interactions between programmed forces and the loading of the limb (Gottlieb, 1993). Theoretical arguments have been made that the existence of a population vector constitutes only weak support for the explicit use of a particular coordinate representation by the motor cortex (Sanger, 1994). Other models (Houk, 1989) have treated the overall premotor network of the arm as a parallel distributed system in which movements are controlled by cooperative neuronal activity distributed in the cerebellum, the red nucleus, motor portions of the thalamus, and the pontine nuclei, as well as in the motor cortex. Finally, it has also been suggested that the search for explicit coding may be diverting us from understanding more distributed neural mechanisms that are more complex and less directly related to explicit movement parameters (Fetz, 1992).

Clearly, many vertebrate nervous systems use population coding to produce a variety of directed movements. However, because nervous systems may control different metrics of movements and because different types of population codes may be used (e.g., winner-take-all, vector summation, and vector averaging), testing the predictions of particular models or hypotheses becomes critical. For example, because cells in columns in the motor cortex tend to have similar preferred directions (Georgopoulos et al., 1984), it should be possible to test the vector summation hypothesis by deactivating a subset of cortical cells coding for a particular direction to see if predictable errors in direction occur, both in the trajectory and endpoint of the movement. In a more general sense, further progress in understanding the role of population coding in the control of movements in vertebrates depends upon developing experimental tests that distinguish one type of population code from another. In such experiments, however, attempts to reconstruct the actual distribution of cells with particular functional properties in various motor areas are important, as are efforts to develop methods for activity-dependent inactivation of cells or for selectively modifying the response properties of particular subsets of functional classes of cells involved in motor control.

Population Codes for Movements in Invertebrates

At first glance, it may seem that animals with relatively simple nervous systems use different strategies for producing behaviors than do animals with more complex nervous systems. Higher vertebrates, with more than 10^{13} neurons, can invest populations of neurons to perform each of their behaviors, whereas animals with less than 10^6 neurons must use each one sparingly. This distinction has bred the expectation that the interneuronal networks in invertebrates would be sparse and simple. It came as a surprise, therefore, when a variety of reflexive movements in invertebrate animals also appeared to use population codes. For instance, cricket and cockroach interneurons that respond to the direction of air movements (and thereby to the direction of an approaching predator) are so broadly tuned that each is activated by inputs from many directions (Miller et al., 1991; Comer and Dowd, 1993; Ritzmann, 1993; Ritzmann and Eaton, chapter 3, this volume). The interneurons responsible for leg reflexes in stick insects are also broadly tuned, both in their responses to mechanosensory input and in the motor effects they produce when stimulated (Baessler, 1993). The simplest segmental bending response of the medicinal leech, caused by light pressure, activates a pool of interneurons whose actions can be mimicked by the sorts of parallel distributed networks generated by neural nets (Lockery et al., 1989; Lockery and Kristan, 1990; Kristan, 1994; see also figure 2.3). In all of these invertebrate systems, the same interneurons can be identified from individual to individual, so are they truly population codes, and, if so, what are their natures? These questions will be addressed in more detail for the leech local-bend reflex and the initial directed turn made by standing cockroaches away from air movement, in anticipation of running away (figure 2.3).

The local-bend reflex and the initial directed turn are similar behaviors in that both are directed responses to mechanical stimuli that may come from anywhere around the animal. In the leech, a touch to the skin around the body surface (top, bottom, left, or right) may be sufficient to activate one or more of the six T (touch) or four P (pressure) cells with overlapping receptive fields in each segment (Kristan et al., 1995). In the cockroach, the activating stimuli are air movements that bend sensory hairs in the posteriorly directed cerci (Kolton and Camhi, 1995), as well as tactile stimuli that activate mechanoreceptors in the anteriorly directed antennae and over the surface of the whole body. Such stimulation activates some of the hundreds of sensory neurons at the bases of the hairs (Ritzmann, 1993). Depending on the size of the cockroach, there are hundreds to thousands of primary mechanoreceptors, plus additional pathways from visual and auditory stimuli that have not yet been as well characterized.

Population Coding in Leech and Cockroach Mechanosensory Interneurons

The mechanosensory interneurons involved in both reflexes respond to stimuli over a broad range. There are about thirty such interneurons per segment in the leech (Lockery and Kristan, 1991). In the cockroach, the major interneurons receiving direct input from the cercal mechanosensors are termed *giant interneurons* (GIs), primarily those with axons located ventrally in the nerve cord, the vGIs (Kolton and Camhi, 1995). There appear to be only two pairs of vGIs (Comer and Dowd, 1993; Levi and Camhi, 1994). In the leech, mechanosensory interneurons make connections directly with motoneurons, whereas the GIs of the cockroach connect with type A thoracic interneurons (TI$_A$s), which in turn alter the excitability of leg motoneurons (Ritzmann, 1993; see also Ritzmann and Eaton, chapter 3 this volume). These leech and cockroach interneurons share several functional properties with those in the primate superior colliculus.

1. Their activity is correlated with the behavior. In both the cockroach and the leech, these interneurons are activated by the same mechanical stimuli that produce motor output (Kristan et al., 1995; Kolton and Camhi, 1995). The broad-tuning curves of the cockroach interneurons are nearly the optimal width and separation from one another to maximize information transfer from primary sensory neurons to interneurons, as established for similar cricket interneurons (Theunissen and Miller, 1991). Most leech local bend interneurons receive input from three or four segmental P cells, the latter being the sensory neurons most strongly responsible for eliciting a local bend (Lockery and Kristan, 1991). As a result, most of the interneuronal receptive fields extend one-half to three-quarters of the way around the animal.

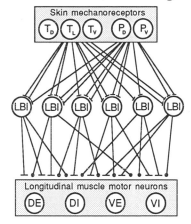

A Leech local bending

Skin mechanoreceptors

T_D T_L T_V P_D P_V

LBI LBI LBI LBI LBI LBI

Longitudinal muscle motor neurons

DE DI VE VI

⊣ = excitatory effect
•— = inhibitory effect

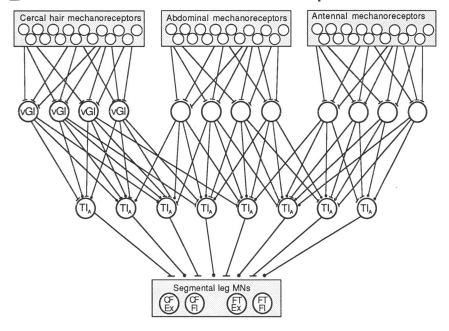

B Cockroach orientation for escape

Cercal hair mechanoreceptors   Abdominal mechanoreceptors   Antennal mechanoreceptors

vGI vGI vGI vGI

TI_A TI_A TI_A TI_A TI_A TI_A TI_A TI_A

Segmental leg MNs

CF Ex   CF Fl   FT Ex   FT Fl

Figure 2.3

Population coding in two invertebrate behaviors. (A) Type of circuit used to produce local bending in the medicinal leech. Two types of mechanoreceptors, the T (touch) and P (pressure) neurons (D, L, and V subscripts indicate dorsal, lateral, and ventral receptive fields), excite local-bend interneurons (LBI), and the LBIs both excite and inhibit the longitudinal muscle motoneurons: dorsal excitors (DE), dorsal inhibitors (DI), ventral excitors (VE), and ventral inhibitors (VI). (B) Types of circuits used to produce the orientation of cockroaches before escape from mechanical stimuli. Three sets of mechanosensory neurons (from the cerci, the abdominal surface, and the anteriorly projecting antennae) make connections with separate sets of interneurons. The best characterized pathway is the one from the cercal mechanoreceptors to the ventral giant interneurons (vGIs), which in turn project to a common set of premotor interneurons in the thoracic ganglia (TI_A). The TI_A layer projects to extensor (Ex) and flexor (Fl) motoneurons at two leg joints, the coxa-femur (CF) and the femur-tibia (FT). This system produces orientation movements away from the stimulus source before the animal starts to run. (For more details, see Ritzmann and Eaton, chapter 3, this volume.) In this figure and in figure 2.4, circles indicate individual neurons and shaded boxes indicate that there is a larger population of each type of cell. Also, the connectivity patterns in both figures are meant to represent the types of connections made and their known effects. The patterns do not necessarily indicate physiologically defined monosynaptic connections.

2. Stimulating individual interneurons produces part of the behavior. Leech interneurons that respond during local bend activate different combinations of motoneurons to the longitudinal muscles (Lockery and Kristan, 1991; Wittenberg and Kristan, 1992). Levi and Camhi (1994 and 1995) discovered that stimulating individual vGIs in cockroaches as they turned in response to air puffs delivered to the cerci produced, for one direction of turning, a bias in the direction of movement away from the source of the stimulus.

3. Removing individual interneurons weakens directional responses. In two studies, leech local bend interneurons were removed transiently by hyperpolarizing them individually while monitoring motoneuronal responses to P-cell stimulation (Lockery and Kristan, 1991; Wittenberg and Kristan, 1992). In fact, only those interneurons whose removal changed motoneuronal responses were considered to be local-bend interneurons. Similarly, killing a single vGI in the nerve cord of a cockroach by injecting a proteolytic enzyme made the animal less likely to turn in the direction of the optimal response of that vGI (Comer and Dowd, 1993).

In summary, both leech local-bending behavior and cockroach orientation are produced by population codes. The nature of the codes can now be investigated in more detail. For instance, is the average firing of the interneurons the only important feature, or do the details of the firing pattern matter? Preliminary findings for cockroach vGIs indicate that the code may be simply a weighted number of spikes in each vGI during the period after an air puff is administered (Liebenthal et al., 1994). Will other features—such as the tonic or phasic nature of the interneuronal responses—turn out to be important, too? Do all the interneurons have the same effects, or are there qualitative differences? Because of the relative simplicity of these invertebrate systems, it should be possible to determine the cellular and network properties important for producing population codes.

Multiplexing by Individual Interneurons

In addition to firing to a broad range of stimuli as part of a coding population, an interneuron can be active during qualitatively different behaviors. For instance, both Dorsal Swim Interneurons (DSI) and Ventral Swim Interneurons (VSI)—identified as members of the central pattern generator (CPG) for swimming in the mollusk *Tritonia*—are also activated in a reflexive withdrawal response (Getting and Dekin, 1985). Which behavior is elicited depends upon what kind of stimulus is given, which interneurons are activated, and possibly modulations of

the properties of the synaptic interactions among the CPG neurons (Katz and Frost, 1995). The number of well-documented cases of multiplexing in which the circuits for both behaviors have been elucidated is, not surprisingly, very small. There is, however, at least one example of a neuron—cell 115 in the leech—that participates both in the population-coded local-bending response and in the CPG for swimming (Lockery and Kristan, 1990; Wittenberg and Kristan, 1992).

The neuronal circuitry controlling leech swimming is largely understood, from stimulation to undulation (Brodfuehrer et al., 1995). It consists of five distinct and hierarchical levels, starting with mechanosensory neurons and moving through two layers of decision-making neurons (*trigger cells* fire a burst at the start of a swimming episode, whereas *gating cells* fire throughout such episodes) to the CPG itself, which in turn connects directly with motoneurons (figure 2.4A). Cell 115 is one of the CPG neurons whose firing centers at 40° in the cycle period; it also contributes to the local-bending response. Cell 115 has several properties that make it suitable for such a dual role. First, it is "premotor," making connections directly to motoneurons, so it *can* participate in local bending, a behavior in which only a single layer of interneurons lies between mechanosensory neurons and motoneurons. Second, cell 115 connects to all motoneurons appropriate for both behaviors: it excites the dorsal longitudinal muscle excitors and inhibits the ventral longitudinal excitors (Lockery and Kristan, 1990), thereby helping to produce a ventral bend useful in both behaviors. Other CPG interneurons are not activated during local bending, and only weak connections exist among any local-bend interneurons. Based on its connections, a reasonable explanation can be given for cell 115's role in these two behaviors. When T and P mechanoreceptors are stimulated at low levels, the swim-activating network is silent, so mechanoreceptors' connections to cell 115 and to other local-bend interneurons produce local bending. At higher stimulus levels, T and P cells excite the swim-activating interneurons strongly, turning on the gating interneurons, so the positive feedback between these gating interneurons and the CPG interneurons produces a prolonged episode of swimming.

In addition, cell 115 is also activated in the whole-body shortening response. There appear to be parallel pathways to the motoneurons for this behavior (figure 2.4B): a fast-conducting system (FCS) and a slower pathway (Shaw and Kristan, 1995). The FCS quickly activates some motoneurons in whole-body shortening. The slower interneuronal pathway responsible for the more prolonged part of the response has not yet been charac-

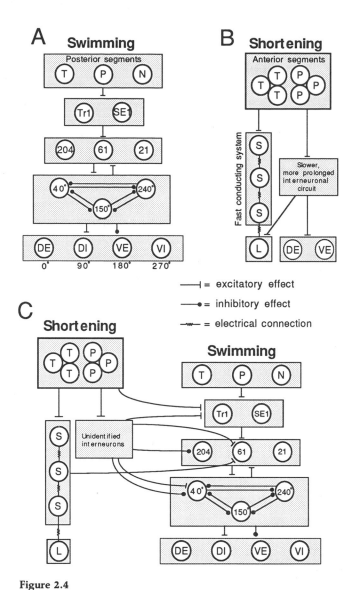

Figure 2.4

Neuronal circuits underlying swimming and whole-body shortening in the medicinal leech. (A) The neuronal circuitry for swimming. The T, P, and N (nociceptive) mechanosensory neurons, particularly those in posterior segments, activate "swim-activator" interneurons (Tr, trigger, SE, swim excitor) in the anterior brain, which excite segmental swim-gating interneurons (paired cells 21 and 61, plus the unpaired cell 204 in many midbody ganglia), which in turn activate the segmental central pattern-generating (CPG) interneurons. The CPG interneurons produce a three-phased oscillatory rhythm and connect to the same longitudinal muscle motoneurons (DE, DI, VE, and VI) used for local bending. (B) Neuronal circuitry for whole-body shortening. T and P mechanoreceptors, especially those in anterior segments, activate two pathways: one is fast, comprising the electrotonically coupled S cells in successive segments, and activates the pairs of segmental L motoneurons; the other is slower and provides more prolonged excitation to the L, DE, and VE motoneurons in each segment. The interneurons in these two pathways have yet to be identified. (C) Excitatory and inhibitory influences from the shortening circuit to neurons in the swimming circuit.

terized in detail, but cell 115's activity may play some role in this response, too.

Behavioral Choice

Some behavioral acts are compatible (e.g., walking and breathing), whereas others are not. For instance, leeches can locally bend while performing a number of other behaviors, but they cannot shorten their whole body and swim at the same time. In several kinds of tests, shortening always dominates swimming. For instance, the same stimulus that reliably elicits shortening in a resting leech (i.e., simultaneous activation of several T and P cells in the front end of the animal) also causes a swimming leech to stop swimming and to shorten. To find the neuronal basis for this behavioral choice, Shaw and Kristan (1997) recorded the neuronal activity at several CNS levels in the swimming hierarchy while delivering shortening-inducing stimuli. Not surprisingly, cell 204—one of the most effective swim-gating interneurons (Brodfuehrer et al., 1995)—is strongly inhibited during shortening, as is cell 208, one of the CPG interneurons (figure 2.4C). Somewhat surprisingly, cell 61, another swim-gating interneuron, is excited during whole-body shortening. Because it is serotonergic, cell 61 may share with other serotonergic neurons (Szczupak and Kristan, 1995) the role of arousing the whole nervous system whenever tactile stimuli are received. Stimulation of cell 61 produces a sensitization of the local bending response, for instance, that can last several minutes (Lockery and Kristan, 1991). The most surprising result of this study, however, was that all the swim-activating neurons at the highest level of the swimming hierarchy are excited by stimuli that produce whole-body shortening. All of these results suggest that the swim-activating interneurons are more likely to be "do something" interneurons, that swimming is just one of several possible outcomes of their activation, and that the decision whether to swim or to shorten is made at the level and below the level of the swim-gating interneurons.

Moreover, the gating neuron, cell 204, may serve a similar function to that proposed for cell C2 in *Tritonia* (Getting and Dekin, 1985): when activated along with other interneurons, swimming occurs; when inhibited while the same (or at least some of the same) interneurons are activated, shortening occurs. In fact, cell 115— the interneuron that functions both in local bending and as a 40° CPG cell in swimming—is also activated during shortening (figure 2.4C), so that it is multiplexed among at least three different behaviors. This neuron and all the other interneurons involved in the population coding of local bending do not appear to participate in the choice of behaviors; the choice is made at a higher hierarchical level. For turtle scratching, the choice of a limb posture to be used to reach a given irritating stimulus is thought to be made by a population-coding scheme (Berkowitz and Stein 1994a, 1994b). All locations within reach of the leg being held in a particular posture are also thought to be determined by a population-coding scheme.

The mechanisms used to make different behavioral choices in different animals may well differ in detail. Given the similarities in the types of neuronal coding mechanisms, however, it seems likely that the general logic of connectivity used to choose between behaviors in virtually all animals will prove to be as similar as are the mechanisms used to code the individual behaviors.

Summary

Neurophysiological findings have forced students of vertebrate and invertebrate behavior to consider the problem of sensorimotor integration from a population-coding perspective. Most sensory signals and motor commands are represented by the spatial and temporal patterns of neural activity in (usually) large populations of sensory, premotor, and motoneurons. It is not a trivial problem to choose among many candidate schemes for extracting signals and/or commands from the spatial and temporal profiles of the ensemble activity. Progress in this area has been most rapid in vertebrate systems in which the sensory singals and motor commands are represented by neural activity within well-defined computational maps and in invertebrate systems in which the neurons involved in the behavior are relatively accessible. Direct manipulations of the spatial and temporal profile of activity (i.e., perturbations of activity within specific regions of a map, or selective activation or inactivation of specific neurons with known functional properties) are necessary to test the predictions of alternative models.

It seems clear that future invertebrate and vertebrate research on this topic will follow a parallel course. Because most population-coding schemes currently proposed generate a single motor output (e.g., a saccade with a particular direction and a particular amplitude), the problems of decision making, behavioral choice, and response selection must be considered in the development of future experimental plans. Preliminary work with vertebrates (e.g., Glimcher and Sparks, 1992) and invertebrates has served to focus the questions, but much additional work is needed before we have a general understanding of the neural mechanisms involved in the selection of particular behavioral responses from a large repertoire of potential actions. Based upon the work already done, it seems likely that decision making or response selection is not the task of a few specialized "command neurons" but arises from consensus in a large population of neurons.

Another problem that has emerged in both vertebrate and invertebrate studies of population coding of movements is the involvement of individual neurons in more than one behavior. For example, the problem of pinpointing the involvement of specific leech neurons in swimming, whole-body shortening, and local bending was discussed in this chapter, but similar problems are emerging in the vertebrate literature as well (i.e., the involvement of neurons in the superior colliculus in movements of both the eyes and head; see Friedman and Sparks, 1994).

Finally, our review has revealed the need for more conceptual work on the use of population coding in the control of movements. In this article, we treated population-coding schemes and pattern generator schemes as separate coding mechanisms, but we ignored the obvious facts that pattern generator circuits involve populations of neurons and that those circuits considered to be the best examples of population codes must generate patterned outputs. More conceptual and computational work is needed as a guide to understanding how the activity of neurons distributed within a motor map is used to generate the temporal pattern of activity required by separate motoneuronal pools, especially when considering the neural control of saccadic eye movements.

Acknowledgments

The research reviewed in this article was supported by an NIH NEI Research Grant (EY01189) and a grant from The McKnight Foundation Endowment Fund for Neuroscience to D. L. Sparks; an NIMH (MH43396) and an NSF Research Grant (IBN11432) to W. B. Kristan Jr.; and an NIH Training Grant (GM08107) to B. K. Shaw.

References

Baessler U (1993) The femur-tibia control system of stick insects: A model system for the study of joint control. *Brain Res Rev* 18:207–226.

Berkowitz A, Stein PSG (1994a) Activity of descending propriospinal axons in the turtle hindlimb enlargement during two forms of fictive scratching: Broad tuning to regions of the body surface. *J Neurosci* 14:5089–5104.

Berkowitz A, Stein PSG (1994b) Activity of descending propriospinal axons in the turtle hindlimb enlargement during two forms of fictive scratching: Phase analyses. *J Neurosci* 14:5105–5119.

Brodfuehrer PD, Debski EA, O'Gara BA, Friesen WO (1995) Neuronal control of swimming. *J Neurobiol* 27:403–418.

Comer CM, Dowd JP (1993) Multisensory processing for movement: Antennal and cercal mediation of escape turning in the cockroach. In: *Biological Neural Networks in Invertebrate Neuroethology and Robotics* (Beer RD, Ritzmann RE, McKenna T, eds.), 89–112. Boston: Academic.

Fetz EE (1992) Are movement parameters recognizably coded in the activity of single neurons? *Behav Brain Sci* 15:679–690.

Freedman EG, Sparks DL (1994) Response properties of saccade-related burst cells in the superior colliculus of the monkey during large, head unrestrained, gaze shifts. *Soc Neurosci Abstr* 20:142.

Georgopoulos AP, Ashe J, Smyrnis N, Taira M (1992) The motor cortex and the coding of force. *Science* 256:1692–1695.

Georgopoulos AP, Kalaska JF, Crutcher MD, Caminiti R, Massey JT (1984) In: *Dynamic Aspects of Neocortical Function* (Edelman GM, Gall WE, Cowan WM, eds.), 501–524. New York: Wiley.

Georgopoulos AP, Kettner RE, Schwartz AB (1988) Primate motor cortex and free arm movements to visual targets in three-dimensional space. II. Coding of the direction of movement by a neuronal population. *J Neurosci* 8:2928–2937.

Georgopoulos AP, Schwartz AB, Kettner RE (1986) Neuronal population coding of movement direction. *Science* 233:1416–1419.

Georgopoulos AP, Taira M, Lukashin A (1993) Cognitive neurophysiology of the motor cortex. *Science* 260:47–52.

Getting PA, Dekin MS (1985) Tritonia swimming: A model system for integration within motor systems. In: *Model Neural Networks and Behavior* (Selverston AI, ed.), 3–20. New York: Plenum.

Glimcher PA, Sparks DL (1992) Movement selection in advance of action: Saccade-related bursters of the superior colliculus. *Nature* 355:542–545.

Glimcher P, Sparks DL (1993) The effects of low frequency stimulation of the superior colliculus on spontaneous and visually guided saccades. *J Neurophysiol* 69:953–964.

Gottlieb GL (1993) A computational model of the simplest motor program. *J Motor Behavior* 25:153–161.

Houk JC (1989) Cooperative control of limb movements by the motor cortex, brainstem, and cerebellum. In: *Models of Brain Function* (Cotterill RMJ, ed.), 309–325. Cambridge, UK: Cambridge University Press.

Humphrey DR, Schmidt EM, Thompson WD (1970) Predicting measures of motor performance from multiple spike trains. *Science* 170:758–762.

Kalaska JF, Crammond DJ (1992) Cerebral cortical mechanisms of reaching movements. *Science* 255:1517–1523.

Katz PS, Frost WN (1995) Intrinsic neuromodulation in the *Tritonia* swim CPG: The serotonergic dorsal swim interneurons act presynaptically to enhance transmitter release from interneuron C2. *J Neurosci* 15:6035–6045.

Kien J, McCrohan CR, Winlow W (1992) *Neurobiology of Motor Programme Selection*. New York: Pergamon.

Kolton L, Camhi JM (1995) Cartesian representation of stimulus direction: Parallel processing by two sets of giant interneurons. *J Comp Physiol (A)* 176:691–702.

Kristan WB Jr (1994) Distributed processing vs dedicated neurons in the production of simple behavioral acts. In: *Emergence of Prerational Intelligence in Biology: From Sensorimotor Intelligence to Collective Behavior* (Cruse H, Dean J, Ritter H, eds.), 37–63. Bielefeld, Germany: ZiF.

Kristan WB Jr, Lockery SR, Lewis JE (1995). Using reflexive behaviors of the medicinal leech to study information processing. *J Neurobiol* 27:380–389.

Latash ML (1993) *Control of Human Movement*. Champaign, Ill: Human Kinetics.

Lee C, Rohrer WH, Sparks DL (1988) Population coding of saccadic eye movements by neurons in the superior colliculus. *Nature* 332:357–360.

Levi R, Camhi JM (1994) Testing for a population vector code for wind direction in the cockroach giant interneurons. *Soc Neurosci Abstr* 20:1025.

Levi R, Camhi JM (1995) Cartesian representation of stimulus direction: Parallel processing by two sets of giant interneurons in the cockroach. *J Comp Physiol (A)* 176:691–702.

Liebenthal E, Uhlmann O, Camhi JM (1994) Critical parameters of the spike trains in a cell assembly: Coding of turn direction by the giant interneurons of the cockroach. *J Comp Physiol (A)* 174:281–296.

Lockery SR, Kristan WB Jr (1990) Distributed processing of sensory information in the leech. II. Identification of interneurons contributing to the local bending reflex. *J Neurosci* 10:1816–1829.

Lockery SR, Kristan WB Jr (1991) Two forms of sensitization of the local bending reflex of the medicinal leech. *J Comp Physiol (A)* 168:165–177.

Lockery SR, Wittenberg G, Kristan WB Jr, Cottrell GW (1989) Function of identified interneurons in the leech elucidated using networks trained by back-propagation. *Nature* 340:468–471.

McIlwain JT (1975) Visual receptive fields and their images in superior colliculus of the cat. *J Neurophysiol* 38:219–230.

Miller JP, Jacobs GA, Theunissen FE (1991) Representation of sensory information in the cricket cercal sensory system. I. Response properties of the primary interneurons. *J Neurophysiol* 66:1680–1689.

Mussa-Ivaldi FA (1988) Do neurons in the motor cortex encode movement direction? An alternative hypothesis. *Neurosci Lett* 91:978–982.

Nusbaum MP, Kristan WB Jr (1986) Swim initiation in the leech by serotonin-containing interneurons, cells 21 and 61. *J Exp Biol* 122:277–302.

Ritzmann RE (1993) The neural organization of cockroach escape and its role in context-dependent orientation. In: *Biological Neural Networks in Invertebrate Neuroethology and Robotics* (Beer RD, Ritzmann RE, McKenna T, eds.), 113–137. Boston: Academic.

Robinson DA (1972) Eye movements evoked by collicular stimulation in the alert monkey. *Vision Res* 12:1795–1808.

Sanger TD (1994) Theoretical considerations for the analysis of population coding in motor cortex. *Neural Comput* 6:29–37.

Schwartz AB (1994) Direct cortical representation of drawing. *Science* 265:540–542.

Schwartz AB, Kettner RE, Georgopoulos AP (1988) Primate motor cortex and free arm movements to visual targets in three-dimensional space. I. Relations between single cell discharge and direction of movement. *J Neurosci* 8:2913–2927.

Shaw BK, Kristan WB Jr (1995) The whole-body shortening reflex of the medicinal leech: motor pattern, sensory basis, and interneuronal pathways. *J Comp Physio (A)* 177:667–681.

Shaw BK, Kristan WB Jr (1997) The neuronal basis of the behavioral choice between swimming and shortening in the leech: Control is not selectively exercised at higher circuit levels. *J Neurosci* 17:786–795.

Sparks DL (1978) Functional properties of neurons in the monkey superior colliculus: Coupling of neuronal activity and saccade onset. *Brain Res* 158:1–16.

Sparks DL, Mays LE (1980) Movement fields of saccade-related burst neurons in the monkey superior colliculus. *Brain Res* 190:39–50.

Sparks DL, Mays LE (1983) Spatial localization of saccade targets. I. Compensation for stimulation-induced perturbations in eye position. *J Neurophysiol* 49:45–63.

Sparks DL, Mays LE (1990) Signal transformations required for the generation of saccadic eye movements. *Ann Rev Neurosci* 13:309–336.

Sparks DL, Holland R, Guthrie BL (1976) Size and distribution of movement fields in the monkey superior colliculus. *Brain Res* 113:21–34.

Sparks DL, Lee C, Rohrer WH (1990) Population coding of the direction, amplitude, and velocity of saccadic eye movements by neurons in the superior colliculus. Cold Spring Harbor Symposia on Quantitative Biology, LV:805–811.

Szczupak L, Kristan WB Jr. (1995) Widespread mechanosensory activation of the serotonergic system of the medicinal leech. *J Neurophysiol* 74:2614–2624.

Theunissen FE, Miller JP (1991) Representation of sensory information in the cricket cercal sensory system. II. Information theoretic calculation of system accuracy and optimal tuning-curve widths of four primary interneurons. *J Neurophysiol* 66:1690–1703.

Van Gisbergen JAM, Van Opstal AJ, Tax AAM (1987) Collicular ensemble coding of saccades based on vector summation. *Neuroscience* 21:541–555.

Van Opstal AJ, Van Gisbergen JAM (1989) A nonlinear model for collicular spatial interactions underlying the metrical properties of electrically elicited saccades. *Biol Cybern* 60:171–183.

Wittenberg G, Kristan WB Jr (1992) Analysis and modeling of the multisegmental coordination of shortening behavior in the medicinal leech. II. Role of identified interneurons. *J Neurophysiol* 68:1693–1707.

Wurtz RH, Goldberg ME (1972) Activity of superior colliculus in behaving monkey. III. Cells discharging before eye movements. *J Neurophysiol* 35:575–586.

3

Neural Substrates for Initiation of Startle Responses

Roy E. Ritzmann and
Robert C. Eaton

Abstract

In both invertebrates and vertebrates, neural systems that mediate startle and escape responses have historically offered technical advantages for cellular analysis because of the presence of large identified neurons, thus making these systems desirable for studies of sensorimotor control. It was often assumed, however, that the associated behavioral responses were perhaps so simple as to be not generally applicable to seemingly more complex, rhythmical locomotor behaviors. Here, we show that this latter point is not correct. We provide detailed examples from two well-studied escape systems, those in the cockroach and the goldfish, and draw upon other examples such as the neural circuits for escape or startle in the crayfish, locust, and mammal to show that the behaviors and underlying neural circuitry in these systems are usually much more complex than is often assumed. This complexity arises from the need to produce accurate escape turns, to control complex peripheral appendages, to time associated biomechanical components properly, to integrate multisensory inputs, and to modulate the escape circuitry appropriate to the environmental context—all factors common to slower cyclical movements. Because escape circuits control muscular apparatus used for other forms of locomotion, studying them may provide important insights into general mechanisms of motor control. For example, during fish escape the pattern of axial muscle contractions resembles that of the agonist and antagonist muscles controlling flexion and extension of vertebrate limb segments. Moreover, well-described functional features of some escape systems, such as pervasive inhibition of conflicting motor acts, should prove with further study to be common to other systems in which these properties are not yet described.

Over the years, neurobiologists have concentrated considerable attention upon various startle responses (Eaton, 1984). Some of the most completely understood neural circuits are those responsible for directing escape behaviors of crayfish, annelid worms, teleost fishes, and various insects. Historically, the feature most responsible for this interest is the inclusion of large interneurons at critical points in the neural circuitry responsible for escape behavior. Such cells as the giant interneurons of crayfish and the Mauthner cell of lower vertebrates provide distinct technical advantages for both mapping out the circuitry and observing cellular activity during the behavior. In addition, the behaviors themselves have typically been considered to be relatively simple, thus lending themselves to the possibility of fairly complete understanding. This simplicity raises a serious concern about escape systems' general usefulness in providing principles for locomotion, however. Do the unique advantages of escape systems limit their usefulness as models for other less approachable neurobiological systems? If the circuits that underlie escape systems are orders of magnitude simpler than other systems, can one assume that they are organized in a manner similar enough to make them useful models for understanding complex systems?

More recent investigations on many escape systems allay this concern. These studies revealed complex properties, including parallel pathways of input or output, large populations of multisensory interneurons for processing sensory information, and neuromodulation of critical synapses to permit reduction or augmentation of responses as conditions require. The ability to identify individual interneurons within such populations provides some very useful systems for studying sensorimotor control (see also Sparks et al., chapter 2, this volume). Moreover, if one considers all of the movements and postural changes necessary for a smooth, efficient, and rapid escape movement, rather than focus on only the simple flexions and extensions associated with the most prominent large neurons, one can appreciate the complexity of these systems. In this chapter, we describe some of the features found in various escape behaviors that are also important to other locomotor systems. We concentrate on the systems most familiar to us (cockroach and teleost fish), but also draw upon other escape systems in which certain features are more easily observed.

The Cockroach Escape System

The American cockroach, *Periplaneta americana*, avoids lunging predators such as toads and lizards by generating a rapid turn away from the approaching predator followed by a more random run (Camhi, 1980). In most cases, the primary signal that evokes the escape turn is a rapidly accelerating wind puff generated by the lunging predator. Latency is minimized by employing rapidly conducting giant interneurons to span the abdomen from the wind-sensitive hairs located on the cerci to the thoracic ganglia. The sensory neurons, which innervate directional hairs on the cerci, synapse with giant interneurons (GIs) in the terminal abdominal ganglion (Callec et al., 1971; Daley and Camhi, 1988). The directional properties of the sensory hairs and the pattern of con-

nection to GIs determine the directional properties of individual GIs (Westin et al., 1977; Kolton and Camhi, 1995). The reproducible wind-receptive fields of GIs divide the surrounding area into front and rear or right and left areas. These fields suggest an assembly code that can then be used to identify the location of the lunging predator and to direct the turning movements (Camhi and Levy, 1989).

The GIs can be divided morphologically and physiologically into two subsets: (1) the three paired dorsal GIs (dGIs) and (2) the four paired ventral GIs (vGIs). Specific lesion experiments indicate that the vGIs in particular play an important role in directing the escape turn. Animals that have had one or more vGIs lesioned by protease injection make significantly greater wrong turns (i.e., toward the wind source rather than away from it) than do normal animals or animals that have had other interneurons changed by injection or other means (Comer, 1985).

The vGIs project to the thoracic ganglia, where they connect to an even larger population of thoracic interneurons called type A thoracic interneurons (TI$_A$s) (Ritzmann and Pollack, 1988). TI$_A$s are found in each thoracic ganglion. Most of them are interganglionic, projecting from their ganglion of origin to both of the other thoracic ganglia and often beyond. To date, 13 TI$_A$s have been identified in each hemiganglion. The fact that they occur in bilateral pairs in each thoracic ganglion accounts for 78 identified TI$_A$s. All TI$_A$s have an axon on the side opposite the soma. Thus, we can describe inputs or outputs to the cell as being relative to the soma side or the axon side.

TI$_A$s can be divided into subclasses based upon their left-right wind bias (Westin et al., 1988). Bilateral cells are equally responsive to wind stimuli either from the right or left side. Unilateral cells are biased to only one side, with the bias either on the soma side or on the axon side. In all cases, the wind field of each TI$_A$ is consistent with the pattern of vGI connections to that particular cell (Ritzmann and Pollack, 1988). That is, bilateral TI$_A$s receive inputs from all vGIs, whereas unilateral TI$_A$s receive vGI inputs only on their preferred side. Moreover, the pattern of vGI connections is indicated by the presence of one or more prominent branches in each TI$_A$ on the ventral side of the ganglion near its midline. These ventral median (VM) branches are believed to be the site of synaptic contact between vGIs and TI$_A$s (Casagrand and Ritzmann, 1991).

Individual TI$_A$s project to motor neurons that control leg joint movements either directly or via local interneurons (Ritzmann and Pollack, 1990). Connections are made on the axon side of the TI_A both in the ganglion of origin and in adjacent thoracic ganglia. To date, all TI_As with dorsal somata were found to make excitatory connections to motor neurons or local interneurons, whereas ventral TI_As made inhibitory connections.

Thus, TI_As make up a network of cells that receive directional activity from vGIs and appear to use this information to direct the leg motor neurons that evoke the appropriate turning movements. They act either directly on the motor neurons or through yet another control circuit made up of local interneurons dedicated to the control movements for each individual leg. Exactly how these decisions are made in the TI_A circuit is still open to question. A reasonable hypothesis is that individual TI_As act independently, however, to form a "congress of cells" similar to that proposed for the primate motor control (Georgopoulos et al., 1988; Grillner et al., chapter 1, this volume; Sparks et al., chapter 2, this volume).

Why is such a large number of thoracic cells, including both TI_As and local interneurons, necessary for controlling the seemingly simple task of turning into one of the four different quadrants around the animal? Several possibilities exist.

Accuracy of Escape Turns

Large populations of broadly tuned cells can serve to generate very accurate orientation movements. In primates, the neurons that control arm movements (Grillner et al., chapter 1, this volume) and eye movements (Sparks et al., chapter 2, this volume) are excellent examples of such systems. The cockroach can escape into one of four different quadrants rather than simply choosing front or back; it can also discriminate signals up to within 40° of each other (Camhi, personal communication). That accuracy may be a product of the TI_A circuit. It is not clear, however, that such accuracy is necessary or even beneficial for an escape system.

The crayfish escape system has a simpler set of giant-to-motor neuron connections. These animals move through water by rapidly contracting their abdominal flexor muscles, creating a forceful swimming movement (Krasne and Wine, 1984). Tactile sensory structures project to the central nervous system, where they excite giant interneurons both directly via electrical synapses and indirectly via a disynaptic chemical path that includes several interneurons, some of which have been identified (Zucker, 1972). Two pairs of giant interneurons exist, the medial pair and the lateral pair. Each inter-

neuron has a large axon, which travels through the nerve cord to the abdominal ganglia, where it excites flexor motor neurons. The most potent flexor motor neurons are the motor giants of each abdominal ganglion that are excited by the giant fibers via electrical synapses (Mittenthal and Wine, 1973). Other flexor motor neurons are excited via two separate pathways: (1) a direct connection from the giant fibers and (2) a polysynaptic connection via a neuron referred to as the segmental giant (Roberts et al., 1982). The latter pathway accounts for nearly 95% of the excitation to the nongiant flexor motor neurons.

Directionality in the initial, giant-mediated tailflip is restricted to either a caudally directed movement or an upwardly directed movement (Wine and Krasne, 1972). The direction of the crayfish's escape movement is dictated by selection of either the medial or lateral giant pair. Medial giant fibers are excited by tactile structures on the anterior regions of the animal and excite flexors in all abdominal segments (Mittenthal and Wine, 1973). The resulting tail flexion causes a rearward movement. The lateral giant fibers, however, are excited by tactile structures on the posterior region and excite flexors only in the first three abdominal segments. As a result, the tail bends in such a way as to direct the escape upward; the upward movement typically results in a somersault that leads to a forward escape. Subsequent tailflip movements can provide additional directionality by virtue of the nongiant-mediated swimming movements that are much more variable than the giant-mediated movements (Schrameck, 1970; Reichert and Wine, 1983).

Like crayfish predators, many of the predators of the cockroach make single ballistic lunges. In order to avoid such attacks, the prey must avoid two fatal errors: (1) remain motionless, the worst error because, once the attack has started, failure to move will almost certainly result in death and (2) escape into the path of the lunging predator because the predator will still make contact with the prey, only more quickly. Thus, the most important consequence of directional escape movements may be to avoid the second error. More accurate movements may be of secondary importance.

Control of a Complex Periphery

Perhaps the greater complexity of the cockroach system is required to control the appendages that generate the movement. The crayfish generates rapid swimming movements by flexing serially homologous muscles of the abdomen. In order to execute turning movements on land, however, the cockroach must generate a coordinated set of movements among the several segments that control three different pairs of legs.

The role of each pair of legs is distinct and changes depending upon the turn direction. Three types of turns have been described (Nye and Ritzmann, 1992). Stimuli from the rear of the animal almost exclusively generate type 1 turns: the hind legs extend and drive the animal forward; in addition, the middle and front legs move back and laterally toward the source of stimulation. For example, a stimulus from the right rear quadrant causes the right middle leg to extend posteriorly and laterally while the left middle leg extends posteriorly and medially. Lateral and medial movements occur as a result of extension of the femur-tibia (FT) joint on the right (ipsilateral) leg and flexion of the FT joint on the left (contralateral) leg. In the type 1 turn, the other important leg joint, the coxa-femur (CF) joint, extends on all six legs and drives the legs rearward. As a result, the animal moves forward while turning through a small angle away from the stimulus source. Stimuli from the side of the animal generate a type 2 turn. In this type of turn, the FT joints make the same movements as those made in type 1 turns, but the CF joints of the contralateral legs flex instead of extending. As a result, the contralateral legs are pulled forward. Because the leg is still in contact with the ground, the contralateral side of the animal moves backward; so the animal pivots in place through a large angle. Executing the type 2 turn is like sharply turning a rowboat by pulling on one oar while pushing on the other. With stimuli from the front, the animal will often generate a type 3 turn. CF joints on both sides of the animal flex, which moves the legs forward and drives the animal backward and away from the stimulus. After the initial type 3 turn, the animal may then execute a type 1 turn to complete an escape to the rear.

Temporal Considerations

When various segmented appendages are used to produce a movement, temporal considerations are also important. Various muscles must contract in a proper sequence in order to produce the appropriate behavior. Temporal factors are particularly apparent in locust escape behavior, in which a series of co-contractions and triggering events result in a movement of the hind leg that is both powerful and rapidly accelerating. Normally, this ability is typically not possible for a single muscle. The locust accomplishes this task by mechanically storing tension from muscle contraction over a relatively long period of time, then rapidly releasing it (Heitler, 1977). The animal generates an isometric contraction by co-contracting the flexor and extensor muscles of the FT joint (Heitler and Burrows, 1977). Exoskeletal specializations provide mechanical advantage to the flexors so that extensor muscles reach a high level of tension. The flexor is then inhibited, thus allowing a sudden release of tension. The period of co-contraction can delay the onset of escape for several hundred milliseconds—in apparent conflict with the necessity for speed in escape systems. What the locust loses in latency, however, it makes up for in acceleration.

The temporal factors critical to a successful locust escape require efficient cocking and triggering control systems. The release of flexor activation must be timed to arrive after the initiation of isometric extensor activation; in addition, peripheral inhibitors must be excited during the triggering event. The entire behavior includes approximately 70 motor neurons activated in concert (Burrows, 1995). Variation of properties in the activation of several motor neurons occurs, in turn causing meaningful variation in the resulting kicks.

Although sensory inputs from the periphery may play some role in setting the sequence of activation, it does not appear to be capable of controlling the behavior by itself. Studies indicate that at least 11 interneurons are activated during either the co-contraction phase or trigger phase of the kick sequence (Gynther and Pearson, 1986).

The C-interneuron, a cell in the mesothoracic ganglion, has projections to the metathoracic ganglion, where it excites both flexor and extensor motor neurons (Pearson and Robertson, 1981). Another cell, the M-interneuron, is excited by many of the cues that can trigger escape jumps; it also makes inhibitory connections to flexor motor neurons (Pearson et al., 1980). Both cells are activated in approximately the correct times to serve in setting the co-contraction phase and triggering the leg kick. However, more recent investigations have suggested that they represent only parts of a more extensive control system. The C-interneuron is not activated until late in the co-contraction phase (Gynther and Pearson, 1986). Moreover, the locust is capable of generating a fully functional kick even after lesioning the connectives between the metathoracic and mesothoracic ganglion (where the C-interneuron originates). Thus, the C-interneuron cannot, by itself, be responsible for the co-contraction phase.

M-interneuron activity typically occurs at the appropriate time for inhibiting the flexor motor neurons and triggering the kick. However, in some kicks, the trigger precedes M-interneuron activation or occurs in the absence of such activation (Gynther and Pearson, 1989). Thus, the M-interneuron may serve as part of the trigger, but it is almost certainly not the only cell involved. At least one other interneuron has been identified that has similar response properties to M-interneurons but does not make direct inhibitory connections with flexor motor neurons. It may contribute to the trigger phase by inhibiting the synaptic drive to flexor activation (Gynther and Pearson, 1989).

Multisensory Inputs

An interneuronal population that receives multiple types of sensory input may serve as a site of multisensory integration. Although wind is a potent stimulus for evoking cockroach escape, it is not the only effective modality. Tactile stimuli to either the antennae or the body cuticle are capable of generating escape turns that are essentially identical to wind-generated escape turns (Comer et al., 1994; Schaefer et al., 1994).

TI$_A$s are equally capable of responding to tactile stimulation to either the antennae or the body cuticle (Ritzmann et al., 1991). When TI$_A$s respond to stimulation to the body cuticle, the left-right bias of the individual TI$_A$s corresponds to the same cell's response to wind (Ritzmann and Pollack, 1994). That is, TI$_A$s that are bilaterally responsive to wind are also unbiased to tactile stimulation, whereas TI$_A$s that are biased to one side for wind are biased to the same side for tactile stimuli. In addition, many TI$_A$s are also responsive to auditory, visual, and proprioceptive stimulation (Ritzmann et al., 1991). In this regard, they are similar to the multisensory cells of the superior colliculus of mammals, the cells which are involved in controlling saccadic eye movements (Meredith and Stein, 1986).

The multisensory response properties of TI$_A$s also allow the TI$_A$ network to factor additional information into the computation for appropriate turn direction. For example, if an animal is standing near a wall at the time of the stimulus, an otherwise appropriate turn away from the wind puff might now cause the animal to crash into the wall. Behavioral observations indicate that this does not happen (Ritzmann et al., 1991), nor does it happen in the Mauthner-initiated escape of the goldfish (Eaton and Emberley, 1991). If the cockroach is close enough to the wall to maintain antennal contact, it modifies its turn decision to escape forward. Thus, the information from the

vGIs is read out by the TI$_A$ network in the context of tactile information from the antennae.

Modulation of Escape Circuitry

Startle responses are not immutable. Many systems can be modulated so that the movement is altered under certain conditions. In crayfish, the threshold of the lateral giant response can be altered by external factors; for example, tactile stimuli to the thoracic cuticle inhibits elements of the escape circuit (Krasne and Wine, 1975). Such inhibition might be an attempt to eliminate futile escape movements when the animal is held by a potentially threatening large animal. Once the grasp is loosened, the system returns to normal sensitivity so that the animal can escape.

Restraint-induced inhibition may occur as a result of neuromodulation. Application of serotonin decreases the amplitude of the chemical component of the lateral giant synaptic response—that is, the response generated over the disynaptic pathway through sensory interneurons (Glanzman and Krasne, 1983). The effect of the amplitude decrease can be powerful enough to prevent the lateral giant from reaching threshold and evoking an action potential. In contrast, application of octopamine augments the disynaptic pathway, thus raising the lateral giant response above threshold. It is possible to lesion selectively serotonergic neurons by injecting 5,7-dihidroxytryptamine (5,7-DHT), a toxic analogue of serotonin, into the hemolymph (Glanzman and Krasne, 1986). Animals treated in this way show little restraint-induced inhibition.

The response to serotonin depends upon the individual animal's social status (Yeh et al., 1996). When crayfish are placed in pairs, they quickly establish a dominance hierarchy. In the subordinate individuals, serotonin reversibly reduces the synaptic strength of the lateral giant input. In dominant animals, however, serotonin enhances the same synapses. The difference appears to be due to the relative efficacy of two different serotonin receptors.

A similar modulatory effect can be found in the cockroach. A quiescent state is generated when a plastic shield is placed in contact with both of the animal's antennae (Watson and Ritzmann, 1994). During the quiescent state, no amount of wind or tactile stimulation can generate an escape response. Moreover, the quiescent state can be achieved only in a well lit room. In darkness, the animal remains responsive. The appropriate conditions for inducing quiescence may mimic an untenable situation in which the cockroach is in a corner and ambient light makes it vulnerable to visual predators.

At least one site at which modulation occurs—the synapses onto TI_As—may account for quiescence. Under the quiescent state, vGI activity remains vigorous (Watson and Ritzmann, 1994); however, such activity fails to generate the typical leg movements. Known neuromodulators can alter the synaptic strength of the connections between vGIs and TI_As (Casagrand and Ritzmann, 1992). As in crayfish, dopamine and octopamine augment the vGI-evoked postsynaptic potentials (PSPs) in TI_As. However, serotonin reduces the amplitude of PSPs. Given the size of the TI_A population, even a small reduction in PSP amplitude in all TI_A inputs might induce a quiescent state.

The Mauthner System

Mauthner neurons trigger the sudden escape response, or C-start, in teleost fish responding to aversive acoustic stimuli caused, for example, by the sudden lunge of an attacking predator. The Mauthner system consists of a bilateral pair of prominent brainstem neurons, the Mauthner cells, and their associated sensory afferents, regulatory interneurons and output followers. In any given escape behavior, only one Mauthner cell is activated, and it fires only one action potential. This seeming simplicity belies the complexity of the entire Mauthner network and the multiple functions it performs in properly organizing the animal's motor response. Indeed, the motor control characteristics of the Mauthner system cannot be understood apart from the reticulospinal system in which it resides because the C-start is too complex to be coordinated by a single interneuron and its followers. Other reticulospinal neurons are also required.

The reticulospinal system is a brainstem network that coordinates complex sequences of body movements, such as orientation and startle, that use the large muscles of the body (McClellan, 1986; Peterson, 1984). The features of the Mauthner cell are characteristic of many types of reticulospinal cells: input from the vestibular or auditory system and from tectum, and output through an axon that serves the spinal cord with widespread excitatory connections on both limb and axial motor neurons (Peterson, 1984). The reticulospinal system is highly conserved throughout evolution (Nissanov and Eaton, 1989) and is organized on a segmental pattern whose

development is regulated by common genetic mechanisms (Guthrie, 1995). Thus, insights into Mauthner-system function may prove important in understanding the general organizational principles of reticulospinal motor function.

General Features of the Mauthner System

There are extensive excitatory and inhibitory inputs to the Mauthner system and widespread consequences of its output. Numerous investigations and reports in the past 30 years have worked out and reviewed the circuitry of the Mauthner system (Eaton and Hackett, 1984; Faber and Korn, 1978; Faber et al., 1991; Fetcho, 1991; Popper and Eaton, 1995).

The known excitatory outputs have been studied mainly from the point of view of activation of the motor neurons excited by the Mauthner axon. Through a disynaptic pathway, activated cranial motor neurons streamline the animal by causing its mouth and operculum to close and its eyes to converge. The Mauthner axon synapses monosynaptically with spinal motor neurons that activate the white fibers of the ipsilateral trunk musculature; in addition, disynaptic activation of the secondary red muscle fibers occurs (Fetcho, 1991). There are accompanying, though less well studied, activations of the fins—including the dorsal fin, which during escape may have a stabilizing or defensive role, and the pectoral fins, which may guide the trajectory or, in some species, assist in propulsion. Thus, virtually the entire motor output of the locomotor spinal circuitry can potentially be activated during the escape response. Because the Mauthner cell has such extensive and direct motor connections, the speed of the escape response is ensured.

From a functional standpoint, the Mauthner system has several well-known types of inhibition, which can be divided into medullary (Faber et al., 1991) and spinal components (Fetcho, 1991). For the medullary part, localized inhibitory circuits serve to ensure proper firing of the appropriate Mauthner cell. These circuits also prevent accidental firing of a Mauthner cell in response to spurious background noise, multiple firings of the same Mauthner cell in response to a complex stimulus, or simultaneous activation of both Mauthner cells in response to a stimulus with an ambiguous location. All of those functions involve the *Passive Hyperpolarizing Potential (PHP) neurons*, which exert a very short latency electronic inhibition on the Mauthner cell at the spike-initiation zone. PHP neurons also produce a slightly longer latency, long duration chemical inhibition due to a chloride conductance change in the Mauthner neuron soma and lateral dendrite.

The PHP cells use the electronic and chemical inhibitions to perform several controlling roles in the network. First, the activation of PHP cells from auditory afferents mediates a monosynaptic, feedforward inhibition that regulates the Mauthner firing threshold (Faber et al., 1991). A connectionist simulation of this function suggests that it may also determine the initial decision to activate either the left or right Mauthner cell in response to a directional stimulus (Eaton et al., 1995a). The second major effect of the PHP cells involves a disynaptic pathway. When one of the Mauthner cells fires, it activates a population of *cranial relay neurons* (CRNs) that activate PHP cells whose terminals inhibit the active Mauthner cell in a feedback mode, thus preventing multiple firing of the Mauthner cell to the same stimulus. Because CRNs have projections to PHP neurons on both sides of the brain, their activation also inhibits the contralateral Mauthner cell. Thus, when one Mauthner cell fires an action potential, the PHP-to-CRN pathway provides not only feedback inhibition, but also reciprocal inhibition, so that only one action potential can be triggered by the two Mauthner cells.

Activation of the spinal inhibitory circuits of the Mauthner system is dictated by the need to turn off competing motor activities. These could arise as a result of a Mauthner cell firing during a conflicting action, such as swimming. For instance, when an escape response was elicited while a sunfish was swimming, there was little or no decrement in escape performance regardless of the initial direction of axial curvature during swimming (Jayne and Lauder, 1993). Thus, Mauthner takes precedence over lower priority motor acts. Its effectiveness is a result of not only its pervasiveness, but also the much higher conduction velocity of the Mauthner axon in comparison with its descending reticulospinal competitors (Eaton et al., 1995b). The network that mediates such effects can be surmised from the well-described reciprocal spinal inhibitory network between the two Mauthner axons.

In each spinal segment, the Mauthner axon makes an electrotonic synapse on a commissural interneuron (CI), whose terminals inhibit the output of the contralateral Mauthner axon. This output includes endings on the contralateral primary motoneurons, on descending premotor interneurons, and on the contralateral CI of the segment in question. Fetcho (1991) has noted the remarkable similarity between the Mauthner inhibitory network and the spinal networks for swimming in the lamprey (Wallen, chapter 6, this volume) and in the em-

bryonic frog (Roberts et al., chapter 7, this volume). In all three networks, excitation of motoneurons and descending premotor interneurons results in a C-like body bend on one side accompanied by the inhibition of similar cells on the opposite side. The CIs that produce the inhibitory effects are all glycinergic. Although some details differ, the basic similarity of the three circuits suggests that they exhibit common organizational principles for vertebrate spinal motor pattern generators (Fetcho, 1991; Kiehn et al., chapter 4, this volume).

Sensorimotor Coordination and Biomechanics of C-Starts

The immediate mono- or disynaptic consequence of Mauthner-system activation in the goldfish is a serial sequence of events proceeding from sensory input to motor output. It takes more circuitry than this, however, to produce the normal variety of escape trajectories that occur when the Mauthner cell fires. As with cockroach escape, the fish does not simply make a random "jump" out of the way. Rather, it orients its body to turn directly away from the predator or aversive stimulus regardless of the angle of the attack. In fact, the escape trajectory angle (ETA) is a linear function of the stimulus angle (SA) relative to the body at the start:

$$ETA = -0.5SA + 154°$$

This equation is the basic input-output relationship to which the underlying sensorimotor processes must conform (Eaton and Emberley, 1991).

To produce the full array of escape angles, the biomechanics require that the fish generate a bilateral sequence of at least two axial muscle contractions. The first is an agonist contraction, on the side opposite the stimulus. The second is an antagonist contraction, on the side opposite the first contraction. Thus, the escape trajectory angle is the sum of the underlying changes in angular orientation caused by two (or sometimes more) underlying muscle contractions.

The example in figure 3.1 shows the relationship between the escape trajectory angle and two subsidiary turns that produced it. Here, the goldfish responded to the stimulus of a ball dropped into the water at the left side of the animal's head. The response consisted of a large initial turn (A1, 140° in figure 3.1C) followed by a smaller counterturn (A2, −20° in figure 3.1C) in the opposite direction. The two turns stabilized the escape trajectory at about 120° relative to the start position. For the fish to produce a large variety of ETAs, A1 and A2 turns will vary widely in relative size and timing.

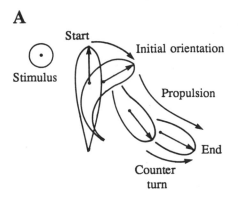

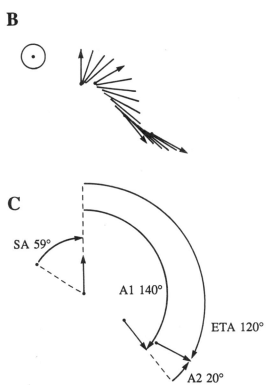

Figure 3.1
(A) Mauthner-initiated C-start of a goldfish responding to a ball dropped into the water at the position marked "stimulus." The behavior consists of an initial rotation and propulsion away from the stimulus. (B) Diagram of the response as measured by a high-speed digital camera and computer system that reproduces the movements of the midlines of the rostral one-third of the body. (C) Angular parameters underlying the kinematic analysis of the behavior: SA, angle of the stimulus relative to the body axis; A1, initial rotation from the stimulus; A2, counterturn rotation between A1 and the end of the response. ETA (escape trajectory angle) = A1 − A2. (From Foreman and Eaton, 1993).

The A1 and A2 turns are produced by correspondingly variable contractions of the axial musculature.

Figure 3.2 shows how the contractions work together to produce two different ETAs. The midline animation in figure 3.2A is from a response typically seen when the stimulus is from a rostral direction. The animal executed a single unilateral motion to the right, nearly reversing its initial orientation. This motion was accompanied by a large agonist electromyogram (EMG) signal in the right axial musculature (top trace, figure 3.2A), but little or no EMG activity on the left side (bottom trace). The eventual result was a turn of about 140° and a displacement of about 4 cm in 100 ms.

Responses to a stimulus from a caudal direction involve both an agonist contraction and an antagonist contraction. As shown in the midline animation of figure 3.2B, the agonist contraction rotated the animal to the right, but this was followed by a strong antagonist contraction, causing a direction change (arrow) so that the fish assumed a rostral trajectory of −20° (that is, slightly to the left of its original orientation). Corresponding to these turns were two major EMG signals in figure 3.2B, an initial one in the right axial musculature (top trace) and a later, prolonged one, in the left axial musculature (arrow, bottom trace). The difference in movements evoked by rostral versus caudal stimuli is reminiscent of the changes in leg movement associated with front versus back stimulation described earlier for cockroach and crayfish escape responses.

The qualitative impressions from figure 3.2 have been confirmed quantitatively by performing multiple regression analysis on the EMG and kinematic data. The following relationship is the result:

$$ETA = S1S2 - LS1LS2$$

(Here, the original equation is simplified; see Foreman and Eaton, 1993, for further details.) In this relationship, the escape trajectory angle, ETA, is a function of (1) *S1S2*—the difference in size between the integrals of the EMG of the agonist contraction and the EMG leading to a direction change, or the antagonist contraction—minus (2) *LS1LS2*, the interval between the agonist and antagonist contractions. For example, if there is no direction change (the antagonist contraction is zero), ETA is large. If the interval between the two contractions is small, ETA is small. Thus, by varying the relative size and timing of the two contractions, the fish can produce any ETA between those extremes.

From such observations, Foreman and Eaton (1993) have proposed that two populations of reticulospinal

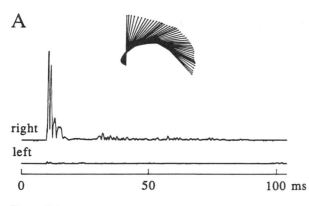

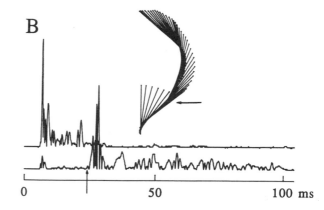

Figure 3.2

Combined midline animations and EMG data from Mauthner-initiated C-starts. (A) A continuous unilateral turn producing a caudal trajectory. (B) A direction change producing a rostral trajectory. Traces are rectified EMG records from the left and right axial musculature. The mid-lines are oriented as in figure 3.1, with the rostrum in the start position indicated by the first vertical line in each animation. (From Foreman and Eaton, 1993.)

neurons activate the agonist and antagonist contractions respectively. The necessary variability in the agonist contraction might be controlled by variable activation of the segmental homologues of the Mauthner cell, MiD2cm and MiD3cm (Lee et al., 1993). These neurons would be excited by sensory inputs from the same side as their somas—thus causing, through their contralateral axonal projections, the initial bend away from the stimulus. Using the same reasoning, a second population of segmental homologues with ipsilateral axonal projections might control the antagonist contraction. Direct evidence in favor of the first part of this hypothesis has been obtained by using a calcium imaging technique with in vivo confocal microscopy on larval zebrafish (O'Malley et al., 1996). These experiments show variable recruitment of MiD2cm and MiD3cm depending on stimulus location. Caudal stimuli, which cause a small agonist contraction, activate only the Mauthner cell; however all three segmental homologues are activated following rostral stimuli that cause a large agonist contraction.

Relevance to the Control of Other Motor Behaviors

The fish escape system may provide clues to the general nature of the descending reticulospinal motor commands for other types of movements. Mauthner cells are prominent in the many vertebrates that have a tailed, aquatic form at some time in their life cycle. In addition to revealing the similarity between the spinal networks for escape and swimming in amniotic vertebrates, recent evidence shows that the Mauthner cells may also activate the rapid hindlimb contraction associated with the diving escape response in some adult frogs, such as

Xenopus (Will, 1991). This evidence suggests that, in the evolutionary developmental of terrestrial vertebrates, Mauthner cells and their homologues have been recruited to other important locomotor functions. Mauthner cells have not yet been found in mammals, and until recently, it was not clear that the reticulospinal system was involved in producing startle responses in the same way it is involved in the generation of C-starts in fish. However, Lingenhöhl and Friauf (1994) recently used intracellular recording and micromarking to define more precisely the basic acoustic startle response circuit in the rat.

Primary interneurons in this circuit are giant reticulospinal cells of the caudal pontine reticular nucleus. They receive convergent input from several auditory brainstem nuclei and, similar to the Mauthner cells (Casagrand et al., 1995), have high firing threshold and broad frequency tuning. These observations lead us to suspect that the neural mechanisms for rapid motor control by the Mauthner system may extend to limbed vertebrates, including mammals.

In motor control research, it is often difficult to know whether descending motor commands specify kinematic parameters (such as position or angle), biomechanical parameters (such as acceleration or force), or other more complex parameters (Fetz, 1992). We can see that for the goldfish C-start, the important movement parameters are the variations in the timing and magnitude of directional control motions—that is, the kinematic parameters. No separate signal specifies forward propulsion or force. Rather, the neural specification of force is embedded in the descending commands to bend the body. Because of the stiffness of the fish anterior and the hydrodynamic resistance of the tail, the angular momentum of the initial turn is transferred into a linear momentum, resulting in a thrust component through the center of mass (Foreman and Eaton, 1993; Webb, 1994).

Because forward propulsion can be ignored, C-start kinematics can be reduced to an analysis of the muscular contractions that cause the simple rotation of the midline; this analysis is similar to those done by others of the rotation of vertebrate limb segments. In fact, as pointed out by Foreman and Eaton (1993), the EMG findings from the goldfish are analogous to the systematic EMG changes in amplitude and timing that occur in rapid limb movements in humans, such as rapid forearm flexion and extension movements (Sherwood et al., 1988). Thus, given the apparent similarity of EMG patterns in systems as diverse as the fish trunk and the primate arm, it could well be that findings from the fish will have implications for understanding the neural mechanisms underlying rapid movements in cases where the anatomical organization of the musculature is quite different.

Conclusion

The examples provided in this chapter clearly describe complex behaviors controlled by equally complex circuitry. Given the common pressure of survival to which every escape behavior must respond, it is not surprising to find commonalities even in animals as diverse as vertebrates and arthropods. Differences certainly exist as a result of different body forms and environments in which each animal lives. We expect, however, that as investigators probe more deeply into the relationship between behavior and circuitry, they will discover more commonalities and more complexities in different sensorimotor systems. For example, it would not be surprising to find that inhibition—as found in the Mauthner system to assure that no competing behaviors are executed during an escape response—will also be found as descending control in the cockroach escape system. Moreover, the necessity for streamlining the body of a fish that results in a concert of additional movements over and above trunk flexion is most certainly also important to the crayfish. As additional behavioral components are studied, the underlying circuitry will also be found to contain additional complexities.

The finding of complex features in escape systems is both a problem and a blessing. The notion that escape is a product of simple systems that we could understand in total may have been comforting but was hardly realistic. The realization that escape behaviors and their under-

lying circuitry are equal in sophistication to other sensorimotor systems, however, brings with it the promise that escape systems will serve as useful models for understanding many less tractable systems. Given that all animals use their limbs, musculature, and related sensory structures in both escape and non-escape forms of locomotion, it is reasonable to expect that they either share some components of the central control systems or have systems that are organized using similar principles.

Acknowledgments

The research described in this paper was supported by grants NS14411 (Ritzmann) and NS22621 (Eaton) from the National Institutes of Health and grants N00014-90-J-1545 (Ritzmann) and N00014-94-1-0380 (Eaton) from the Office of Naval Research.

References

Burrows M (1995) Motor patterns during kicking movements in the locust. *J Comp Physiol (A)* 176:289–305.

Callec JJ, Guillet JC, Pichon Y, Boistel J (1971) Further studies on synaptic transmission in insects. II. Relations between sensory information and its synaptic integration at the level of a single giant axon in the cockroach. *J Exp Biol* 55:123–149.

Camhi JM (1980) The escape system of the cockroach. *Sci Am* 243(6):158–172.

Camhi JM, Levy A (1989) The code for stimulus direction in a cell assembly in the cockroach. *J Comp Physiol (A)* 165:83–97.

Casagrand JL, Guzik AL, Eaton RC (1995) Frequency dependence of auditory PSPs in the goldfish Mauthner cell. *Soc Neurosci Abstr* 21:399.

Casagrand JL, Ritzmann RE (1991) Localization of ventral giant interneuron connections to the ventral median branch of thoracic interneurons in the cockroach. *J Neurobiol* 22:643–658.

Casagrand JL, Ritzmann RE (1992) Biogenic amines modulate synaptic transmission between identified giant interneurons and thoracic interneurons in the escape system of the cockroach. *J Neurobiol* 23:644–655.

Comer CM (1985) Analyzing cockroach escape behavior with lesions of individual giant interneurons. *Brain Res* 335:342–346.

Comer CM, Mara E, Murphy KA, Getman M, Mungy MC (1994) Multisensory control of escape in the cockroach *Periplaneta americana*. II. Patterns of touch-evoked behavior. *J Comp Physiol (A)* 174:13–26.

Daley DL, Camhi JM (1988) Connectivity pattern of the cercal-to-giant interneuron system of the American cockroach. *J Neurophysiol* 60:1350–1368.

Eaton RC (1984) *Neural Mechanisms of Startle Behavior*. New York: Plenum.

Eaton RC (1991) Neuroethology of the Mauthner system. *Brain Behav Evol* 37:245–332.

Eaton RC, Canfield JG, Guzik AL (1995a) Left-right discrimination of sound onset by the Mauthner system. *Brain Behav Evol* 46:165–179.

Eaton RC, Emberley DS (1991) How stimulus direction determines the trajectory angle of the Mauthner initiated escape response in a teleost fish. *J Exp Biol* 161:469–487.

Eaton RC, Hackett JT (1984) The role of the Mauthner cell in fast-starts involving escape in teleost fishes. In: *Neural Mechanisms of Startle Behavior* (Eaton RC, ed.), 213–266. New York: Plenum.

Eaton RC, Hofve JC, Fetcho JR (1995b) Beating the competition: The reliability hypothesis for Mauthner axon size. *Brain Behav Evol* 45:183–194.

Faber DS, Korn H (1978) Electrophysiology of the Mauthner cell: Basic properties, synaptic mechanisms, and associated networks. In: *Neurobiology of the Mauthner Cell* (Faber DS, Korn H, eds.), 47–131. New York: Raven.

Faber DS, Korn H, Lin J-W (1991) The role of medullary networks and postsynaptic membrane properties in regulating Mauthner cell responsiveness to sensory excitation. *Brain Behav Evol* 37:286–297.

Fetcho JR (1991) The spinal network of the Mauthner cell. *Brain Behav Evol* 37:298–316.

Fetz EE (1992) Are movement parameters recognizably coded in the activity of single neurons? *Behav Brain Sci* 15:679–690.

Foreman MB, Eaton RC (1993) The direction change concept for reticulospinal control of goldfish escape. *J Neurosci* 13:4101–4113.

Georgopoulos AP, Kettner RE, Schwartz AB (1988) Primate motor cortex and free arm movements to visual targets in three-dimensional space II. Coding of the direction of movement by a neuronal population. *J Neurosci* 8:2928–2937.

Glanzman DL, Krasne FB (1983) Serotonin and octopamine have opposite modulatory effects on the crayfish's lateral giant escape reaction. *J Neurosci* 3:2263–2269.

Glanzman DL, Krasne FB (1986) 5,7-Dihydrotryptamine lesions of crayfish serotonin-containing neurons: Effect on the lateral giant escape reaction. *J Neurosci* 6:1560–1569.

Guthrie S (1995) The status of the neural segment. *Trends Neurosci* 18:74–79.

Gynther IC, Pearson KG (1986) Intracellular recordings from interneurones and motoneurones during bilateral kicks in the locust: Implications for mechanisms controlling the jump. *J Exp Biol* 122:323–343.

Gynther IC, Pearson KG (1989) An evaluation of the role of identified interneurons in triggering kicks and jumps in the locust. *J Neurophysiol* 61(1):45–57.

Heitler WJ (1977) The locust jump. III. Structural specializations of the metathoracic tibiae. *J Exp Biol* 67:29–36.

Heitler WJ, Burrows M (1977) The locust jump. I. The motor programme. *J Exp Biol* 66:203–219.

Jayne BC, Lauder GV (1993) Red and white muscle activity and kinematics of the escape response of the bluegill sunfish during swimming. *J Comp Physiol (A)* 173:495–508.

Kolton L, Camhi JM (1995) Cartesian representation of stimulus direction: Parallel processing by two sets of giant interneurons in the cockroach. *J Comp Physiol (A)* 176:691–702.

Krasne FB, Wine JJ (1975) Extrinsic modulation of crayfish escape behaviour. *J Exp Biol* 63:433–450.

Krasne FB, Wine JJ (1984) The production of crayfish tailflip responses. In: *Neural Mechanisms of Startle Behavior* (Eaton RC, ed.), 179–212. New York: Plenum.

Lee RKK, Eaton RC, Zottoli SJ (1993) Segmental arrangement of reticulospinal neurons in the goldfish hindbrain. *J Comp Neurol* 327:1–18.

Lingenhöhl K, Friauf E (1994) Giant neurons in the rat reticular formation: A sensorimotor interface in the elementary acoustic startle circuit. *J Neurosci* 14:1176–1194.

McClellan AD (1986) Command system for initiating locomotion in fish and amphibians parallels to initiation systems in mammals. In: *Neurobiology of Vertebrate Locomotion* (Grillner S, Stein PSG, Stuart DG, Forssberg H, Herman RM, eds.), 3–20. London: Macmillan.

Meredith MA, Stein BE (1986) Visual, auditory, and somatosensory convergence on cells in superior colliculus results in multisensory integration. *J Neurophysiol* 56(3):640–662.

Mittenthal JE, Wine JJ (1973) Connectivity patterns of crayfish giant interneurons: Visualization of synaptic regions with cobalt dye. *Science* 179:182–184.

Nissanov J, Eaton RC (1989) Reticulospinal control of rapid escape turning in fishes. *Am Zool* 29:103–121.

Nye SW, Ritzmann RE (1992) Motion analysis of leg joints associated with escape turns of the cockroach, *Periplaneta americana*. *J Comp Physiol (A)* 171:183–194.

O'Malley DM, Kao Y-H, Fetcho JR (1996) Imaging the functional organization of zebrafish hindbrain segments during escape behaviors. *Neuron* 17:1145–1155.

Pearson KG, Heitler WJ, Steeves JD (1980) Triggering of locust jump by multimodal inhibitory interneurons. *J Neurophysiol* 43:257–278.

Pearson KG, O'Shea M (1984) Escape behavior of the locust: The jump and its initiation by visual stimuli. In: *Neural Mechanisms of Startle Behavior* (Eaton RC, ed.), 93–131. New York: Plenum.

Pearson KG, Robertson RM (1981) Interneurons coactivating hindleg flexor and extensor motoneurons in the locust. *J Comp Physiol* 144:391–400.

Peterson BW (1984) The reticulospinal system and its role in the control of movement. In: *Brain Stem Control of Spinal Cord Function* (Barnes CD, ed.), 27–86, New York: Academic.

Popper AN, Eaton RC (1995) Mauthner cells and their auditory interactions. *Brain Behav Evol* 46:121–180.

Reichert H, Wine JJ (1983) Coordination of lateral giant and non-giant systems in crayfish escape behavior. *J Comp Physiol* 153:3–15.

Ritzmann RE (1993) The neural organization of cockroach escape and its role in context-dependent orientation. In: *Biological Neural Networks in Invertebrate Neuroethology and Robotics* (Beer RD, Ritzmann RE, McKenna T, eds.), 113–138. Boston: Academic.

Ritzmann RE, Pollack AJ (1988) Wind activated thoracic interneurons of the cockroach: II. Patterns of connection from ventral giant interneurons. *J Neurobiol* 19:589–611.

Ritzmann RE, Pollack AJ (1990) Parallel motor pathways from thoracic interneurons of the ventral giant interneuron system of the cockroach, *Periplaneta americana. J Neurobiol* 21:1219–1235.

Ritzmann RE, Pollack AJ (1994) Responses of thoracic interneurons to tactile stimulation in the cockroach, *Periplaneta americana. J Neurobiol* 25:1113–1128.

Ritzmann RE, Pollack AJ, Hudson SE, Hyvonen A (1991) Convergence of multi-modal sensory signals at thoracic interneurons of the escape system of the cockroach, *Periplaneta americana. Brain Res* 563:175–183.

Roberts AM, Krasne FB, Hagiwara G, Wine JJ, Kramer AP (1982) Segmental giant: Evidence for a driver neuron interposed between command and motor neurons in the crayfish escape system. *J Neurophysiol* 47:761–781.

Schaefer PL, Kondagunta GV, Ritzmann RE (1994) Motion analysis of escape movements evoked by tactile stimulation in the cockroach, *Periplaneta americana. J Exp Biol* 190:287–294.

Schrameck JE (1970) Crayfish swimming: Alternating motor output and giant fiber activity. *Science* 169:698–700.

Sherwood DE, Schmidt RA, Walter CB (1988) Rapid movements with reversals in direction. II. Control of movement amplitude and inertial load. *Exp Brain Res* 69:355–367.

Watson JT, Ritzmann RE (1994) The escape response versus the quiescent response of the American cockroach: Behavioural choice mediated by physiological state. *Anim Behav* 48:476–478.

Webb PW (1994) Exercise performance of fish. In: *Advances in Veterinary Science and Comparative Medicine* (Jones JH, ed.), 38B, 1–49. Orlando: Academic.

Westin J, Langberg JJ, Camhi JM (1977) Responses of giant interneurons of the cockroach *Periplaneta americana* to wind puffs of different directions and velocities. *J Comp Physiol* 121:307–324.

Westin J, Ritzmann RE, Goddard DJ (1988) Wind activated thoracic interneurons of the cockroach. I. Responses to controlled wind stimulation. *J Neurobiol* 19:573–588.

Will U (1991) Amphibian Mauthner cells. *Brain Behav Evol* 37:317–332.

Wine JJ, Krasne FB (1972) The organization of escape behaviour in the crayfish. *J Exp Biol* 56:1–18.

Yeh S-R, Fricke FA, Edwards DH (1996) The effect of social experience on serotonergic modulation of the escape circuit of crayfish. *Science* 271:366–369.

Zucker RS (1972) Crayfish escape behavior and central synapses. I. Neural circuit exciting lateral giant fiber. *J Neurophysiol* 35:599–620.

Part II

Generation and Formation of Motor Patterns: Cellular and Systems Properties

4

Basic Building Blocks of Vertebrate Spinal Central Pattern Generators

Ole Kiehn, Jørn Hounsgaard, and Keith T. Sillar

Abstract

Neuronal circuits intrinsic to the vertebrate spinal cord can generate rhythmic motor patterns that drive locomotory movements even in the absence of sensory feedback or descending inputs from higher brain centers. These central pattern generators produce coordinated motor rhythms, which result in the patterns of motoneuron discharge that generate the actual behavior. The aim of this review is to describe the basic building blocks of vertebrate spinal locomotor central pattern generators, to discuss limitations in our understanding of the basis for rhythm and pattern generation in spinal motor systems, and to describe the locomotor networks in a range of vertebrate preparations. Although we know more about the neuronal organization of central pattern generators in lower vertebrates, some emerging general principles offer the hope that at least the elementary features of rhythm and pattern generation have been conserved during vertebrate evolution. For example, both N-methyl-D-aspartate (NMDA) and non-NMDA types of excitatory amino acids receptors seem ubiquitously present in the membranes of spinal motoneurons and are activated during locomotor rhythm generation. In addition, the reciprocal inhibition that ensures alternating activity between functionally antagonistic motoneuron pools is mediated, for the main part, by glycine acting at strychnine-sensitive receptors that gate a Cl^- conductance. Ion channels controlling spike-frequency regulation and non-linear membrane properties are present in both lower and higher vertebrate motoneurons and interneurons. Those properties, which include intrinsic bursting properties and Ca^{2+}-dependent plateau potentials, are conditional upon the activation of receptors for certain transmitters—including NMDA, serotonin, noradrenaline, and several peptides. The functional role of nonlinear membrane properties for rhythm and pattern generation and their role in cellular information processing is also discussed in this review.

Neuronal circuits intrinsic to the vertebrate spinal cord can generate rhythmic motor patterns subserving loco-motory movements even in the absence of sensory feedback or descending inputs from higher brain centers. These *central pattern generators* (CPGs), produce coordinated motor outputs that are reflected in the patterns of motoneuron discharge that generate the actual behavior.

Early progress toward defining the locomotor circuits of the spinal cord originated from studies of locomotor-like behavior in decerebrated or spinal cats in vivo. Although such studies have contributed a great deal, they do not lend themselves to detailed analysis of the electrophysiological and pharmacological properties of the CPG elements. Alternatively, in vitro techniques offer more control of the extracellular medium and easy drug access, and they are more amenable to quantitative analysis. In order to foster realistic hopes of progress toward understanding the cellular and synaptic mechanisms of overall CPG function, use must be made of relatively simple and accessible animal preparations. This need has spurred the search for model systems that fulfill those criteria. Foremost among such systems are the lamprey (Wallén, chapter 6, this volume) and the *Xenopus* embryo (Roberts et al., chapter 7, this volume; Dale, chapter 8, this volume), with valuable information more recently coming from the use of frog and chick embryos, the neonatal rat, the adult turtle, and the mud puppy. Evidence to this point suggests that certain basic mechanisms of CPG function are ontogenetically and phylogenetically conserved, such that a multipreparation approach facilitates the quest for a general understanding of the locomotor CPGs of the vertebrate spinal cord.

Here, we review insights gained into the nature of the basic building blocks of vertebrate spinal locomotor CPGs and discuss the limitations in our understanding of the basis for *rhythm generation* (the production of repetitive cyclical motoneuron activity) and *pattern generation* (the actual timing and coordination of agonist and antagonist muscles). Both the rhythm and the pattern are subject to chemical modulation (Sillar et al., chapter 17, this volume).

The Locomotor Pattern

During locomotion, the basic pattern of motoneuron discharge involves the reciprocal activation of functionally antagonist muscles—the extensor and flexor muscles within and between the limbs of vertebrates. In addition, the pattern also applies to left/right coordination of axial muscles during aquatic locomotion. Graham Brown (1911) showed the fundamental organization of the locomotor pattern early in the twentieth century, using acute spinal and deafferented cats. He proposed a simple *half-center model* to explain the reciprocal activation of extensors and flexors (Stein and Smith, chapter 5, this volume). Each half-center was thought to excite either flexors or extensors, and the two half-centers were thought to be mutually connected by reciprocal inhibition to ensure that when one center is active, the other is silent. Later, Lundberg, Jankowska, and collaborators (e.g., Jankowska et al., 1967a, 1967b) described a spinal network organization in cats that incorporated the basic features of Brown's half-center model. They found that,

following intravenous injection of L-DOPA, stimulation of ipsi- and contralateral high-threshold sensory afferents cause "late L-DOPA reflexes" in flexor and extensor motoneurons, respectively. When the ipsi- and contralateral stimulation was combined and appropriately sequenced in time, the flexor and extensor pathways mutually inhibited each other at a premotoneuronal level, as proposed in Brown's half-center scheme. Interestingly, when L-DOPA is combined with low doses of a monoamine oxidase inhibitor, high-threshold sensory afferent stimulation elicits short periods of alternating efferent discharges, not unlike those which occur during locomotor activity (see Gossard and Hultborn, 1991). Higher doses of a monoamine oxidase inhibitor and L-DOPA induce prolonged spinal locomotor-like activity, suggesting that the late DOPA reflexes and DOPA-induced spinal locomotion share the same neuronal networks (the CPGs) and that these networks are organized in a half-center fashion (Lundberg, 1979).

In its most extreme version, the half-center organization implies that the locomotor CPGs generate a simple alternating activity of all extensors and flexors (Lundberg, 1979). Such an organization is clearly not compatible with experimental observations showing that (1) locomotor activity can display distinct timing of individual flexors and extensors in the absence of afferent inputs (Grillner and Zangger, 1979; Pearson and Rossignol, 1991; Kiehn and Kjærulff, 1996), and (2) spinal locomotor CPGs are distributed over several segments, each containing oscillatory units (Grillner and Zangger, 1979; Gelfand et al., 1988; Ho and O'Donovan, 1993; Kjærulff and Kiehn, 1996; Stein et al., 1995; Cowley and Schmidt, 1997; cf., however, Cazalets et al., 1995, and Wheatley et al., 1994). These observations support the alternative view that spinal motor networks are composed of several unit burst generators, which can be recruited into a reciprocally organized common network (Grillner, 1981). Such a design allows for maximal flexibility of the spinal locomotor CPGs and accommodates the basic organization of the much better understood CPGs underlying undulatory swimming behavior in the *Xenopus* embryo and the lamprey. In these animals, spinal CPGs are thought to be distributed along the cord with a pair of half-center unit generators in each segment generating reciprocal activation of the two sides of the cord (Arshavsky et al., 1993; Grillner and Matsushima, 1991).

At the motoneuron level the reciprocal organization is produced by alternating excitation and inhibition in each cycle of rhythmic motor output. In the next section, we consider how this alternation and the rhythm itself might be generated.

Initiation of Rhythmic Activity

In intact animals, spinal CPGs are thought to be activated by an unpatterned (i.e., tonic) descending drive from the brain. Experimentally, this situation can be mimicked by tonic stimulation of discrete areas in the brain stem or the midbrain (Grillner et al., chapter 1, this volume), stimulation of relatively high-threshold skin afferents, or replacement of the descending drive with exogenous application of excitatory transmitters. Although the first two methods activate synaptic pathways, more or less directly implicated in locomotor control, the third method is clearly unphysiological. It cannot, therefore, always be inferred that phenomena elicited by external drug application have a functional role in the intact animal. Two potential problems must be acknowledged in evaluating transmitter-induced studies of CPG activity. First, receptors for the exogenous agonist may not normally be subject to continuous activation; also, where the receptors allow Ca^{2+} entry (e.g., N-methyl-D-aspartate [NMDA] receptors), the long-term consequences for CPG function are unpredictable and unknown. Second, many spinal neurons that are not components of the basic CPG (e.g., sensory pathway neurons, neuromodulatory fibers), but which possess the appropriate receptors, could be activated and contribute, unphysiologically, to the motor pattern. Nevertheless, exogenous transmitter application is a convenient method used to elicit continuous rhythmic activity for experimental manipulation.

Monoamines and Acetylcholine

It has long been known that intravenous injection of the catecholamine precursor, L-DOPA, can evoke locomotion in the spinal cat (Jankowska et al., 1967a, 1967b; Forssberg and Grillner, 1973) and the rabbit (Viala and Buser, 1969). Pharmacological analysis indicates that the DOPA effects on the spinal cord are mainly mediated by activation of noradrenergic receptors (for discussion, see Grillner, 1981, and Conway et al., 1988). This conclusion is further supported by the fact that intravenous injection of the alpha-agonist clonidine in the acute (Forssberg and Grillner, 1973) and chronic (Barbeau and Rossignol, 1991) spinal cat, or intrathecal application of noradrenaline in the acute spinal cat (Kiehn et al., 1992), can evoke locomotion. The role of dopamine cannot be entirely discounted, however, because recent experiments have shown that it can initiate spinal locomotion in the neonatal rat (Smith et al., 1988; Kiehn and Kjærulff, 1996).

5-hydroxytryptamine (5-HT or serotonin) is another transmitter that appears to play a role in the initiation of locomotion in some vertebrates. In both the rabbit (Viala and Buser, 1969) and the neonatal rat (Cazalets et al., 1990, 1992; Kiehn and Kjærulff, 1996), 5-HT induces alternating rhythmic flexor and extensor discharges. There seem to be species differences in 5-HT's effect because it cannot initiate locomotion in the cat (Barbeau and Rossignol, 1991), the lamprey (Harris-Warrick and Cohen, 1985), or the tadpole (Sillar et al., 1992). In vertebrates studied to this point, however, 5-HT exerts powerful modulatory control over rhythm generation. The ability of 5-HT to modulate the ongoing rhythm is considered further in a separate chapter (Sillar et al., chapter 17, this volume).

Finally, acetylcholine can cause a strong activation of spinal CPGs in the tadpole (Panchin et al., 1991) and the neonatal rat (Smith et al., 1988; Cowley and Schmidt, 1994, 1995).

Excitatory Amino Acids

Using an in vitro preparation of the lamprey spinal cord, Cohen and Wallén (1980) and Poon (1980) were the first to show that excitatory amino acids (EAAs), such as glutamate, can activate locomotory movements in vertebrates. Later studies by Grillner and colleagues (Grillner et al., 1981; Brodin et al., 1985; for additional references see Grillner and Matsushima, 1991) suggested that the EAAs primarily activated the CPGs through the NMDA and kainate receptor sites. Similar conclusions have been reached for swimming in the amphibian embryo (Dale and Roberts, 1984; 1985). Furthermore, in the lamprey, selective activation of either NMDA or kainate receptors produces either slow (0.1 to 2–3 Hz) or fast (1–8 Hz) fictive swimming, respectively. Thus, activation of these two receptor subtypes in combination can account for the entire behavioral frequency range of lamprey swimming (Grillner and Matsushima, 1991). More recent experiments have provided evidence for the additional involvement of quisqualate, acting on the AMPA receptor site, in the generation of swimming in the lamprey (Alford and Grillner, 1990). In contrast, bath-applied quisqualate in the *Xenopus* embryo evokes a motor pattern inappropriate for swimming (Dale and Roberts, 1984). In higher vertebrates, including the chick embryo (Barry and O'Donovan, 1987), the neonatal rat (Smith and Feldman, 1987; Kudo and Yamada, 1987), the adult rabbit (Fenaux et al., 1991), the mouse (Hernadez et al., 1991), the mud puppy (Wheatley and Stein, 1992), the cat (Douglas et al., 1993), and the monkey (Hultborn et al., 1993), bath-applied NMDA is used as one of the primary tools to activate spinal CPGs that control various forms of locomotion. In these preparations, however, kainate/AMPA receptor agonists produce a weaker and less stable rhythm than does NMDA (Smith et al., 1988, Kudo and Yamada, 1987; Cazalets et al., 1992; Douglas et al., 1993). Nevertheless, both NMDA and kainate/AMPA receptors seem to be involved in the generation of locomotory movements elicited by the stimulation of brainstem or peripheral sensory afferents. Thus, blocking either NMDA or kainate/AMPA receptors suppresses or abolishes the stimulation-evoked rhythmicity in a variety of preparations (McClellan and Grillner, 1984; Brodin and Grillner, 1985; Dale and Roberts, 1984; Barry and O'Donovan, 1987; Smith et al., 1988; Fenaux et al., 1991; Douglas et al., 1993).

Taken together, the above described experiments suggest that several receptors for a given transmitter (e.g., glutamate) and several transmitters can be involved in the initiation of vertebrate locomotion. Selected transmitters most likely act on different subcomponents of spinal CPGs and are thereby able to reconfigure the network. Such selectivity is analogous to that found in invertebrate motor systems (Harris-Warrick et al., chapter 19, this volume; Kupfermann et al., chapter 20, this volume). However, the necessity or sufficiency of any of these transmitters and transmitter-receptor combinations has yet to be determined. Taking into account the fact that EAA, monoamine, and acetylcholine receptors are widely distributed in the spinal cord, the global effect of activating a selected transmitter-receptor may reflect an additional and secondary activation of other transmitter-receptors (e.g., a 5-HT-induced glutamate release from segmental interneurons).

Components, Connections, and Transmitters in Spinal CPGs

Once initiated, CPG circuitry provides temporally coded synaptic inputs to the motoneurons to ensure an appropriate sequencing of their rhythmic firing during locomotory movement. The synaptic inputs to a given motoneuron in each cycle of motor activity comprise (1) excitatory drive during one phase of the cycle to generate action potentials and (2) inhibition during the opposite phase to ensure that action potentials do not occur when antagonist motoneuron pools are active. In this section, we consider which intrinsic spinal neuron classes are responsible for the synaptic drive and what transmitters they use.

Reciprocal Inhibition

The reciprocal organization of spinally generated locomotor activity indicates a role for inhibitory transmission in the shaping of the patterns. A wealth of experimental evidence from a wide range of preparations supports the conclusion that glycinergic neurotransmission is the principal mechanism underlying the reciprocal organization of the locomotor pattern. Blocking glycine receptors with strychnine during locomotion in the tadpole (Soffe, 1987, 1989), the neonatal rat (Kudo et al., 1991; Cowley and Schmidt, 1995), the adult lamprey (Cohen and Harris-Warrick, 1984), and the cat (Noga et al., 1993) disrupts left/right alternation or midcycle inhibition; it also causes co-activation of flexor and extensor muscles in legged animals. However, when interpreting such data, it is well to recall that strychnine can also block various ion channels (for references see Dale, 1995) and gamma-aminobutyric acid (GABA) receptors (Tauck et al., 1988) at concentrations (1–20 μM) usually used to block glycine-mediated reciprocal inhibition. This issue illustrates the need for further investigation of inhibitory components of spinal CPGs in vertebrates.

Phasic inhibition in motoneurons is mainly mediated by an increase in a strychnine-sensitive (and thus presumably) glycinergic Cl^- conductance (for references see Soffe, 1989). Paired intracellular recordings in the tadpole and the lamprey have shown that interneurons with crossed axons elicit strychnine-sensitive inhibitory postsynaptic potentials (IPSPs) in and fire out of phase with contralateral motoneurons (Buchanan, 1982; Buchanan and Cohen, 1982; Dale, 1985; Buchanan and Grillner, 1987). The crossed-axon neurons may therefore be responsible for the phasic inhibition observed during swimming. More recent studies (Buchanan and Grillner, 1988) describe a new class of inhibitory interneurons that project to ipsilateral motoneurons. These latter cells might also be part of the segmental CPGs that operate in lamprey swimming. In higher vertebrates, the source of the inhibitory drive during locomotion is unknown. Ia interneurons (one of the few well-characterized groups of spinal interneurons; for a review, see Jankowska, 1992) are rhythmically active during locomotion (Pratt and Jordan, 1987) and have the appropriate reciprocal connections to provide inhibition of antagonist muscles. They are not, however, considered part of the rhythm-generating network (Pratt and Jordan, 1987), although they might be important for shaping the final motoneuronal output from the spinal cord. One potential group of inhibitory interneurons within the actual locomotor CPG might be those commissural neurons that project segmentally to the contralateral side (for references, see Silos-Santiago and Snider, 1992). The axons of the commissural neurons cross to the opposite side in front of the central canal (Silos-Santiago and Snider, 1992), and recent experiments indicate that lesioning of the axons abolishes left/right coordination in the neonatal rat (Kjærulff and Kiehn, 1996).

The role of the inhibitory transmitter GABA in reciprocal inhibition is less clear. In the neonatal rat, Cazalets and others (1994) found that the GABA$_A$ receptor blocker, bicuculline, did not prevent the reciprocal inhibition, but rather increased the cycle frequency of the locomotion. These findings are in keeping with early studies on the tadpole (Soffe, 1987) and lamprey (Grillner and Wallén, 1980; Tegner et al., 1993), but are in contrast with recent observations on neonatal rats by Cowley and Schmidt (1995), who showed that bicuculline produces a complete block of reciprocal inhibition. At present, no one has explained this diversity of findings for bicuculline, but non-specific effects of high concentrations of this GABA$_A$ antagonist cannot be ruled out as a contributing factor. It is also likely that GABA may play roles at early stages in development that subsequently disappear. For example, in the developing embryonic motor system of the chick spinal cord, inhibitory neurons generate depolarizing IPSPs in sartorius (flexor) motoneurons that limit the extent of their firing in each half cycle of locomotor activity. Slightly later in development, the depolarizing IPSP input disappears, thereby allowing the neurons to fire in a different temporal sequence. The loss of this inhibitory input coincides with the disappearance of spinal interneurons with GABA immunoreactivity (O'Donovan et al., 1992). On the other hand, it is clear that both GABA$_A$ and GABA$_B$ receptors can cause inactivation of locomotor CPGs in both the lamprey (Tegner et al., 1993) and the neonatal rat (Cazalets et al., 1994; Cowley and Schmidt, 1995), an effect mediated either by local spinal neurons or, possibly, by descending systems.

Experiments such as those cited in the previous paragraph suggest that rhythm generation itself is not dependent on glycinergic inhibition because the rhythm can continue in its absence (cf., however, studies done by Grillner and Wallén, 1980). The primary locomotor function of glycinergic neurons is probably to ensure a strict alternation between rhythmically active half-centers and antagonist motoneurons. A supplementary function may be to facilitate rebound firing as neurons recover from mid-cycle inhibition (see Roberts et al., chapter 7, this volume). A primary function of GABA systems may be to serve as a brake on the locomotor

CPGs, although some contribution to shaping the reciprocal alternation cannot be entirely excluded. In the *Xenopus* embryo, a clear-cut function for reticulospinal neurons of the hindbrain in the termination of swimming has been described: the descending GABA neurons are activated by primary sensory afferents of the rostral cement gland to ensure that swimming behaviour stops upon contact with obstacles in the environment (see Roberts et al., chapter 7, this volume).

Excitatory Components of the CPG

In both the lamprey and the tadpole, a major part of the excitatory drive within the locomotor CPGs and onto motoneurons is due to the release of an EAA that excites both NMDA and non-NMDA receptors (Dale and Roberts, 1985; Dale and Grillner, 1986; Dale, 1986). In both animals, the excitatory drive is thought to be generated by small interneurons that have monosynaptic connections to and fire rhythmically in phase with ipsilateral motoneurons (Dale and Roberts, 1985; Buchanan and Grillner, 1987; Buchanan et al., 1989). When active, these small interneurons release an EAA that co-activates postsynaptic NMDA and non-NMDA receptors to produce slow rise-and-fall excitatory postsynaptic potentials (EPSPs) and fast rise-and-fall EPSPs, respectively. The resulting "dual-component" excitations are fast-rise and slow-fall EPSPs (Dale and Roberts, 1985). The slow EPSPs have important consequences for rhythm generation in the *Xenopus* embryo because they last 200 msec, which thereby exceeds the duration of the swimming cycle period (50 to 100 msec). As a result, the NMDA potentials summate over consecutive cycles to provide a tonic (background) excitation in both motoneurons and interneurons. This drive—a feature of most vertebrate locomotor systems—has been attributed to the tonic firing of descending neurons from the brain stem. In at least the spinal cord of *Xenopus*, there is no need for a tonic drive from descending systems after the initial phase of activation. Furthermore, it has been proposed that in *Xenopus* the pool of excitatory spinal interneurons participate in feedback re-excitation as a means of sustaining rhythm generation (Arshavsky et al., 1993). At the moment, it is not known whether similar mechanisms are present in higher vertebrates, although it is clear that the excitatory drive to motoneurons is mediated by both NMDA and non-NMDA receptors (Brownstone et al., 1994; Cazalets et al., 1996). The interneuronal source of this excitation has not been identified, however. Recent research has attempted to identify a group of first-order interneurons in a locomotor-related group Ib pathway (Gossard et al., 1994; Fedirchuk et al., 1994), but the function of such cells in the spinal CPG operation is not yet known.

In summary, a detailed characterization of CPG networks is available to this point only for the tadpole and the lamprey (see also Roberts et al., chapter 7, this volume, and Wallén, chapter 6, this volume). It is possible, at least in the more complicated lamprey spinal cord, that networks are composed of more elements than were hitherto anticipated. Future research should offer a more detailed understanding of locomotor CPGs in higher vertebrates, particularly in terms of the properties of their neurons and interconnections. Given the complexity of the spinal cord, such an understanding will not be easily obtained and will require the use of multiple techniques. Recent use of activity-dependent labeling with c-*fos* (Dai et al., 1990; Barajon et al., 1992) and fluorescent dyes (Kjærulff et al., 1994), field potential mapping (Noga et al., 1995), lesion studies (Ho and O'Donovan, 1993; Kjærulff and Kiehn, 1996; Cowley and Schmidt, 1997), and Ca^{2+} imaging (O'Donovan et al., 1994) has suggested that the intermediate zone of and the areas around the central canal of the spinal cord are important for rhythm and pattern generation in birds and mammals. The recent introduction of tight-seal, whole-cell recordings from interneurons in the vertebrate cord (Sernagor and O'Donovan, 1991; Hochman et al., 1994a; Raastad et al., 1996; Kiehn et al., 1996) has allowed recordings from small interneurons that were previously inaccessible. Hopefully, recordings, in combination with anatomical techniques and stimulation of peripheral sensory afferents known to perturb the locomotor CPG (see Pearson and Ramirez, chapter 21, this volume), will advance understanding of some key elements of CPGs, even in the mammalian spinal cord.

Postsynaptic Mechanisms for Rhythm and Pattern Generation

The final motor output generated by any neuronal network depends not only on the synaptic connections within the network, but also on their interactions with the intrinsic membrane properties of the component neurons. In this section, we consider the possible postsynaptic mechanisms that contribute to rhythm and pattern generation. The discussion is somewhat hampered by our limited knowledge of the actual composition of the CPGs in higher vertebrates; it is also difficult, in all preparations, to establish criteria that define a particular cell as a member of the CPG and to assess the relative contribution of electroresponsive properties and synaptic inputs to the overall network function. Even though motoneurons are not normally considered a member of the CPG (cf., however, Roberts et al., chapter 7, this volume), we start by discussing their intrinsic response properties.

Motoneuron Conductances

Detailed information on the conductances responsible for the intrinsic response properties of spinal motoneurons is available for the tadpole (Dale, 1993; Wall and Dale, 1993, 1994), the neonatal rat (Harada and Takahashi, 1983; Takahashi, 1990a, 1990b), the adult cat (Schwindt and Crill, 1984), and the turtle (Hounsgaard et al., 1988b; Hounsgaard and Mintz, 1988). In these species, motoneurons are capable of repetitive firing during sustained depolarization (but see Soffe, 1990).

Repetitive firing requires that Na$^+$ channels be rescued from inactivation in the interval between spike discharges. In spinal motoneurons, repetitive firing is controlled by the slow afterhyperpolarization (sAHP) following action potentials, as was first shown for repetitive firing in motoneurons of the cat (see Schwindt and Crill, 1984) and subsequently in motoneurons of the frog (Barrett and Barrett, 1976), the neonatal rat (Harada and Takahashi, 1983), the turtle (Hounsgaard et al., 1988b), and the lamprey (Wallén et al., 1989). In motoneurons of these species, the sAHP is mediated by a Ca^{2+}-dependent K$^+$ current recruited by activation of high-threshold Ca^{2+} channels during the action potential (Barrett and Barrett, 1976; Harada and Takahashi, 1983; Schwindt and Crill, 1984; Hounsgaard et al., 1988b). At least part of the current underlying the sAHP is apamin sensitive (Zhang and Krnjevic, 1987; Hounsgaard et al., 1988b; Hill et al., 1992; Meer and Buchanan, 1992). Because the size of the AHP is a major factor in determining spike frequency and adaptation, a change in the profile of the sAHP will dramatically influence the response to synaptic inputs.

Other conductances involved in repetitive firing include a hyperpolarization-activated inward, mixed K$^+$/Na$^+$ conductance sensitive to extracellular Cs$^+$ (I$_h$; Hounsgaard et al., 1988b; Takahashi, 1990b); a transient, outward current sensitive to 4-aminopyridine (I$_A$); and a sustained, delayed rectifier (I$_{KD}$) sensitive to tetra-ethylammonium (Schwindt and Crill, 1984; Hounsgaard et al., 1988b; Hounsgaard and Mintz, 1988; Takahashi, 1990a; Wall and Dale, 1993). Although I$_{KD}$ and I$_A$ may contribute to the repolarization of the Na$^+$ spike (Schwindt and Crill, 1984; Takahashi, 1990a), the exact role of I$_h$ has not yet been determined. In many neurons, it contributes to the resting membrane potential and to rebound burst discharges (see Kiehn and Harris-Warrick, 1992).

Finally, Ca^{2+} conductances also contribute to repetitive firing. The Ca^{2+} influx during action potentials, which activates the sAHP, is mediated by a high-threshold Ca^{2+} conductance (Barrett and Barrett, 1976; Harada and Takahashi, 1983; Hounsgaard et al., 1988b). This conductance is insensitive to dihydropyridines and may be mediated by N- and/or P-type Ca^{2+} channels, as are found in hypoglossal neurons of the neonatal rat (Umemiya et al., 1994). Also described in this preparation is a low-threshold, transient Ca^{2+} current (T-type), which may be important for burst discharges (Berger and Takahashi, 1990).

Transmitter-Modulation of Spinal Motoneurons

The actions of 5-HT have been studied the most (Kiehn, 1991a, 1991b; Wallis, 1994), but other transmitter actions have also been described (Hultborn and Kiehn, 1992). The most common mechanism is a decrease of outward currents with a resulting increase in excitability. More rarely, 5-HT transmitters reduce excitability by opening K^+ channels (Kiehn, 1991b; Wallis, 1994).

Tonic depolarization   In the embryonic and neonatal rat, 5-HT evokes strong depolarization of spinal motoneurons (Takahashi and Berger, 1990; Berger and Takahashi, 1990; Ziskind-Conhaim et al., 1993; Wallis, 1994). Although the effect is clear, there are conflicting reports on the ionic basis of the 5-HT-mediated depolarization. Some researchers have suggested a reduction in a K^+ current (for references see Ziskind-Conhaim et al., 1993). A more rigorous voltage-clamp study has shown that 5-HT enhances I_h (which has a reversal potential more depolarized than the resting membrane potential) and enhances a low-threshold, transient Ca^{2+} current (T-type; Berger and Takahashi, 1990). In rat motoneurons, it is conceivable that 5-HT does indeed regulate all three currents. The 5-HT-mediated tonic depolarization provides a background for synaptic modulation, and it might be an important component of rhythm generation in spinal interneurons.

Reduction of sAHP   The effect of 5-HT on I_h and the T-type Ca^{2+} current has not been studied in detail in species other than the rat. However, a strong reduction in the sAHP has been reported (for references, see Kiehn 1991b), which means that a given excitatory input will elicit more action potentials after 5-HT administration than before. In other words, 5-HT increases the gain of the conversion from synaptic input to spike-coded output. The functional significance of the ability to block the sAHP for the locomotor cycle frequency and motoneuronal burst duration is discussed in a later chapter (Sillar et al., chapter 17, this volume).

Induction of intrinsic plateau potentials and oscillatory membrane potential properties   In addition to enhancing excitability, transmitters can change the balance between voltage-activated, intrinsic current generators. This fundamental effect of transmitters is dramatically illustrated by the bistability induced by 5-HT in motoneurons of the cat (Hounsgaard et al., 1988a) and the turtle (Hounsgaard and Kiehn, 1989). In those species, 5-HT uncovers a plateau potential mediated by an L-type Ca^{2+} channel sensitive to dihydropyridine (Hounsgaard and Kiehn, 1989). Although this effect was originally attributed to a reduction in the sAHP, pharmacological blocks of other outward K^+ currents also uncover the plateau potential in turtle motoneurons (Hounsgaard and Mintz, 1988). Plateau potentials in cat motoneurons are also promoted by activation of noradrenergic receptors (Conway et al., 1988). Furthermore, it has been shown in the turtle that muscarine (Hounsgaard and Mintz, unpublished; Svirskis and Hounsgaard, 1995) and tACPD, an agonist of G-protein-coupled metabotropic glutamate receptors (Svirskis and Hounsgaard, 1995 and unpublished), can elicit plateau potentials. Moreover, evidence demonstrates that plateau potentials are recruited in decerebrated cats during brainstem-induced locomotion (Brownstone et al., 1994). Although plateau potentials may contribute mainly to tonic motor output (Eken and Kiehn, 1989; Kiehn, 1991a, 1991b), they also enhance and boost rhythmic synaptic inputs, thereby shaping the duration and enhancing the amplitude of the final motoneuronal output (Kiehn, 1991a).

NMDA-induced, TTX-resistant voltage oscillations in the membrane potential of motoneurons have been reported in lamprey (Sigvardt et al., 1985; Grillner and Wallén, 1985; Wallén and Grillner, 1987), *Rana* tadpole (Sillar and Simmers, 1994), neonatal rat (Hochman et al., 1994b), and turtle motoneurons (J. Hounsgaard and I. Mintz, unpublished). The induced intrinsic oscillations change frequency and amplitude in a limited voltage window (cf., however, Hochman et al., 1994b), and as in other neurons, they result from the induction of a negative slope region in the current-voltage relationship caused by a Mg^{2+}-activated, voltage-sensitive block of the activated NMDA receptor ionophore (Novak et al., 1984). Unlike the plateau potential elicited by 5-HT and noradrenaline, the NMDA-induced depolarization is periodically self-terminating, most likely because of an intracellular accumulation of Ca^{2+} that results in activation of $K_{(Ca)}$ channels and in subsequent inactivation of the NMDA ionophore (Grillner and Wallén, 1985).

Muscarine also induces oscillations in the membrane potential of a proportion of turtle motoneurons. The depolarizing phase of each burst is mediated by L-type Ca^{2+} channels. The termination involves an interaction with intracellular Ca^{2+} sequestering because the hyperpolarizing phase is blocked by caffeine and ryanodine (Hounsgaard and Mintz, unpublished observations).

In summary, we now have substantial knowledge about ionic conductances of motoneurons and about the transmitter modulation of individual conductances. However, we do not fully understand the functional role of some of these properties during locomotion (see, however, Sillar et al., chapter 17, this volume for the role of 5-HT modulation during locomotion). For example, the locomotor role of intrinsic membrane potential oscillations in motoneurons remains relatively unclear. However, it is likely that the main role of plateau and bursting properties is to shape the duration and to enhance the amplitude of the final motoneuronal output. The synaptic processing might take place in the dendrites of motoneurons. In turtle motoneurons, Ca^{2+} channels and $K^+_{(Ca)}$ channels have been detected distally on the dendrites (Hounsgaard and Kiehn, 1993), and the local application of NMDA onto a distal dendrite has been shown to induce phasic response properties exclusively in that dendrite (Skydsgaard and Hounsgaard, 1994).

Interneuron Response Properties

Even more limited information is available on the response properties of interneurons in the locomotor CPGs of the vertebrate spinal cord. To date, there is no systematic description of the electroresponsive repertoire of any of the identified spinal interneurons of the lamprey or the tadpole (see, however, Dale, 1995, for data on cultured neurons). As a result, modeling studies of CPG networks often assume that all neurons in the network have the same membrane properties (Roberts and Tunstall, 1990; Wallén et al., 1992), an assumption that ignores differences in membrane properties between classes of interneurons, as well as between interneurons and motoneurons, which must surely exist and be important for the overall network function.

The sAHP in lamprey interneurons is as sensitive to apamin and 5-HT as motoneurons are (Meer and Buchanan, 1992; Hill et al., 1992). A reduction in the sAHP may play an important role in the 5-HT-induced slowing

of the rate of swimming in the lamprey and the tadpole (see Sillar et al., chapter 17, this volume). The same population of interneurons also acquire TTX-resistant, membrane potential oscillations in the presence of NMDA (Sigvardt et al., 1985; Grillner and Wallén, 1985; Wallén and Grillner, 1987). As in motoneurons, the oscillation frequency can be determined by the level of membrane polarization. Also, the duration of the depolarizing phase can be prolonged by reducing $I_{K(Ca)}$ with apamin (El Manira et al., 1994). The NMDA oscillations are blocked in zero Mg^{2+} (Grillner and Wallén, 1985), which also removes the negative slope region from the current-voltage relationship. In a thin slice preparation of the neonatal rat spinal cord (segments L5–S1), Hochman and others (1994a) demonstrated that high concentrations of NMDA induce TTX-resistant, membrane potential oscillations in a small percentage of neurons located around the central canal. Because there was no network rhythmicity in the slice, the cells' oscillations could not be correlated with ventral root activity. However, NMDA-induced membrane potential oscillations and muscarine-induced plateau properties have recently been demonstrated in locomotor-related cells located in the intermediate zone and around the central canal in the spinal cord of a relatively intact, neonatal rat spinal cord preparation (Kiehn et al., 1996). Endogenous bursting properties were found in a relatively minor percentage of these neurons. Whether these properties play a significant role in rhythm generation itself remains to be determined not only for the mammalian spinal cord, about whose network structure we know so little, but also for the lower-vertebrate spinal cord. It is thus somewhat surprising that the tadpole (Soffe and Roberts, 1989), lamprey (Brodin and Grillner, 1986) and neonatal rat spinal cord (Kiehn et al., unpublished) can all generate transmitter-induced locomotor activity in zero Mg^{2+} salines, which abolish the NMDA-induced membrane potential oscillations (but not the EAA-mediated EPSPs). This set of findings suggests that NMDA oscillations might not be necessary for the rhythm generation and accommodates the possibility that NMDA, muscarine, and possibly other transmitters may amplify and enhance synaptic inputs, thereby regulating pattern generation by the spinal CPG. These effects may be brought about by the transmitter-induced negative slope region in the current-voltage relationship, which in a certain voltage window will enhance and amplify synaptic inputs in a nonlinear way.

In the turtle, subpopulations of interneurons in the ventral and dorsal horn display plateau potentials mediated by L-type Ca^{2+} channels, as well as membrane potential oscillations even in the absence of exogenously applied transmitters (Hounsgaard and Kjærulff, 1991; Russo and Hounsgaard, 1994; Russo and Hounsgaard, 1996a). Another distinct group of dorsal interneurons produce tonic firing when depolarized from resting voltage. However, they exhibit burst firing when activated from more hyperpolarized levels. These effects are due to the presence of a T-type Ca^{2+} channel (Russo and Hounsgaard, 1996b). Again, however, it is not known if the interneurons so far characterized in the turtle are part of the locomotor CPG.

Conclusions

A functional understanding of vertebrate CPGs requires identification of the component neurons, mapping of their synaptic connectivity, description of the membrane properties of individual neurons, and elucidation of the modulation of synaptic transmission and cellular conductances. Such a complete understanding has not yet been obtained, even in the *Xenopus* embryo and in the adult lamprey. Nevertheless, some general principles have emerged, despite the strong possibility that substantial interspecies differences exist in selected aspects of the motor patterns driving distinct behaviors. The following general principles suggest that at least some elementary features of rhythm and pattern generation have been conserved during vertebrate evolution.

First, the transmitters used by spinal interneurons to produce the basic pattern of motor output appear to be the same, independent of phylogenetic position or ontogenetic stage. EAA receptors seem ubiquitously present in the membrane of spinal motoneurons, and they are activated during generation of locomotion. Furthermore, both NMDA and non-NMDA receptors are apparently responsible for the excitatory drive during locomotion. Second, the reciprocal inhibition that ensures alternating activity between functionally antagonistic motor pools appears to be mediated mainly by the amino acid glycine, which acts on strychnine-sensitive receptors that gate a Cl^- conductance. The evidence supporting both principles is strongest in the tadpole and the lamprey. However, a block of locomotor rhythm generation by EAA antagonists and an interruption of reciprocal coupling by strychnine during locomotion have been observed in many vertebrate species.

Certain similarities have also emerged in the ensemble of ionic conductances that convert presynaptic inputs into patterned motor outputs. Ion channels controlling spike-frequency regulation and nonlinear membrane properties, such as intrinsic bursting capability and plateau potentials, are present in lower and higher vertebrate motoneurons and interneurons alike. Clearly, however, substantial differences exist between animals, not only in the complexity of the neural circuitry, but also in the response properties of their constituent neuronal elements. For example, the spiking capability of *Xenopus* neurons is apparently less well developed when compared to the capability of mature neurons (Soffe, 1990; Sillar et al., 1992). Furthermore, differences in the balance of ionic conductances will have important implications for the neuromodulation and timing of synaptic events within the different CPG networks.

NMDA-induced oscillatory behavior has attracted much attention in vertebrate CPG research. However, in no preparation has a causal link been established between the presence of transmitter-induced intrinsic membrane potential oscillations in interneurons and rhythm generation itself. Modeling studies in *Xenopus* have shown that neurons with Hodgkin-Huxley-type membrane properties, and with the two types of synaptic interaction described above, are sufficient to reproduce a rhythmic motor pattern similar to that seen during swimming. Perhaps the presence of intrinsic bursting capability and plateau properties serve no crucial role in rhythm generation per se, but instead act as *boosting* mechanisms that amplify and shape synaptic inputs in the CPG network.

Although we have a wealth of information on the overall structure of spinal CPGs in higher vertebrates, our understanding of their operation is still quite superficial, largely because of the complexity of the spinal cord in higher vertebrates. Identification of the component neurons of higher-vertebrate CPGs and the mapping of their synaptic connectivity will no doubt remain problematic for the immediate future. The recent introduction of a variety of new techniques that allow recordings from small neurons or simultaneously from several neurons, as well as identification of specific sensory afferent inputs to CPG components, raises hopes for identifying key neurons in the more complex spinal CPGs. However, at this time we should not restrict ourselves to rigorous network studies without continuing the study of individual interneurons and their membrane properties, of synaptic processing, and of neuromodulation in both lower and higher vertebrates. Such studies will undoubtedly reveal new and general principles about the function of the brain.

Acknowledgments

We thank the following for their support of research carried out in our laboratories: the Novo Nordic Foundation and the Danish MRC (Kiehn and Hounsgaard); the Royal Society (London), the BBSRC, and the Wellcome Trust (Sillar). Ole Kiehn is a Hallas Møller Senior Research Fellow.

References

Alford S, Grillner S (1990) CNQX and DNQX block non-NMDA synaptic transmission but not NMDA-evoked locomotion in lamprey spinal cord. *Brain Res* 506:297–302.

Arshavsky Y, Orlovsky GN, Panchin Y, Roberts A, Soffe SR (1993) Neuronal control of swimming locomotion: Analysis of the pteropod mollusc *Clione* and embryos of the amphibian *Xenopus*. *Trends Neurosci* 16:227–233.

Barajon I, Gossard JP, Hultborn H (1992) Induction of *fos* expression by activity in the spinal rhythm generator for scratching. *Brain Res* 588:168–172.

Barbeau H, Rossignol S (1991) Initiation and modulation of the locomotor pattern in the adult chronic spinal cat by noradrenergic, serotonergic, and dopaminergic drugs. *Brain Res* 546:250–260.

Barrett EF, Barrett JN (1976) Separation of two voltage sensitive potassium currents, and demonstration of a tetrodotoxin-resistent calcium current in frog motoneurones. *J Physiol* 304:737–774.

Barry M, O'Donovan MJ (1987) The effects of excitatory amino acids and their antagonists on the generation of motor activity in the isolated chick cord. *Dev Brain Res* 36:271–276.

Berger AJ, Takahashi T (1990) Serotonin enhances a low-voltage-activated calcium current in rat spinal motoneurons. *J Neurosci* 10:1922–1928.

Brodin L, Grillner S (1985) The role of putative excitatory amino acid neurotransmitters in the initiation of locomotion in the lamprey spinal cord. I. The effects of excitatory amino acid antagonists. *Brain Res* 360:139–148.

Brodin L, Grillner S (1986) Effects of magnesium on fictive locomotion induced by activation of N-methyl-D-aspartate (NMDA) receptors in the lamprey spinal cord in vitro. *Brain Res* 380:244–252.

Brodin L, Grillner S, Rovainen CM (1985) N-Methyl-D-aspartate (NMDA), kainate and quisqualate receptors and the generation of fictive locomotion in the lamprey spinal cord. *Brain Res* 325:302–306.

Brown TG (1911) The intrinsic factors in the act of progression in the mammal. *Proc Roy Soc Lond* B84:308–319.

Brownstone RM, Gossard J-P, Hultborn H (1994) Voltage-dependent excitation of motoneurones from spinal locomotor centres in the cat. *Exp Brain Res* 102:34–44.

Buchanan JT (1982) Identification of interneurons with contralateral, caudal axons in the lamprey spinal cord: Synaptic interactions and morphology. *J Neurophysiol* 47:961–975.

Buchanan JT, Cohen AH (1982) Activities of identified interneurons, motoneurons, and muscle fibers during fictive swimming in the lamprey and effects of reticulospinal and dorsal cell stimulation. *J Neurophysiol* 47:948–960.

Buchanan JT, Grillner S (1987) Newly identified "glutamate interneurons" and their role in locomotion in the lamprey spinal cord. *Science* 236:312–314.

Buchanan JT, Grillner S (1988) A new class of small inhibitory interneurones in the lamprey spinal cord. *Brain Res* 438:404–407.

Buchanan JT, Grillner S, Cullheim S, Risling M (1989) Identification of excitatory interneurons contributing to generation of locomotion in lamprey: Structure, pharmacology, and function. *J Neurophysiol* 62:59–69.

Cazalets JR, Borde M, Clarac F (1995) Localization and organization of the central pattern generator for hindlimb locomotion in newborn rats. *J Neurosci* 15:4943–4951.

Cazalets JR, Borde M, Clarac F (1996) The synaptic drive from the spinal locomotor network to motoneurons in the newborn rat. *J Neurosci* 16:298–306.

Cazalets JR, Grillner P, Menard I, Cremieux J, Clarac F (1990) Two types of motor rhythm induced by NMDA and amines in an in vitro spinal cord preparation of neonatal rat. *Neurosci Letts* 111:116–121.

Cazalets JR, Sqalli-Houssaini Y, Clarac F (1992) Activation of the central pattern generators for locomotion by serotonin and excitatory amino acids in neonatal rat. *J Physiol* 455:187–204.

Cazalets JR, Sqalli-Houssaini Y, Clarac F (1994) GABAergic inactivation of the central pattern generators for locomotion in isolated neonatal rat spinal cord. *J Physiol* 474:173–181.

Cohen AH, Harris-Warrick R (1984) Strychnine eliminates alternating motor output during fictive locomotion in the lamprey. *Brain Res* 293:164–167.

Cohen AH, Wallén P (1980) The neuronal correlate of locomotion in fish: "Fictive swimming" induced in an in vitro preparation of the lamprey spinal cord. *Exp Brain Res* 41:11–18.

Conway BA, Hultborn H, Kiehn O, Mintz I (1988) Plateau potentials in alpha-motoneurones induced by intravenous injection of L-dopa and clonidine in the spinal cat. *J Physiol* 405:369–384.

Cowley KC, Schmidt BJ (1994) A comparison of motor patterns induced by N-methyl-D-aspartate, acetylcholine, and serotonin in the in vitro rat spinal cord. *Neurosci Letts* 171:147–150.

Cowley KC, Schmidt BJ (1995) Effects of inhibitory amino acids antagonists on reciprocal inhibitory interactions during rhythmic motor activity in the in vitro neonatal rat spinal cord. *J Neurophysiol* 74:1109–1117.

Cowley KC, Schmidt BJ (1997) Regional distribution of the locomotor pattern-generating network in the neonatal rat spinal cord. *J Neurophysiol* 77:247–259.

Dai X, Douglas JR, Nagy JI, Noga BR, Jordan LM (1990) Localization of spinal neurons activated during treadmill locomotion usig c-*fos* immunohistochemical method. *Soc Neurosci Abstr* 16:889.

Dale N (1985) Reciprocal inhibitory interneurones in the *Xenopus* embryo spinal cord. *J Physiol* 363:61–70.

Dale N (1986) Excitatory synaptic drive for swimming mediated by amino acid receptors in the lamprey. *J Neurosci* 6:2662–2675.

Dale N (1993) A large, sustained Na$^{(+)}$- and voltage-dependent K$^+$ current in spinal neurons of the frog embryo. *J Physiol* 462:349–372.

Dale N (1995) Experimentally derived model for the locomotor pattern generator in the *Xenopus* embryo. *J Physiol* 489(2):489–510.

Dale N, Grillner S (1986) Dual-component synaptic potentials in the lamprey mediated by excitatory amino acid receptors. *J Neurosci* 6: 2653–2661.

Dale N, Roberts A (1984) Excitatory amino acid receptors in *Xenopus* embryo spinal cord and their role in the activation of swimming. *J Physiol* 348:527–543.

Dale N, Roberts A (1985) Dual-component amino-acid-mediated synaptic potentials: Excitatory drive for swimming in *Xenopus* embryos. *J Physiol* 363:35–59.

Douglas JR, Noga BR, Dai X, Jordan LM (1993) The effects of intrathecal administration of excitatory amino acid agonists and antagonists on the initiation of locomotion in the adult cat. *J Neurosci* 13:990–1000.

Eken T, Kiehn O (1989) Bistable firing properties of soleus motor units in unrestrained rats. *Acta Physiol Scand* 136:383–394.

El Manira A, Tegner J, Grillner S (1994) Calcium-dependent potassium channels play a critical role for burst termination in the locomotor network in lamprey. *J Neurophysiol* 72:1852–1861.

Fedirchuk B, Noga B, Carr P, Jordan LM, Hultborn H (1994) Candidate first-order interneurons in a locomotor-related group Ib pathway from hindlimb extensors in the cat. *Eur J Neurosci Suppl* 7:166.

Fenaux F, Corio M, Palisses R, Viala D (1991) Effects of a NMDA-receptor antagonist, MK-801, on central locomotor programming in the rabbit. *Exp Brain Res* 86:392–401.

Forssberg H, Grillner S (1973) The locomotion of the acute spinal cat injected with clonidine i.v. *Brain Res* 50:184–186.

Gelfand IM, Orlowsky GN, Shik ML (1988) Locomotion and scratching in tetrapods. In: *Neural Control of Rhythmic Movements in Vertebrates* (Cohen AH, Rossignol S, Grillner S, eds.), 285–332. New York: Wiley.

Gossard J-P, Brownstone RM, Barajon I, Hultborn H (1994) Transmission in a locomotor-related group Ib pathway from hindlimb extensor muscles in the cat. *Exp Brain Res* 98:213–228.

Gossard J-P, Hultborn H (1991) The organisation of spinal rhythm generation in locomotion. In: *Plasticity of Motoneuronal Connections* (Wernig A, ed.), 385–404. Amsterdam: Elsevier Science.

Grillner S (1981) Control of locomotion in bipeds, tetrapods, and fish. In: *Handbook of Physiology* (Brooks VB, ed.), 1179–1236. Bethesda, Md.: American Physiological Society.

Grillner S, Matsushima T (1991) The neural network underlying locomotion in lamprey: Synaptic and cellular mechanisms. *Neuron* 7:1–15.

Grillner S, McClellan A, Sigvardt K, Wallén P, Wilen M (1981) Activation of NMDA-receptors elicits "fictive locomotion" in lamprey spinal cord in vitro. *Acta Physiol Scand* 113:549–551.

Grillner S, Wallén P (1980) Does the central pattern generation for locomotion in lamprey depend on glycine inhibition? *Acta Physiol Scand* 110:103–105.

Grillner S, Wallén P (1985) The ionic mechanisms underlying N-methyl-D-aspartate receptor-induced, tetrodotoxin-resistant membrane potential oscillations in lamprey neurons active during locomotion. *Neurosci Letts* 60:289–294.

Grillner S, Zangger P (1979) On the central generation of locomotion in the low spinal cat. *Exp Brain Res* 34:241–261.

Harada Y, Takahashi T (1983) The calcium component of the action potential in spinal motoneurones of the rat. *J Physiol* 335:89–100.

Harris-Warrick R, Cohen AH (1985) Serotonin modulates the central pattern generator for locomotion in the isolated lamprey spinal cord. *J Exp Biol* 116:27–46.

Hernandez P, Elbert K, Droge MH (1991) Spontaneous and NMDA evoked motor rhythms in the neonatal mouse spinal cord: An in vitro study with comparisons to in situ activity. *Exp Brain Res* 85:66–74.

Hill R, Matsushima T, Schotland J, Grillner S (1992) Apamin blocks the slow AHP in lamprey and delays termination of locomotor bursts. *Neuroreport* 3:943–945.

Ho S, O'Donovan MJ (1993) Regionalization and intersegmental coordination of rhythm-generating networks in the spinal cord of the chick embryo. *J Neurosci* 13:1354–1371.

Hochman S, Jordan LM, MacDonald JF (1994a) N-methyl-D-aspartate receptor-mediated voltage oscillations in neurons surrounding the central canal in slices of rat spinal cord. *J Neurophysiol* 72:565–577.

Hochman S, Jordan LM, Schmidt BJ (1994b) TTX-resistant NMDA receptor-mediated voltage oscillations in mammalian lumbar motoneurons. *J Neurophysiol* 72:2559–2562.

Hounsgaard J, Hultborn H, Jespersen B, Kiehn O (1988a) Bistability of alpha-motoneurones in the decerebrate cat and in the acute spinal cat after intravenous 5-hydroxytryptophan. *J Physiol* 405:345–367.

Hounsgaard J, Kiehn O (1989) Serotonin-induced bistability of turtle motoneurones caused by a nifedipine-sensitive calcium plateau potential. *J Physiol* 414:265–282.

Hounsgaard J, Kiehn O (1993) Calcium spikes and calcium plateaux evoked by differential polarization in dendrites of turtle motoneurones in vitro. *J Physiol* 468:245–259.

Hounsgaard J, Kiehn O, Mintz I (1988b) Response properties of motoneurones in a slice preparation of the turtle spinal cord. *J Physiol* 398: 575–589.

Hounsgaard J, Kjærulff O (1991) Ca^{2+}-mediated plateau potentials in a subpopulation of interneurons in the ventral horn of the turtle spinal cord. *Eur J Neurosci* 4:183–188.

Hounsgaard J, Mintz I (1988) Calcium conductance and firing properties of spinal motoneurones in the turtle. *J Physiol* 591–603.

Hultborn H, Kiehn O (1992) Neuromodulation of vertebrate motor neuron membrane properties. *Cur Opin Neurobiol* 2:770–775.

Hultborn H, Petersen N, Brownstone R, Nielsen J (1993) Evidence of fictive spinal locomotion in the marmoset (*callithrix Jacchus*). *Soc Neurosci Abstr* 19:539.

Jankowska E (1992) Interneuronal relay in spinal pathways from proprioception. *Prog Neurobiol* 38:335–378.

Jankowska E, Jukes MG, Lund S, Lundberg A (1967a) The effect of DOPA on the spinal cord. 5. Reciprocal organization of pathways

Basic Building Blocks of Vertebrate Spinal CPGs

transmitting excitatory action to alpha motoneurones of flexors and extensors. *Acta Physiol Scand* 70:369–388.

Jankowska E, Jukes MG, Lund S, Lundberg A (1967b) The effect of DOPA on the spinal cord. 6. Half-centre organization of interneurones transmitting effects from the flexor reflex afferents. *Acta Physiol Scand* 70:389–402.

Kiehn O (1991a) Plateau potentials and active integration in the "final common pathway" for motor behaviour. *TINS* 14:68–73.

Kiehn O (1991b) Electrophysiological effects of 5-HT on vertebrate motoneurones. In: *Aspects of Synaptic Transmission: LTP, Galanin, Opioids, Autonomic, and 5-HT* (Stone TW, ed.), 330–357. London: Taylor & Francis.

Kiehn O, Harris-Warrick R (1992) 5-HT modulation of hyperpolarization-activated inward current and calcium-dependent outward current in a crustacean motor neuron. *J Neurophysiol* 68:496–508.

Kiehn O, Hultborn H, Conway BA (1992) Spinal locomotor activity in acutely spinalized cats induced by intrathecal application of noradrenaline. *Neurosci Letts* 143:243–246.

Kiehn O, Johnson BR, Raastad M (1996) Plateau properties in mammalian spinal interneurons during transmitter-induced locomotor activity. *Neuroscience* 75:263–273.

Kiehn O, Kjærulff O (1996) Spatiotemporal characteristics of 5-HT and dopamine-induced hindlimb locomotor activity in the in vitro neonatal rat. *J Neurophysiol* 75:1472–1482.

Kjærulff O, Barajon I, Kiehn O (1994) Sulphorhodamine-labelled cells in the neonatal rat spinal cord following chemically induced locomotor activity in vitro. *J Physiol* 478:265–273.

Kjærulff O, Kiehn O (1996) Distribution of networks generating and coordinating locomotor activity in the neonatal rat spinal cord in vitro: A lesion study. *J Neurosci* 16:5777–5794.

Kudo N, Ozaki S, Yamada T (1991) Ontogeny of rhythmic activity in the spinal cord of the rat. In: *Neurobiological Basis of Human Locomotion* (Shimanura M, Grillner S, Edgerton VR, eds.), 3–20. Tokyo: Japan Scientific Societies.

Kudo N, Yamada T (1987) N-methyl-D,L-aspartate-induced locomotor activity in a spinal cord—hindlimb muscles preparation of the newborn rat studied in vitro. *Neurosci Letts* 75:43–48.

Lundberg A (1979) Multisensory control of spinal reflex pathways. In: *Reflex Control of Posture and Movement* (Granit R, Pompeiano O, eds.), 11–28. Amsterdam: Elsevier Biomedical.

McClellan AD, Grillner S (1984) Activation of "fictive swimming" by electrical microstimulation of brainstem locomotor regions in an in vitro preparation of the lamprey central nervous system. *Brain Res* 300:357–361.

Meer DP, Buchanan JT (1992) Apamin reduces the late afterhyperpolarization of lamprey spinal neurons, with little effect on fictive swimming. *Neurosci Letts* 143:1–4.

Noga BR, Cowley KC, Huang A, Jordan LM, Schmidt BJ (1993) Effects of inhibitory amino acids antagonists on locomotor rhythm in the decerebrate cat. *Soc Neurosci Abst* 19:540.

Noga BR, Fortier PA, Kriellaars DJ, Dai X, Detillieux GR, Jordan LM (1995) Field potential mapping of neurons in the lumbar spinal cord activated following stimulation of the mesencephalic locomotor region. *J Neurosci* 15:2203–2217.

Novak L, Bregestovski P, Ascher P, Herbet A, Prochinatz A (1984) Magnesium gates glutamate-activated channels in mouse central neurones. *Nature* 307:462–465.

O'Donovan M, Sernagor E, Sholomenko G, Ho S, Antal M, Yee W (1992) Development of spinal motor networks in the chick embryo. *J Exp Zool* 261:261–273.

O'Donovan M, Ho S, Wayne Y (1994) Calcium imaging of rhythmic activity in the developing spinal cord of the chick embryo. *J Neurosci* 14:6354–6369.

Panchin YV, Perrins RJ, Roberts A (1991) The action of acetylcholine on the locomotor central pattern generator for swimming in *Xenopus* embryos. *J Exp Biol* 161:527–531.

Pearson KG, Rossignol S (1991) Fictive motor patterns in chronic spinal cats. *J Neurophysiol* 66:1874–1887.

Poon M (1980) Induction of swimming in lamprey by L-DOPA and amino acids. *J Comp Physiol* 136:337–344.

Pratt CA, Jordan LM (1987) Ia inhibitory interneurons and Renshaw cells as contributors to the spinal mechanisms of fictive locomotion. *J Neurophysiol* 57:56–71.

Raastad M, Johnson BR, Kiehn O (1996) The number of postsynaptic currents necessary to produce locomotor-related cyclic information in neurons in the neonatal rat spinal cord. *Neuron* 17:729–738.

Roberts A, Tunstall MJ (1990) Mutual re-excitation with postinhibitory rebound: A simulation study on the mechanism for locomotor rhythm generation in the spinal cord of *Xenopus* embryos. *Eur J Neurosci* 2:11–23.

Russo RE, Hounsgaard J (1994) Short-term plasticity in turtle dorsal horn neurons mediated by L-type Ca^{2+} channels. *Neurosci* 61:191–197.

Russo RE, Hounsgaard J (1996a) Plateau generating neurones in the dorsal horn in an in vitro preparation of the turtle spinal cord. *J Physiol* 493:39–54.

Russo RE, Hounsgaard J (1996b) Burst generating neurones in the dorsal horn studied an in vitro preparation of the turtle spinal cord. *J Physiol* 493:55–66.

Schwindt PC, Crill WE (1984) Membrane properties of cat spinal motoneurones. In: *Handbook of the Spinal Cord* (Davidoff RA, ed.), 199–242. New York, Basel: Marcel Dekker.

Sernagor E, O'Donovan MJ (1991) Whole cell patch clamp of rhythmically active neurons in the isolated spinal cord of the chick embryo. *Neurosci Letts* 128:221–226.

Sigvardt KA, Grillner S, Wallén P, Van DP (1985) Activation of NMDA receptors elicits fictive locomotion and bistable membrane properties in the lamprey spinal cord. *Brain Res* 336:390–395.

Sillar KT, Simmers AJ (1994) Oscillatory membrane properties of spinal cord neurons that are active during fictive swimming in *Rana temporaria* embryos. *Eur J Morph* 32:185–192.

Sillar KT, Wedderburn JF, Simmers AJ (1992) Modulation of swimming rhythmicity by 5-hydroxytryptamine during post-embryonic development in *Xenopus laevis*. *Proc Roy Soc Lond* B250:107–114.

Silos-Santiago I, Snider WD (1992) Development of commissural neurons in the embryonic rat spinal cord. *J Comp Neurol* 325:514–526.

Skydsgaard M, Hounsgaard J (1994) Spatial integration of local transmitter responses in motoneurones of the turtle spinal cord in vitro. *J Physiol* 479:223–246.

Smith JC, Feldman JL (1987) In vitro brainstem–spinal cord preparations for study of motor systems for mammalian respiration and locomotion. *J Neurosci Meth* 21:321–333.

Smith JC, Feldman JL, Schmidt BJ (1988) Neural mechanisms generating locomotion studied in mammalian brainstem–spinal cord in vitro. *FASEB J* 2:2283–2288.

Soffe SR (1987) Ionic and pharmacological properties of reciprocal inhibition in *Xenopus* embryo motoneurones. *J Physiol* 382:463–473.

Soffe SR (1989) Roles of glycinergic inhibition and N-methyl-D-aspartate receptor mediated excitation in the locomotor rhythmicity of one half of the *Xenopus* embryo central nervous system. *Eur J Neurosci* 1:561–571.

Soffe, SR (1990) Active and passive membrane properties of spinal neurons that are rhythmically active during swimming in *Xenopus* embryos. *Eur J Neurosci* 2:1–10.

Soffe SR, Roberts A (1989) The influence of magnesium ions on the NMDA mediated responses of ventral rhythmic neurons in the spinal cord of *Xenopus* embryos. *Eur J Neurosci* 1:507–515.

Stein PSG, Victor JC, Field EC, Currie SN (1995) Bilateral control of hindlimb scratching in the spinal turtle: Contralateral spinal circuitry contributes to the normal ipsilateral motor pattern of fictive rostral scratching. *J Neurosci* 15:4343–4355.

Svirskis G, Hounsgaard J (1995) Depolarization-induced facilitation of L-type Ca channels underlies slow kinetics of plateau potentials in turtle motoneurons. *Soc Neurosci Abst* 21:65.

Takahashi T (1990a) Membrane currents in visually identified motoneurones of neonatal rat spinal cord. *J Physiol* 423:27–46.

Takahashi T (1990b) Inward rectification in neonatal rat spinal motoneurones. *J Physiol* 423:47–62.

Takahashi T, Berger AJ (1990) Direct excitation of rat spinal motoneurones by serotonin. *J Physiol* 423:63–76.

Tauck DL, Frosch MP, Lipton SA (1988) Characterization of GABA- and glycine-induced currents of solitary rodent retinal ganglion cells in culture. *Neurosci* 27:193–203.

Tegner J, Matsushima T, El Manira A, Grillner S (1993) The spinal GABA system modulates burst frequency and intersegmental coordination in the lamprey: Differential effects of $GABA_A$ and $GABA_B$ receptors. *J Neurophysiol* 69:647–657.

Umemiya N, Berger AJ (1994) Properties and function of low- and high-voltage-activated Ca^{2+} channels in hyperglossal motoneurons. *J Neurosci* 14:5652–5660.

Viala D, Buser P (1969) The effects of DOPA and 5-HTP on rhythmic efferent discharges in hindlimb nerves in the rabbit. *Brain Res* 12:437–443.

Wall MJ, Dale N (1993) $GABA_B$ receptors modulate glycinergic inhibition and spike threshold in *Xenopus* embryo spinal neurones. *J Physiol* 469:275–290.

Wall MJ, Dale N (1994) A role for potassium currents in the generation of the swimming motor pattern of *Xenopus* embryos. *J Neurophysiol* 72:337–348.

Wallén P, Buchanan JT, Grillner S, Hill RH, Christenson J, Hökfelt T (1989) Effects of 5-hydroxytrytamine on the afterhyperpolarization, spike frequency regulation, and oscillatory membrane properties in lamprey spinal cord neurons. *J Neurophysiol* 61:759–768.

Wallén P, Ekeberg Ö, Lansner A, Brodin L, Tråvén H, Grillner S (1992) A computer model for realistic simulations of neural networks. II. The segmental network generating locomotor rhythmicity in the lamprey. *J Neurophysiol* 68:1939–1950.

Wallén P, Grillner S (1987) N-methyl-D-aspartate receptor-induced, inherent oscillatory activity in neurons active during fictive locomotion in the lamprey. *J Neurosci* 7:2745–2755.

Wallis DI (1994) 5-HT receptors involved in initiation or modulation of motor patterns: Opportunities for drug development. *Trends Pharmacol Sci* 15:288–292.

Wheatley M, Jovanovic K, Stein RB, Lawson V (1994) The activity of interneurons during locomotion in the in vitro *Necturus* spinal cord. *J Neurophysiol* 71:2025–2032.

Wheatley M, Stein RB (1992) An in vitro preparation of the mud puppy for simultaneous intracellular and electromyographic recording during locomotion. *J Neurosci* 42:129–137.

Zhang L, Krnjevic K (1987) Apamin depresses selectively the afterhyperpolarization of cat spinal motoneurones. *Neurosci Lett* 74:58–62.

Ziskind-Conhaim L, Seebach BS, Gao BX (1993) Changes in serotonin-induced potential during spinal cord development. *J Neurophysiol* 69:1338–1349.

5

Neural and Biomechanical Control Strategies for Different Forms of Vertebrate Hindlimb Motor Tasks

Paul S. G. Stein and Judith L. Smith

Abstract

Patterns of motor output, kinematics, and kinetics observed during vertebrate hindlimb cyclic movement, such as cat locomotion and turtle scratching, demonstrate considerable complexity. Analyses of these patterns during movement provide support for hypotheses concerning the modular organization of motor circuitry. Patterns of motor output recorded from spinal, immobilized vertebrates demonstrate that spinal circuits generate these complex outputs; in addition, they provide further insight into the modular organization of these circuits.

The set of spinal cord neurons responsible for generating the normal patterns of motor output for a specific form of a behavior is termed the *central pattern generator* for that form. Experimental evidence gathered during cyclic motor behaviors—for example, cat locomotion and turtle scratching—support the concept that neural elements in the central pattern generator for one form may be shared with neural elements in the central pattern generator for a different form or even for a different behavior. Therefore, the shared circuitry may be part of a multitask processor involved in the generation of each of several tasks.

A motor task is classified by its goal. For example, the goal of locomotion is to move the center of mass of an organism from one location in space to another while maintaining equilibrium and appropriate postures. The goal of scratching is to exert force against a site on the body surface that has received a tactile stimulus. A given task may be performed in several ways, each way termed a *form* of the task (Stein et al., 1986). This chapter emphasizes several forms of cat locomotion (Zernicke and Smith, 1996) and turtle scratching (Stein, 1989).

The movement pattern for a form is the temporal sequence of kinematic variables observed during the expression of the behavior. An excellent set of kinematic variables for the vertebrate hindlimb is the array of hindlimb joint angles (hip, knee, ankle) measured as a function of time. For each form, there is a characteristic movement pattern—that is, a distinct set of relative timings of these variables. The joint-torque pattern (hip, knee, ankle) for a form is the temporal sequence of kinetic variables observed during the behavior. The motor pattern for a form is the temporal sequence of muscle or motoneuron activations, obtained either from electromyographic (EMG) recordings from a selected set of muscles or from electroneurographic (ENG) recordings from the corresponding set of nerves innervating these muscles. For the muscles of the vertebrate hindlimb, there is a 1:1 temporal correspondence between each motoneuron action potential and each muscle action potential. Key features of the motor pattern may correspond to key features of the movement patterns (the *kinematics*) and joint-torque patterns (the *kinetics*; see Smith and Zernicke, 1987).

ENG recordings are also obtained from immobilized preparations under neuromuscular blockade with a nicotinic, acetylcholine antagonist. In the immobilized preparation, the motor pattern is activated with an appropriate stimulus; for example, tactile stimulation of a site in a scratch form's receptive field activates the ENG motor pattern for that scratch form. The ENG motor pattern is also termed the *fictive* motor pattern.

For many behaviors, the fictive motor pattern exhibits many features of the EMG motor pattern recorded during movement (e.g., rhythmic alternation between agonists and antagonists). Such observations establish that the basic features of the motor pattern are generated within the central nervous system (CNS). The set of CNS neurons that generate the fictive motor pattern for a form is the central pattern generator (CPG) for that form. For some behaviors, key features of the EMG motor pattern are not observed in the ENG motor pattern; for example, the relative duration of extensor activity in the cat scratch observed during actual scratching (Kuhta and Smith, 1990) is greater than that observed in the immobilized preparation (Deliagina et al., 1981). These differences are used to assess the nature of the CPG modulation by motion-related sensory feedback (see also Pearson and Ramirez, chapter 21, this volume).

Spinal preparations are also utilized to study movement and motor patterns: the spinal cord is completely transected at a specific level. The spinal vertebrate can perform several specific forms of a motor task with a limb caudal to the segmental level of the transection. The resulting behaviors often have motor patterns and limb motions relatively similar to those observed in intact animals, establishing that supraspinal neuronal circuitry is not required for these forms of a task. Differences between intact and spinal preparations may be used to assess the extent of modulation of the spinal CPG from supraspinal centers. For many tasks, fictive motor patterns obtained from immobilized, spinal vertebrates (figure 5.1) show important similarities with the EMG motor pattern recorded from the corresponding

muscles during actual behavior. These observations establish that key elements of the CPG are programmed by spinal circuitry at a level caudal to the transection. This chapter uses information gathered from limb motion and motor pattern analyses to discuss working hypotheses concerning the organization of the neural circuitry of spinal CPGs for cyclical motions of the vertebrate hindlimb.

Levels of Coordination of Vertebrate Limb Motor Patterns

Coordination within the motor pattern for a given task occurs at multiple levels. At the lowest level, the elements of a motor pool are the set of motoneurons that innervate a single muscle. An ENG recording from a nerve that innervates a single muscle can serve as a monitor of the activity of an entire motor pool, (e.g., the hip flexor motor pool). For a given task, co-activation of motoneurons occurs within a single motor pool. For many movements—e.g., forward locomotion at different speeds in the cat (Zernicke and Smith, 1996) and rostral scratching in the turtle (Robertson et al., 1985; Robertson and Stein, 1988)—an orderly sequence of motoneurons is recruited and then de-recruited. This orderly recruitment pattern may contribute to the characteristic shape of the motor pool's ENG burst—for example, the fusiform shape of the hip flexor ENG during rostral scratching in the turtle (see figure 5.1).

The next level of coordination is between motor pools at a single degree of freedom (e.g., between hip flexor and hip extensor activation). Most cyclical tasks have a rhythmic alternation between agonist and antagonist (figure 5.1C gives an example during rostral scratching). In some situations, there may be "deletions": several bursts of agonist activity occur with no intervening bursts of antagonist activity—for example, hip extensor deletion during downslope walking of the cat (Smith and Carlson-Kuhta, 1995) and the hip extensor deletion variation of turtle rostral scratching (see the first part of figure 5.1A; Robertson and Stein, 1988; Stein et al., 1995b).

Another level of coordination is the regulated intralimb timing of an agonist at one degree of freedom with respect to an agonist at another degree of freedom. For each form, there is a regulated intralimb timing between degrees of freedom. Some behaviors, such as cat forward walking (figure 5.2; Buford and Smith, 1990) and turtle pocket scratching (Robertson et al., 1985), have mainly

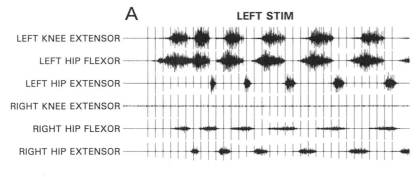

A   **LEFT STIM**

LEFT KNEE EXTENSOR

LEFT HIP FLEXOR

LEFT HIP EXTENSOR

RIGHT KNEE EXTENSOR

RIGHT HIP FLEXOR

RIGHT HIP EXTENSOR

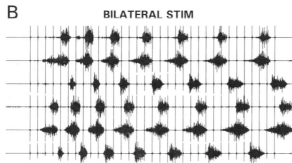

B   **BILATERAL STIM**

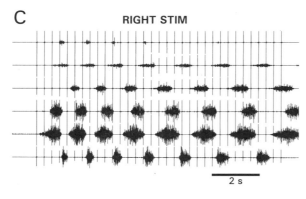

C   **RIGHT STIM**

2 s

Figure 5.1

Bilateral ENG motor patterns during fictive rostral scratching in the turtle. This preparation had a complete transection of the spinal cord. (A and C) Unilateral stimulation of the left and the right rostral scratch receptive field, respectively. (B) Bilateral stimulation of both the left and the right rostral scratch receptive fields. (From Stein et al., 1995b.)

conventional synergies: extensors at one joint are activated during activation of extensors at a nearby joint. Other behaviors, such as cat paw shaking (Smith et al., 1985; Pearson and Rossignol, 1991) and turtle rostral scratching (see figure 5.1; Robertson et al., 1985), have mixed synergies: extensors at one joint are co-activated with flexors at another joint.

A different level of coordination is the regulated interlimb timing of an agonist at one degree of freedom in the left hindlimb—e.g., left hip flexors—with respect to the homologous agonists in the right hindlimb. For many behaviors, such as cat forward walking (Grillner, 1981) and turtle rostral scratching (figure 5.1; Field and Stein, 1994; Field, 1995; Stein et al., 1995b), left hip flexors

alternate with right hip flexors. This is an example of out-of-phase coordination. For other behaviors, such as cat galloping (Grillner, 1981) and some episodes of turtle bilateral caudal scratching (Field, 1995; Field and Stein, 1997), left hip flexors are active at, or nearly at, the same time as right hip flexors. This is an example of in-phase coordination.

Each level of coordination has been studied in intact, behaving animals as well as in spinal, immobilized animals. This chapter focuses on experiments that examine the different levels of coordination in cats and turtles; data from these experiments are used to examine specific models of organization of spinal cord circuitry.

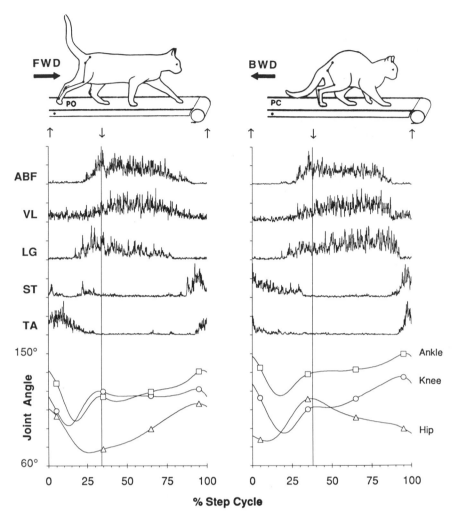

Figure 5.2
Cat posture, hindlimb kinematics, and motor patterns for two walking forms. Top drawings show forward walking (FWD) with the cat's right hindlimb at paw off (PO) and backward walking (BWD) with the same limb at paw contact (PC). Middle traces show EMGs from three extensors: ABF, anterior biceps femoris (hip); VL, vastus lateralis (knee); LG, lateral gastrocnemius (ankle); as well as from two flexors, ST, semitendinosus (knee); and TA, tibialis anterior (ankle). Lowest records illustrate joint displacements for the ankle (anterior angle measured in degrees), knee (posterior angle), and hip (anterior angle) joints for 10 normalized and averaged step cycles, beginning and ending with paw lift off (up arrow). Paw contact is marked by the downward arrow and the vertical line. Swing occurred to the left of the vertical line, and stance to the right. (Adapted from Zernicke and Smith, 1996.)

Cat Hindlimb Motor Patterns as a Model System

The neuronal organization proposed for the control of quadrupedal locomotion includes a spinal CPG for each limb modulated by output from supraspinal centers and motion-related feedback (Grillner, 1981; Rossignol, 1996). Interlimb coordination is organized by propriospinal neuron arrays that set limb couplings for different forms of locomotion (Grillner, 1981; Cowley and Schmidt, 1995). Several forms of locomotion on a level surface have been studied: three speed-related forward gaits (walk, trot, gallop) and backward walking. In addi-

tion, slope walking in the forward direction has been studied (Zernicke and Smith, 1996).

Traditionally, interlimb coordination, limb kinematics, and motor patterns for each locomotor form have been assessed. Recent research on limb kinetics has concentrated on understanding the role of muscle contraction in counteracting external and internal joint forces that arise during the step cycle (see review in Zernicke and Smith, 1996). Knowledge of limb kinetics has led to predictions about form-dependent motor patterns and to insights about the requirements for mutable motor patterns. The key points of these studies are reviewed in the next three sections.

Stance-Related Activity

During forward walking, extensor muscles across the hindlimb are co-active during most of stance to counteract ground-reaction forces that tend to flex the joints (Perell et al., 1993). Extensor synergy is typical of forward and backward walking (Buford and Smith, 1990), as well as of trotting and galloping (Engberg and Lundberg, 1969; Smith et al., 1993). Although extensor synergy is robust for all but downslope walking, most extensor muscles have a distinct burst profile of EMG activity and slightly different onsets and offsets for each form. These details are illustrated in figure 5.2, especially for knee (e.g., VL) and ankle (e.g., LG) extensors during forward and backward walking; see the figure legend for specific muscle names.

Whether the joint extends or flexes during the extensor contraction phase of stance depends on the kinetics. During both forward and backward walking, for example, recruitment of uniarticular hip extensors (ABF in figure) opposes the hip flexor torque generated by ground-reaction forces during the first half of stance (Perell et al., 1993). During forward walking, hip extensor contraction is sufficient to overcome the external forces, and the hip extends as these muscles undergo a shortening contraction. Recruitment of the same muscles during backward walking is not sufficient to effect hip extension, so the rate of hip flexion is decelerated by a lengthening contraction.

For downslope walking at inclines of 15°–45°, hip and ankle extensor activity is largely replaced by hip and ankle flexor activity during stance (Smith and Carlson-Kuhta, 1995; Trank and Smith, 1995). As shown in figure 5.3B the hip flexors (IP) are active at the onset of stance, whereas the ankle flexors (TA, EDL) are active around midstance. Why is there a predominance of flexor activity at the hip and ankle joints during the stance phase of downslope walking? During flexor contraction, the hip and ankle joints extend, presumably due to an extensor torque generated by ground-reaction forces (Smith and Carlson-Kuhta, 1995; Trank and Smith, 1995). A flexor muscle torque may be required at each joint to decelerate the rate of extension.

Changes in stance-related activity reported for key hindlimb muscles are illustrated in figure 5.3B. Uniarticular knee extensors are not represented because the timing of their stance-related activity appears to be independent of the locomotor form. Although ankle extensors always have stance-related activity, the duration of their activity is mutable: longest for backward walking and shortest for downslope walking (see LG, FHL, and PLT in figure 5.3B). Uniarticular hip extensors are active during most of stance for all forms of locomotion except downslope walking (see ABF and ASM in figure 5.3B). Biarticular hip extensors, such as the semitendinosus (ST—a hip extensor, knee flexor), are not usually active during the weight-bearing portion of stance. During upslope walking, however, the ST may be active during the first half of stance when the cat walks or gallops up inclines greater than 15° (see figures 5.3B and 5.3C). Perhaps the recruitment of these biarticular muscles is necessary to augment the extensor muscle torque at the hip during stance.

The rectus femoris (RF—a hip flexor, knee extensor) is recruited later than other stance-related muscles and is active around midstance during forward on level surfaces and upslope walking (figure 5.3B). The onset of RF activity coincides with the development of a flexor muscle torque at the hip joint from midstance to paw liftoff (Perell et al., 1993). RF activity shifts to the first half of the stance phase for downslope walking. In contrast, during backward walking the RF is active throughout stance, its activity associated with a continuous flexor muscle torque at the hip (Pratt et al., 1996).

Swing-Related Activity

Muscles with swing-related activity have either one or two bursts of activity during swing (figure 5.3A). During all forms of walking, the cat's hip (IP) and ankle (TA) flexor muscles exhibit one burst of activity, and the burst is associated with a flexor muscle torque at each joint. For forward and slope walking, these muscles are active during most of swing (see figure 5.2). During backward walking, their EMGs peak just before paw lift-off, and then the EMG amplitude markedly declines (e.g., TA in figure 5.2). Oddly, the decline in uniarticular flexor activity is associated with an increase in the magnitude of the flexor muscle torque at both joints (Perell et al., 1993; their figure 2). Biarticular muscles, however, continue to contract and contribute to the flexor muscle torques. These muscles include the medial sartorius (a hip flexor, knee flexor; Pratt et al., 1996) and the extensor digitorium longus (an ankle flexor, toe extensor; Trank and Smith, 1996).

The ST has two EMG bursts during the swing phase of forward walking; one occurs around paw lift-off and the other precedes paw contact (figure 5.3C). Changes in the duration and amplitude of both bursts are closely tied to changes in the magnitude and duration of the flexor muscle torque at the knee joint (Smith et al., 1993).

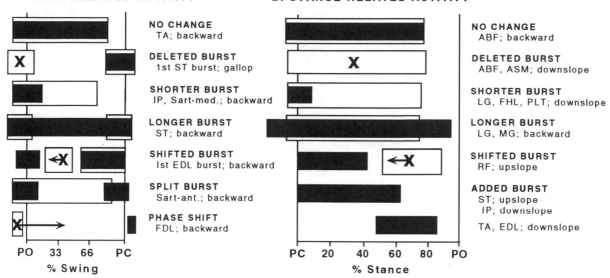

A. SWING-RELATED ACTIVITY

	NO CHANGE TA; backward
X	DELETED BURST 1st ST burst; gallop
	SHORTER BURST IP, Sart.-med.; backward
	LONGER BURST ST; backward
←X	SHIFTED BURST 1st EDL burst; backward
	SPLIT BURST Sart.-ant.; backward
X →	PHASE SHIFT FDL; backward

PO   33   66   PC
% Swing

B. STANCE-RELATED ACTIVITY

	NO CHANGE ABF; backward
X	DELETED BURST ABF, ASM; downslope
	SHORTER BURST LG, FHL, PLT; downslope
	LONGER BURST LG, MG; backward
←X	SHIFTED BURST RF; upslope
	ADDED BURST ST; upslope IP; downslope
	TA, EDL; downslope

PC   20   40   60   80   PO
% Stance

C. FORM-RELATED SEMITENDINOSUS (ST) ACTIVITY

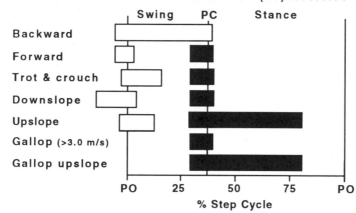

Swing   PC   Stance

Backward
Forward
Trot & crouch
Downslope
Upslope
Gallop (>3.0 m/s)
Gallop upslope

PO   25   50   75   PO
% Step Cycle

Figure 5.3

Mutable activity patterns of several hindlimb muscles during the two phases of the cat's step cycle. (A and B) Unshaded bars represent the timing of EMG activity during forward walking, whereas the shaded bars represent the timing of activity during other forms of locomotion (indicated to the right). Each X marks a deleted or time-shifted burst. Muscle names, in addition to those identified in figure 5.2, are flexor muscles in A: EDL, extensor digitorium longus (ankle), Sart.-med., medial sartorius (hip and knee flexor), Sart.-ant., anterior sartorius (hip flexor and knee extensor), FDL, flexor digitorium longus (toe); as well as extensor muscles in B: ASM, anterior semimembranosus (hip), FHL, flexor hallicus longus, PLT, plantaris, MG, medial gastrocnemius (ankle), RF, rectus femoris (knee extensor, hip flexor). (C) The timing of ST activity is represented for several forms of locomotion. Shaded bars depict flexor-related activity, whereas unshaded bars show extensor-related activtiy. For sloped walking, see Smith and Carlson-Kuhta (1995) for changes in the duration of ST stance activity related to inclines that are greater than or less than the grade specified.

Consider, for example, the ST burst that accompanies paw lift-off. As walking and trotting speeds increase, the knee flexor muscle torque shows a linear increase that is speed related (Wisleder et al., 1990) and correlated with increases in the duration and amplitude of the paw-off burst and the duration of knee flexion at the onset of swing (Smith et al., 1993). During the gallop, however, the same ST burst is markedly reduced or absent because knee flexion at the onset of swing is controlled mainly by inertial forces due to leg angular acceleration and hip linear velocity.

Changes in swing-related activity reported for several hindlimb muscles are illustrated in figure 5.3A. For muscles with one EMG burst during forward swing, the burst duration may increase, decrease, or be interrupted (split) during the swing phase of other forms of locomotion. For muscles with two EMG bursts, the bursts appear to be controlled independently: one of the two bursts may be absent (e.g., the first ST burst during fast gallop; Smith et al., 1993) or shifted in time (e.g., the first EDL burst during backward walking; Trank and Smith, 1996). Lastly, one of the toe flexors (FDL) has a brief burst before paw lift-off during forward and slope walking, but this burst is delayed until after paw contact during backward walking (Trank and Smith, 1995, 1996).

Shared CPGs and Mutable Patterns for Different Locomotor Forms

Motor patterns recorded during fictive locomotion from acutely spinal, decerebrate, or decorticate cats are usually described in terms of extensor- and flexor-related activity. The motor output to many muscles is similar for all three preparations; for some muscles, however, the output depends on the preparation. For example, ENGs of VL are usually co-active with other extensor motor pools, regardless of the preparation. In contrast, ENGs of ST may be extensor- or flexor-related, depending on the preparation; similarly, EMGs of ST may be swing- or stance-related, depending on the form of locomotion (figure 5.3C). During spontaneous fictive walking of decorticate cats, the ST is co-active with other extensor ENGs (Perret and Cabelguen, 1980), mimicking ST activity during upslope galloping. In acutely spinal cats, the ST is coactive with the TA during DOPA- and clonidine-induced fictive walking (Grillner and Zangger, 1979; Pearson and Rossignol, 1991), mimicking ST activity during backward walking. In decerebrate cats with hindlimb deafferentation, the ST has a flexor-related burst and a prolonged extensor-related burst (Grillner and Zangger, 1984), mimicking ST activity during upslope walking.

The fact that ST activity is preparation specific during fictive locomotion suggests that spinal networks may be reconfigured by different arrays of supraspinal input, even in the absence of motion-related feedback from the limbs. Central reconfiguration might be accomplished by descending fibers that set connections among unit-burst generators (Grillner, 1981) or alter the phasing between circuit elements (Harris-Warrick et al., chapter 19, this volume). In this way, a single network may provide the spinal organization for all locomotor forms. Generation of form-specific output, however, may require supraspinal guidance to set muscle synergies, general posture, and feedback modulation (see discussion of Buford and Smith, 1990).

With regard to feedback modulation, it has been demonstrated that facilitation of the extensor phase of the locomotor CPG is decreased and facilitation of the flexor phase is increased when ankle extensors are unloaded and the hip joint is extended (Pearson and Ramirez, chapter 21, this volume). This set of proprioceptive inputs occurs at the end of stance during forward walking. Proprioceptive inputs are markedly different, however, at the end of stance during backward walking; the hip joint is flexed and the contractile tension of the gastrocnemius (an ankle extensor, knee flexor) is just reaching its peak. Nonetheless, the same switch—extensors off and flexors on—must occur. Thus, the effect of feedback modulation may be form dependent and may require specific instructions from supraspinal centers.

Turtle Hindlimb Scratching Motor Patterns as a Model System

Motor Output Ipsilateral to the Site of Stimulation

The spinal turtle exhibits three forms of hindlimb scratching: rostral, pocket, and caudal (Mortin et al., 1985). During rostral scratching, the dorsum of the foot rubs a site on the shell bridge in the midbody region; during pocket scratching, the side of the knee rubs a site in the pocket region; and during caudal scratching, the heel or side of the foot rubs a site near the tail. Other vertebrates also display multiple forms of scratching: for example, a human will use an elbow-over-shoulder strategy to scratch the upper back, but an elbow-under-shoulder strategy to scratch the lower back.

The ENG fictive motor pattern for each form of turtle hindlimb scratching is a replica of the corresponding EMG motor pattern during actual scratching (Robertson et al., 1985). Common to the normal patterns for all three forms is rhythmic alternation between hip flexor activity and hip extensor activity (e.g., the fictive rostral scratch in figure 5.1C). During hip extensor deletion rostral scratching, however, successive bursts of hip flexor activity occur without intervening hip extensor activity (initial part of figure 5.1A; see also Robertson and Stein, 1988). Distinct for each form is the timing of the uniarticular knee extensor within the cycle of hip motor activity. During both normal and hip extensor deletion rostral scratching, the uniarticular knee extensor is active during the latter portion of each burst of hip flexor activity (figure 5.1A and 5.1C); during pocket scratching, the uniarticular knee extensor is active during hip extensor activity; and during caudal scratching, the uniarticular knee extensor is active near the termination of hip extensor activity.

Bilateral and Shared Organization of Spinal Circuitry for Scratching

Scratching is usually considered to be a unilateral activity: stimulation of an ipsilateral site on the body surface activates a scratch reflex in the ipsilateral limb. Contralateral motor activity does take place, however, during scratching of an ipsilateral limb (Currie and Stein, 1989; Berkowitz and Stein, 1994a, 1994b; Stein et al., 1995b). During fictive rostral scratching (figure 5.1A and 5.1C) and fictive pocket scratching, contralateral hip flexor activity is out-of-phase with ipsilateral hip flexor activity.

Single-unit recordings from the axons of individual descending propriospinal interneurons during fictive rostral and fictive pocket scratching reveal that many individual neurons have a receptive field that includes both left and right rostral and left and right pocket scratch receptive fields (Berkowitz and Stein, 1994a, 1994b). Most of these neurons are phasically active during a particular portion of the fictive scratch cycle. In many cases, the neuron's preferred phase during ipsilateral rostral scratching is similar to the neuron's preferred phase during ipsilateral pocket scratching, contralateral rostral scratching, and contralateral pocket scratching. Each propriospinal interneuron that has a bilateral receptive field is activated during either left hindlimb or right hindlimb scratching. Therefore, a bilateral set of spinal cord neurons is activated by stimulation of a single site in a scratch receptive field. These results support the conclusion that members of the bilateral set are "shared", that is, they are activated during the ipsilateral as well as the contralateral rostral scratch and during the ipsilateral as well as the contralateral pocket scratch.

Modular Organization of Spinal Circuitry for Scratching

Intracellular recordings from individual motoneurons involved in each form of fictive scratching reveal excitatory postsynaptic potentials (EPSPs) during activation of each motoneuron and its motor pool, alternating with inhibitory postsynaptic potentials (IPSPs) during quiescence of that motoneuron and its motor pool (Robertson and Stein, 1988). Hip extensor activation occurs during hip flexor quiescence; EPSPs in hip extensor motoneurons occur when IPSPs in hip flexor motoneurons occur. During hip extensor deletion rostral scratching, there is no hip extensor activation, no EPSPs in hip extensor motoneurons, no corresponding quiescence in hip flexors, and no corresponding IPSPs in hip flexor motoneurons. Similar deletions have been observed during cat fictive locomotion (Jordan, 1991).

These observations of deletions support the concept of a *modular* organization of spinal circuitry (Jordan, 1991; Stein et al., 1995b).

The concept of a module that controls agonist motoneurons at a hindlimb joint is a generalization of the concept of a module proposed for the circuitry controlling lateral bending of the body of the lamprey (Wallén, chapter 6, this volume) and the tadpole (Roberts et al., chapter 7, this volume). Based on this generalization, at least three classes of neurons per module have been identified for an agonist function: (1) agonist motoneurons, (2) excitatory interneurons that produce EPSPs onto agonist motoneurons as well as onto other members of the agonist and synergist modules, and (3) inhibitory interneurons that produce IPSPs onto members of antagonist modules (see figure 5.4). During right hindlimb hip extensor deletion rostral scratching, no activity has been detected in three classes of neurons that comprise the right hip extensor module: right hip extensor motoneurons, right hip extensor excitatory interneurons that produce EPSPs in hip extensor motoneurons, and right hip extensor inhibitory interneurons that produce IPSPs in hip flexor motoneurons.

Stein and colleagues (1995b) developed the hemi-enlargement preparation in which the left halves of the spinal segments comprising the hindlimb enlargement were removed and the hindlimb motor output to the right hindlimb was recorded. In this preparation, the midbody spinal segments innervating the left and right rostral scratch receptive fields were left intact and in communication with the remaining right halves of the segments of the hindlimb enlargement. Two possible pathways for this communication include descending propriospinal neurons with axons in the white matter on the right side of the hindlimb enlargement that have somata in the right halves of midbody spinal segments, and other descending propriospinal neurons that have somata in the left halves of these segments (Berkowitz and Stein, 1994c). In the hemi-enlargement preparation, stimulation of a site in the right rostral scratch receptive field elicited rhythmic activity in right hip flexor motoneurons, but no activity in the right hip extensor motoneurons (hip extensor deletion rostral scratching). This experiment establishes that (1) neural circuitry in the left hindlimb enlargement is required to generate the normal pattern of rostral scratching in right hindlimb motoneurons in response to stimulation in the right rostral scratch receptive field, and (2) multiple cycles of rhythmic right hip flexor activity can be generated in the absence of right hip extensor activity. Moreover, stimulation of a site in the left rostral scratch receptive field elicited

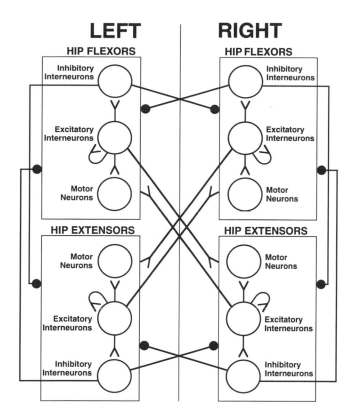

Figure 5.4
Sketch of proposed modular organization of the bilateral shared core of neurons involved in the production of rostral scratching in the turtle. For further details, see text. (From Stein et al., 1995b.)

LEFT RIGHT

HIP FLEXORS

Inhibitory Interneurons

Excitatory Interneurons

Motor Neurons

HIP EXTENSORS

Motor Neurons

Excitatory Interneurons

Inhibitory Interneurons

HIP FLEXORS

Inhibitory Interneurons

Excitatory Interneurons

Motor Neurons

HIP EXTENSORS

Motor Neurons

Excitatory Interneurons

Inhibitory Interneurons

rhythmic activity in right hip extensor motoneurons, establishing that there is a hip extensor rhythm generator in hindlimb enlargement circuitry contralateral to the stimulation site.

Stein and colleagues (1995b) suggested that, in a preparation with an intact hindlimb enlargement, neurons in the ipsilateral hip flexor and hip extensor modules interact with neurons in the contralateral hip flexor and hip extensor modules to generate the normal pattern of rostral scratching in right hindlimb motoneurons. According to this point of view, the ipsilateral rostral scratch CPG includes both ipsilateral and contralateral modules. Moreover, they cited single-unit recordings of propriospinal neurons with bilateral receptive fields (Berkowitz and Stein, 1994a, 1994b) to suggest that some elements of the right hindlimb rostral scratch CPG are also elements of the left hindlimb rostral scratch CPG; that is, each hindlimb's rostral scratch CPG contains a bilateral shared core of neurons that are activated during either left rostral scratching or right rostral scratching. A sketch of the modular organization of this proposed bilateral shared core is presented in figure 5.4.

Simultaneous Bilateral Stimulation of Left and Right Scratch Receptive Fields

Bilateral scratching can be activated by stimulation of one site in a left scratch receptive field and of a second site in a right scratch receptive field. Stimulation of mirror-image sites elicits bilateral same-form scratching; stimulation of a left site in one scratch receptive field and a right site in a scratch receptive field for a different form elicits bilateral mixed-form scratching. There is an out-of-phase kinematic relationship between left hip and right hip angles during actual bilateral rostral scratching, during bilateral pocket scratching, and during ipsilateral rostral and contralateral pocket scratching (Field and Stein, 1994, 1997; Field, 1995). Bilateral stimulation in caudal scratch receptive fields elicits bilateral caudal scratching (Field, 1995; Field and Stein, 1997). Some episodes of bilateral caudal scratching exhibit an out-of-phase coordination pattern; other episodes exhibit an in-phase coordination pattern.

In immobilized animals, bilateral stimulation of mirror-image sites in the left and right rostral scratch receptive fields activates fictive rostral scratching in both left and right hindlimb motoneurons. Left hip flexor motoneurons are out-of-phase with right hip flexor motoneurons (see figure 5.1B; also see Stein et al., 1995b). In a preparation with the left half of the hindlimb enlargement removed, (1) right rostral scratch receptive field stimulation elicits right hip flexor rhythms; (2) left rostral scratch receptive field stimulation elicits right hip extensor rhythms; and (3) bilateral stimulation elicits the normal rostral scratching motor pattern of rhythmic alternation between hip flexor bursts and hip extensor bursts (Stein et al., 1995a). These results support the hypothesis that one function of descending activity is to set the excitability level of individual modules. The resulting behavior is therefore a dynamic consequence of the interactions among each of the individual modules.

Conceptual Models of Organization of Spinal CPG Circuitry

Data from a number of different preparations have been used to support conceptual models of the organization of spinal CPGs. These conceptual models have been influential and have served as important paradigms for investigators in the field of spinal cord motor control. The models discussed in this section are not computational models, however (see computational models of Marder et al., Lansner et al., Frost et al., in chapters 13, 15, and 16 of this volume, respectively).

Brown's half-center model (1911, 1914) and its expansion by Lundberg (Jankowska et al., 1967; Lundberg, 1981) have been important and influential conceptual models of the CPG for hindlimb cyclic motor output. The half-center model is unilateral, bipartite, shared, and modular. All the neurons related to the flexors of one limb are lumped into the flexor module; all the neurons related to extensors of the same limb are lumped into the extensor module. Reciprocal inhibition between modules is hypothesized to be the main mechanism for rhythm generation. Such a formulation implies that, when one module is quiescent, the other module does not generate a rhythm—that is, each half-center by itself is not a rhythm generator (see also Calabrese and Feldman, chapter 11, this volume). It is also hypothesized that the elements of the flexor module are shared and involved in the generation of both forward stepping and the flexion reflex. The half-center model can account for selected aspects of behaviors with conventional synergies: for example, co-activation of all extensors of a limb that alternate with co-activation of all flexors of a limb. However, the half-center model fails to account for behaviors with mixed synergies in which there is co-activation of the flexors at one joint with extensors at another joint. It also fails to account for deletions—rhythmic bursts of activation of an agonist during quiescence of the antagonist.

Grillner's unit burst generator model (1981) is an important refinement and expansion of the half-center model. The unit burst generator model is unilateral, multipartite, shared, and modular. Each unit burst generator (1) controls an agonist at a single joint of a hindlimb; (2) can produce rhythmic bursts of output even when the generator of its antagonist is quiescent; and (3) is "shared"—each generator may participate in the production of each of several behaviors. In 1985 Robertson and colleagues suggested that the unit burst generator hypothesis could be extended to account for motor patterns during the three forms of turtle scratching. In the unit burst generator model, conventional synergies may be produced by neurons in the extensor unit burst generator at one joint that excite neurons in the extensor unit burst generator at another joint; mixed synergies may be produced by neurons in the extensor unit burst generator at one joint that inhibit neurons in the extensor unit burst generator at an adjacent joint. Thus, the unit burst generator model can account for both conventional and mixed synergies as well as deletions.

In his formulation of the unit burst generator hypothesis, Grillner (1981) suggested that backward walking in the cat resulted from a mixed synergy, with hip extensors co-active with knee and ankle flexors. Buford and Smith (1990) established that this was not the case: hip extensors are co-activated with other extensors during stance of backward walking to counteract contact forces. Other cyclic motions of the cat's hindlimb are characterized by a mixed synergy—for example, paw shaking (Smith et al., 1985; Pearson and Rossignol, 1991). Thus, a modification of the unit burst model has been used to suggest the configuration necessary for the co-activation of the knee extensor and ankle flexor typical of the paw shake (Koshland and Smith, 1989). Other modifications may be used to suggest the reconfigurations needed to switch muscles such as the TA and ST from flexor- to extensor-related activity depending on the form of locomotion (see the section titled "Swing-Related Activity").

The concept of the module for limb motor control introduced by Jordan (1991) allows for important modifications of both the half-center model and the unit burst generator model (see "Modular Organization of Spinal Circuitry for Scratching" for a description of the set of neurons comprising a module). Both the half-center of Brown and the unit burst generator of Grillner are modules according to Jordan's formulation. The modular concept of Jordan focuses upon the neurons that generate a pattern of activity. A module controlling the agonists at a given joint may or may not be able to generate rhythmic bursts of activity when the module controlling its antagonist is quiescent. Each agonist module that can generate rhythmic bursts of activity during antagonist quiescence may be classified as a *burst generator* or a *rhythm generator module*. The modular concept is therefore a more neutral concept than the unit burst generator concept because it allows the experimenter to determine which modules are rhythm generators (e.g., the hip flexor module during turtle hip extensor deletion rostral scratching), and which modules are simply pattern generators but not rhythm generators (e.g., see figure 10 in Koshland and Smith, 1989).

Grillner's unit burst generator model also suggests that a change in the sign of synaptic interactions (e.g., from excitation to inhibition) between unit burst generators may lead to a change in the intralimb coordination pattern. Descending input from supraspinal centers may select the appropriate connections required for the form that matches the animal's behavioral goal—for example, level walking versus downslope walking. Conventional synergies may be facilitated for level walking;

in contrast, mixed synergies may be facilitated for down-slope walking (Smith and Carlson-Kuhta, 1995). Furthermore, it is possible that proprioceptive feedback from the moving limb reinforces the appropriate connections once the behavior begins.

Berkowitz and Stein (1994b) have suggested an alternate point of view to account for several forms of turtle scratching. They proposed that conventional pocket scratch synergies are produced by a population of hip extensor excitatory interneurons that also excite knee extensors, and suggested that these excitatory interneurons are maximally activated by pocket stimulation. They further proposed that mixed rostral scratch synergies are produced by a population of hip flexor excitatory interneurons that also excite knee extensors, and suggested that these excitatory interneurons are maximally activated by rostral stimulation. Lastly, they suggested that the precise timing of knee extensor activity in the cycle of hip motor activity is the result of summed synaptic activity in knee extensor motoneurons (see also Robertson and Stein, 1988). This point of view is consistent with population-coding hypotheses advanced for other motor systems (Grillner et al.; Sparks et al.; Ritzmann and Eaton, chapters 1–3, this volume), and suggests that selection of a specific form of movement ("decision") is a function distributed among a population of neurons.

Perret and Cabelguen (1980) advanced a similar hypothesis for the control of bifunctional muscles (such as the ST) that may have extensor- or flexor-related activity (or both) during locomotion (see their figure 10). They proposed that the motor pool of a bifunctional muscle receives commands from both the flexor and extensor half-centers, and that the combined strength of the two inputs—influenced by afferent and supraspinal input—determines the phasing of the muscle's activity. Thus, the ST might have pure extensor or flexor activity, or some combination of the two. Perret and Cabelguen also noted that not all muscles need the multiple input. For example, a muscle such as VL, active during only one phase of a movement (extension in this case), receives input from only one half-center.

All models discussed to this point in this section are unilateral models: neurons responsible for generating the motor rhythm for the right hindlimb are located on the right side of the spinal cord, and those responsible for the rhythm of the left hindlimb are located on the left side. Coordination between the left and the right hindlimbs is hypothesized to occur as the result of interactions between the left set of modules (half-centers or unit burst generators) and the right set of modules. In contrast, the bilateral shared core hypothesis (see figure 5.4; see also Stein et al., 1995b) suggests that some left-side neurons involved in left hindlimb rhythm generation also participate in the production of the normal motor rhythm for the right hindlimb, and vice versa. From this point of view, some components of interlimb coupling are embedded within each limb's bilateral CPG.

The proposed bilateral shared core hypothesis explains aspects of turtle scratching. However, its applicability to the neuronal control of multi-limbed locomotion in other vertebrates is not yet known in the preparations studied to date. Locomotor rhythms for one limb persist when the cord is split or chemically decoupled (Kiehn et al., chapter 4, this volume; Cowley and Schmidt, 1995), but the full details of potential changes in the locomotor pattern have yet to be described. We still do not know whether the neural network responsible for the programming of intralimb locomotor coordination in one hindlimb depends upon the network that controls the contralateral limb. Future experiments are required to reveal which hypotheses of spinal motor control offer the best insights into the organization of spinal circuits responsible for the generation of rhythmic limb movements in vertebrates.

Acknowledgments

Research in the Stein Laboratory is supported by NIH Grant NS-30786; research in the Smith Laboratory is supported by NIH Grant NS-19864.

References

Berkowitz A, Stein PSG (1994a) Activity of descending propriospinal axons in the turtle hindlimb enlargement during two forms of fictive scratching: Broad tuning to regions of the body surface. *J Neurosci* 14:5089–5104.

Berkowitz A, Stein PSG (1994b) Activity of descending propriospinal axons in the turtle hindlimb enlargement during two forms of fictive scratching: Phase analyses. *J Neurosci* 14:5105–5119.

Berkowitz A, Stein PSG (1994c) Descending propriospinal axons in the hindlimb enlargement of the red-eared turtle: Cells of origin and funicular courses. *J Comp Neurol* 346:321–336.

Brown TG (1911) The intrinsic factors in the act of progression in the mammal. *Proc R Soc Lond Biol* 84:308–319.

Brown TG (1914) On the nature of the fundamental activity of the nervous centres; together with an analysis of the conditioning of rhythmic activity in progression, and a theory of evolution of function in the nervous system. *J Physiol* (Lond) 48:18–46.

Buford JA, Smith JL (1990) Adaptive control for backward quadrupedal walking. II. Hindlimb muscle synergies. *J Neurophysiol* 64:756–766.

Cowley KC, Schmidt BJ (1995) Effects of inhibitory amino acid antagonists on reciprocal inhibitory interactions during rhythmic motor activity in the in vitro neonatal rat spinal cord. *J Neurophysiol* 74:1109–1117.

Currie SN, Stein PSG (1989) Interruptions of fictive scratch motor rhythms by activation of cutaneous flexion reflex afferents in the turtle. *J Neurosci* 9:488–496.

Deliagina TG, Orlovsky GN, Perret C (1981) Efferent activity during fictitious scratch reflex in the cat. *J Neurophysiol* 45:595–604.

Engberg I, Lundberg A (1969) An electromyographic analysis of muscular activity in the hindlimb of the cat during unrestrained locomotion. *Acta Physiol Scand* 75:614–630.

Field EC (1995) Spinal cord control of hindlimb coordination in the turtle. Doctoral thesis. Washington University, St. Louis, Missouri.

Field EC, Stein PSG (1994) Spinal cord control of bilateral hindlimb coordination in the turtle. *Soc Neurosci Abstr* 20:1754.

Field EC, Stein PSG (1997) Spinal cord coordination of hindlimb movements in the turtle: Interlimb temporal relationships during bilateral scratching and swimming. *J Neurophysiol* in press.

Grillner S (1981) Control of locomotion in bipeds, tetrapods, and fish. In: *Handbook of Physiology*, sec. 1, vol. 2 (Brooks VB, ed.), 1179–1236. Bethesda, Md.: American Physiological Society.

Grillner S, Zangger P (1979) On the central generation of locomotion in the low spinal cat. *Exp Brain Res* 34:241–261.

Grillner S, Zangger P (1984) The effect of dorsal root transection on the efferent motor pattern in the cat's hindlimb during locomotion. *Acta Physiol Scand* 120:393–405.

Jankowska E, Jukes MG, Lund S, Lundberg A (1967) The effect of DOPA on the spinal cord. 5. Reciprocal organization of pathways transmitting excitatory action to alpha motoneurones of flexors and extensors. *Acta Physiol Scand* 70:369–388.

Jordan LM (1991) Brainstem and spinal cord mechanisms for the initiation of locomotion: Single limb analysis. In: *Neurological Basis of Human Locomotion* (Shimamura M, Grillner S, Edgerton VR, eds.), 3–20, Tokyo: Japan Scientific Societies.

Jordan LM, Brownstone RM, Kriellaars DJ, Noga BR (1986) Spinal modules for walking movements revealed in fictive locomotion experiments. *Soc Neurosci Abstr* 12:877.

Koshland GF, Smith JL (1989) Mutable and immutable features of pawshake responses after hindlimb deafferentation in the cat. *J Neurophysiol* 62:162–173.

Kuhta PC, Smith JL (1990) Scratch responses in normal cats: Hindlimb kinetics and muscle synergies. *J Neurophysiol* 64:1653–1667.

Lundberg A (1981) Half-centres revisited. *Adv Physiol Sci* 1:155–167.

Mortin LI, Keifer J, Stein PSG (1985) Three forms of the scratch reflex in the spinal turtle: Movement analyses. *J Neurophysiol* 53:1501–1516.

Mortin LI, Stein PSG (1989) Spinal cord segments containing key elements of the central pattern generators for three forms of scratch reflex in the turtle. *J Neurosci* 9:2285–2296.

Pearson KG, Rossignol S (1991) Fictive motor patterns in chronic spinal cats. *J Neurophysiol* 66:1874–1887.

Perell KL, Gregor RJ, Buford JA, Smith JL (1993) Adaptive control for backward quadrupedal walking. IV. Hindlimb kinetics during stance and swing. *J Neurophysiol* 70:2226–2240.

Perret C, Cabelguen J-M (1980) Main characteristics of the hindlimb locomotor cycle in the decorticate cat with special reference to bifunctional muscles. *Brain Res* 187:333–352.

Pratt CA, Buford JA, Smith JL (1996) Adaptive control for backward quadrupedal walking. V. Mutable activation of bifunctional thigh muscles. *J Neurophysiol* 75:832–842.

Robertson GA, Mortin LI, Keifer J, Stein PSG (1985) Three forms of the scratch reflex in the spinal turtle: Central generation of motor patterns. *J Neurophysiol* 53:1517–1534.

Robertson GA, Stein PSG (1988) Synaptic control of hindlimb motoneurones during three forms of the fictive scratch reflex in the turtle. *J Physiol* (Lond) 404:101–128.

Rossignol S (1996) Neural control of stereotypic limb movements. In: *Handbook of Physiology*, sec. 12, (Rowell LB, Shepherd JT, eds.), 173–216, New York: Oxford University.

Smith JL, Carlson-Kuhta P (1995) Unexpected motor patterns for hindlimb muscles during slope walking in the cat. *J Neurophysiol* 74:2211–2215.

Smith JL, Chung SH, Zernicke RF (1993) Gait-related motor patterns and hindlimb kinetics for the cat trot and gallop. *Exp Brain Res* 94:308–322.

Smith JL, Hoy MG, Koshland GF, Phillips DM, Zernicke RF (1985) Intralimb coordination of the paw-shake response: A novel mixed synergy. *J Neurophysiol* 54:1271–1281.

Smith JL, Zernicke RF (1987) Predictions for neural control based on limb dynamics. *Trends Neurosci* 10:123–128.

Stein PSG (1989) Spinal cord circuits for motor pattern selection in the turtle. *Ann NY Acad Sci* 563:1–10.

Stein PSG, Mortin LI, Robertson GA (1986) The forms of a task and their blends. In: *Neurobiology of Vertebrate Locomotion* (Grillner S, Stein PSG, Stuart DG, Forssberg H, Herman RM, eds.), 201–216. London: Macmillan.

Stein PSG, Victor JC, Field EC (1995a) Modular organization of rhythm generating circuitry for rostral scratching in the hemisected hindlimb enlargement of the spinal turtle. *Soc Neurosci Abstr* 21:1764.

Stein PSG, Victor JC, Field EC, Currie SN (1995b) Bilateral control of hindlimb scratching in the spinal turtle: Contralateral spinal circuitry contributes to the normal ipsilateral motor pattern of fictive rostral scratching. *J Neurosci* 15:4343–4355.

Trank TV, Smith JL (1995) Paw dynamics for slope walking at different grades. *Soc Neurosci Abstr* 21:419.

Trank TV, Smith JL (1996) Adaptive control for backward quadrupedal walking. VI. Metatarsophalangeal joint dynamics and motor patterns of toe muscles. *J Neurophysiol* 75:678–694.

Wisleder D, Zernicke RF, Smith JL (1990) Speed-related changes in hindlimb intersegmental dynamics during the swing phase of cat locomotion. *Exp Brain Res* 79:651–660.

Zernicke RF, Smith JL (1996) Biomechanical insights into neural control of movement. In: *Handbook of Physiology*, sec 12 (Rowell LB, Shepherd JT, eds.), 293–330. New York: Oxford University.

6

Spinal Networks and Sensory Feedback in the Control of Undulatory Swimming in Lamprey

Peter Wallén

Abstract

In the study of the cellular basis of vertebrate locomotion, the reductionist approach has resulted in two "simple" model systems that have been analyzed in considerable detail: the lamprey system, the subject of this review (see also Grillner et al.; Marder et al.; Lansner et al.; Nusbaum et al.; MacPherson et al.; chapters 1, 13, 15, 22, and 23 of this volume), and the *Xenopus* system described elsewhere (Roberts et al.; Dale; Sillar et al.; chapters 7, 8, and 17 of this volume). The two systems share several common features, including some very striking similarities in principal organization of the pattern-generating circuitry, which are made evident in this chapter and the one by Roberts and colleagues (chapter 7, this volume). This chapter also emphasizes the modulatory control of the locomotor pattern exerted by sensory, movement-related feedback signals (see also Pearson and Ramirez, chapter 21, this volume).

The lamprey system constitutes the only vertebrate preparation for which the neuronal mechanisms underlying the sensory feedback control have been analyzed on the cellular level. Two separate sensory control systems for the lamprey have been described: one signals the undulatory movements of the trunk during swimming and involves intraspinal stretch receptor neurons and their specific synaptic interactions with the segmental network; and the other—a recently identified sensory feedback circuit—controls the movements of the dorsal fin during locomotion and incorporates monosynaptic connections between sensory dorsal cells and fin motoneurons. Both sensory control systems display characteristics similar to those of the mammalian muscle spindle and its associated stretch reflex feedback control system.

Mechanisms of Rhythm Generation in the Segmental Circuitry

During swimming, the lamprey passes waves of muscle contractions along its body, which cause undulatory movements of the trunk that propel the animal forward. The muscle activation pattern is characterized by bursts of activity that alternate between the left and right sides of each myotomal segment. In addition, a constant intersegmental phase lag occurs between bursts of activity in successive segments along the body (Grillner et al., 1991, 1993, 1995; see this volume Lansner et al., chapter 15; Marder et al., chapter 13). This locomotor pattern with bursts is similar to that of the *Xenopus* larva (Sillar et al., chapter 17, this volume), but different from that of the *Xenopus* embryo (Roberts et al., chapter 6, this volume).

Initiation of Locomotion

The initiation of swimming is normally controlled from the brain stem and mediated by glutamatergic excitation of the spinal circuitry from reticulospinal neurons (Ohta and Grillner, 1989; Grillner et al., chapter 1, this volume). The reticulospinal neurons are specialized brainstem cells that provide descending control, as they do in higher vertebrates. They activate both AMPA/kainate- and NMDA-type glutamate receptors on the cells of the locomotor network. In the in vitro spinal cord preparation, the spinal network can be activated to produce its rhythmic output—that is, fictive locomotion—by perfusing the preparation with glutamate receptor agonists. Activation of NMDA receptors results in burst activity in the lower end of the frequency range (0.1–3 Hz), whereas an activation of AMPA/kainate receptors gives burst rates between 1 and 8 Hz (Grillner et al., 1981b; Brodin et al., 1985; Grillner et al., 1991). The combined activation of the different types of glutamate receptors may thus produce rates of fictive locomotion that correspond to the natural range of swimming speeds.

The Segmental Network

The segmental network responsible for generating the basic locomotor rhythm has been characterized in several previous reports (Buchanan and Grillner, 1987; Grillner et al., 1991, 1995) and is schematically depicted in figure 6.1A. Following activation from areas corresponding to the mesencephalic and diencephalic locomotor regions (MLR, DLR; see Grillner et al., chapter 1, this volume), the brainstem reticulospinal neurons excite all neurons of the bilaterally organized segmental circuitry (boxes). The network consists of glutamatergic excitatory (E), and glycinergic inhibitory (I, L) interneurons, with cholinergic motoneurons (M) as the output elements (Wallén and Lansner, 1984). Reciprocal inhibitory connections between the two parts of the network ensure that the left and right sides of the myotomal segment are alternately activated. Intraspinal stretch receptor neurons (SR-E, SR-I) provide sensory feedback from the undulatory movements to the network. Figure 6.1B shows, in diagrammatic form, the patterns of activity of the different cell types on one side of the spinal segment. All cell types on one side are, to a first approximation, active in phase with each other, except for the subclass of motoneurons that innervate the dorsal fin (fMN), which are active in antiphase (Buchanan and Cohen, 1982; Shupliakov et al., 1992).

Cellular Properties Controlling Burst Onset and Termination

Several different cellular and network properties act in concert to shape the rhythmic output of the network, and different modulatory systems (GABA, 5-HT, dopamine) exert a fine-tuning action by influencing these properties. The mechanisms of these modulatory systems fall beyond the scope of this brief review, but they have been recently detailed elsewhere (Grillner et al., 1995; see also Sillar et al., chapter 17, this volume). Figure 6.1C summarizes the different factors that control the onset and termination of each burst in a network neuron. The onset of a burst results from disinhibition from the contralateral side in combination with a background excitatory drive that activates the different network interneurons. The E-interneurons further excite the other neurons in the network (see figure 6.1A). In addition, the depolarization may be enhanced by the activation of voltage-dependent NMDA receptor channels and low-voltage-activated (LVA) Ca^{2+} channels (Wallén and Grillner, 1987; Matsushima et al., 1993; Grillner et al., 1995). The activity is terminated when the influx of calcium through these channels activates calcium-dependent K^+ channels (K_{Ca}) that, in turn, causes a progressive hyperpolarization and closure of the NMDA receptor channels, all of which contribute to the termination of the depolarized phase and its action potentials. Spike-frequency adaptation due to summation of the K_{Ca}-dependent afterhyperpolarizations during the burst can also contribute to its termination. In addition, activation of stretch receptor neurons during body undulations contributes to burst onset and termination (see figure 6.1A).

Cellular Mechanisms and Calcium Influx

Calcium entry into the different network neurons upon activation of NMDA channels and various types of voltage-activated Ca^{2+} channels has a number of roles essential for the operation of a multitude of cellular mechanisms: NMDA-mediated plateau potentials, spike afterhyperpolarizations, and postinhibitory rebound depolarization. Our present knowledge of the spatial and

A Segmental network

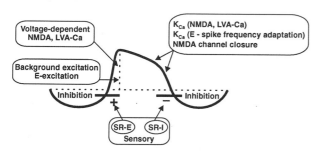

Excitatory, Glutamate
Inhibitory, Glycine

B Neuronal activity on one side

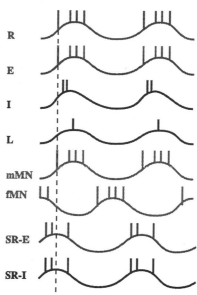

R
E
I
L
mMN
fMN
SR-E
SR-I

C Factors controlling burst onset and termination

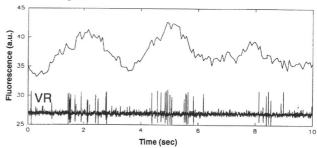

Voltage-dependent
NMDA, LVA-Ca

Background excitation
E-excitation

Inhibition

Inhibition

K_{Ca} (NMDA, LVA-Ca)
K_{Ca} (E - spike frequency adaptation)
NMDA channel closure

SR-E   SR-I
Sensory

D Calcium fluctuations in motoneuron dendrite during fictive locomotion

VR

Figure 6.1

Characteristics of the segmental network that generates the basic loco-motor rhythm in the lamprey. (A) Schematic representation of the seg-mental circuitry. Glutamatergic interneurons (E) excite inhibitory, glycinergic network interneurons (I, L) as well as the output motoneu-rons (M). In addition, E interneurons on one side excite other E inter-neurons on the same side. All cell symbols denote populations of neurons. The crossing I interneurons mediate reciprocal inhibition be-tween the left and right sides (boxes) of the circuitry, ensuring alternat-ing activity. Brainstem reticulospinal neurons excite all segmental neurons and receive ascending rhythmic feedback from the spinal net-work. Excitatory and inhibitory intraspinal stretch receptor neurons (SR-E, SR-I) excite ipsilateral network neurons and inhibit contralateral neurons, respectively, providing movement-related sensory feedback from the undulatory movements of the trunk during swimming. (B) Schematic of the activity patterns of the different neuron types during rhythmic locomotor activity. Activity on only one side is depicted for clarity. All neurons are active approximately in phase in relation to each other, except the subclass of motoneurons that innervates the dorsal fin musculature (fMN), which is active out of phase relative to the myotomal motoneurons (mMN). A phasic reticulospinal neuron (R) is depicted in the top trace. (C) Different cellular factors controlling the onset and termination of the locomotor burst. One and a half cycles are shown, with spikes omitted for clarity. See text for further explanation. (D) Rhythmic influx of calcium in a motoneuron distal dendrite during fictive locomotion. Fluctuations of free intracellular calcium was mea-sured after injection of the fluorescent calcium indicator Fluo-3, using video-rate confocal microscopy. Ordinate denotes changes in fluo-rescence (in arbitrary units) of the region of the dendrite being imaged and is thus a monitor of fluctuations of intracellular calcium levels. Fluctuations occur in phase with the ongoing locomotor rhythm, which is shown in the ventral root record (VR) below. (Modified from Bacskai et al., 1995.)

temporal dynamics of calcium influx in different neuron types and their components is, however, very scarce. To provide such information, which is needed for the continued cellular analysis of the network, fluorescent calcium indicators and fast-scanning confocal microscopy have been used to measure intracellular calcium fluctuations in motoneurons during different forms of activation (Bacskai et al., 1995; cf. Tsien and Bacskai, 1995). Figure 6.1D shows rhythmic fluctuations of calcium levels in a distal dendrite of a motoneuron during fictive locomotion. The calcium level oscillates in relation to the ongoing rhythmic activity of the network (cf. the ventral root record below); the fluctuations occur in dendrites, which presumably receive phasic synaptic input from network interneurons. Accordingly, a local increase of intracellular calcium has been recorded in distal motoneuron dendrites in response to synaptic excitatory input evoked by stimulation of reticulospinal axons (Bacskai et al., 1995). The calcium increase occurred even when the excitation was subthreshold for eliciting a spike in the postsynaptic cell and was only partially blocked by the NMDA-receptor antagonist APV, suggesting that calcium entered the dendrite through LVA-type Ca^{2+} channels as well as through NMDA channels (Bacskai et al., 1995).

Sensory Feedback Control of Body Undulations during Swimming

During active swimming movements, the locomotor network in the lamprey spinal cord is subject to sensory feedback signals evoked by the lateral undulations of the body. Indeed, if swimming movements are mimicked by experimentally imposing lateral movements to the caudal part of the in vitro spinal cord preparation, the centrally generated rhythm is efficiently entrained to follow the rhythm of the movement, at frequencies both above and below its "resting" frequency (Grillner et al., 1981a; Andersson et al., 1981; see also figure 6.2A). Such a powerful, movement-related sensory control has been previously demonstrated in several other invertebrate and vertebrate systems and thus constitutes a general organizational feature of sensorimotor integration.

The Intraspinal Control Circuit for Sensory Feedback

That the strong sensory influence remained in the isolated spinal cord preparation, deprived of skin and muscle, was at first unexpected. Grillner and colleagues (1984) subsequently found that the receptive elements are intraspinal stretch receptor neurons located close to

the lateral margin of the flattened lamprey spinal cord and therefore eminently suited to signal lateral bending movements of the body when the cord margin is stretched. Similar marginal cells, probably with a stretch receptor function, have also been described in the spinal cord of several other vertebrates—for example, elasmobranch fish (Anadon et al., 1995), amphibians (Schroeder and Egar, 1990), and snakes (Schroeder, 1986). Two types of intraspinal stretch receptor neurons have been identified in the lamprey (Viana Di Prisco et al., 1990; see also figure 6.1A): one, ipsilaterally projecting (SR-E) and exciting network neurons on the same side; and the other, contralaterally projecting (SR-I) and inhibiting network neurons on that side. This arrangement of synaptic connections between stretch receptor neurons and the network, established with paired intracellular recordings (Viana Di Prisco et al., 1990), can account for the sensory control of the network activity during swimming movements, a finding that has also been corroborated in computer modeling studies (Grillner et al., 1991; Tråvén et al., 1993; Lansner et al., chapter 15, this volume). When, for instance, a burst on the right side of the body segment causes a contraction, the left side of the spinal cord becomes stretched, activating the stretch receptors of the left cord margin. This activation leads to excitation of left side network neurons that, in turn, contribute to the onset of burst activity on the left side. At the same time, the network neurons on the right side are inhibited, thus contributing to the termination of the ongoing burst on the right side (see figures 6.1A and 6.1C).

The control circuit for the sensory feedback during undulatory swimming movements, characterized at the cellular level in the lamprey, thus includes stretch-sensitive neurons located within the spinal cord itself. The stretch-sensitive neurons have direct excitatory and inhibitory connections to the ipsi- and contralateral parts of the segmental network, and the connections ensure a fast and reliable transmission of feedback signals to the central pattern generator (CPG) at the appropriate phase of the ongoing movement. In addition to their effects on segmental network interneurons, the intraspinal stretch receptor neurons (SR-E) also directly excite myotomal motoneurons on the ipsilateral side (see figure 6.2B; see also Viana Di Prisco et al., 1990). This arrangement is similar to the monosynaptic stretch reflex in mammals in its simplest form. Indeed, when the isolated spinal cord preparation is bent to one side (figure 6.2B, lower panels), motoneurons on the side being stretched receive a massive barrage of excitatory synaptic potentials during the stretch.

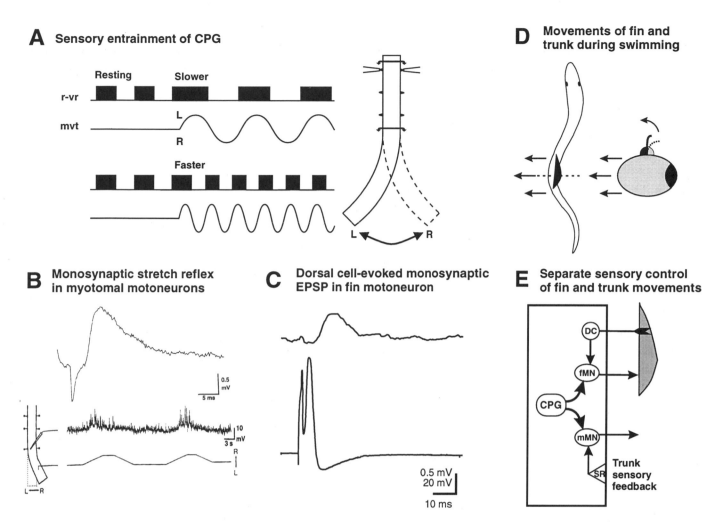

Figure 6.2
Mechanisms for sensory feedback control during locomotion in lamprey. (A) Schematic illustration of entrainment of the central pattern-generating network evoked by imposed lateral movements of the isolated spinal cord preparation, mimicking swimming movements. Imposed movement to the left (L) and right (R) sides is depicted by the trace (mvt) below the burst activity pattern in a ventral root on the right side (r-vr). The centrally generated rhythm can be entrained to follow burst rates above as well as below the resting rate. (B) Intracellular stimulation of an intraspinal stretch receptor neuron can evoke a monosynaptic EPSP in an ipsilateral myotome motoneuron—that is, a monosynaptic stretch reflex. Lateral bending of the spinal cord elicited excitatory potentials in a motoneuron located on the side being stretched (lower panels). (Modified from Viana Di Prisco et al., 1990.) (C) Monosynaptic EPSP in a fin motoneuron, evoked by intracellular stimulation of a sensory dorsal cell. (D) Schematic drawing illustrating the laterally directed movements of the trunk and dorsal fin upon activation of the myotomal musculature on the right side, causing movement toward the left. Black portions in the cross-section depict simultaneous activity of the right myotome and left dorsal fin musculature. See text for further explanation. (E) Summarizing diagram depicting the two separate circuits providing sensory feedback control for the movements of the trunk and fin, respectively, during swimming. (C–E modified from El Manira et al., 1996.)

Efferent Control of Stretch Receptor Neurons

Like mammalian muscle spindles, stretch receptor neurons are subject to an efferent control from the pattern-generating network. During locomotor activity, they are phasically modulated with alternating periods of excitation and inhibition (Buchanan and Cohen, 1982; Barthe at al., 1992; Vinay et al., 1996). Peak depolarization occurs towards the end of the ipsilateral ventral root burst, which compensates for the unloading of the stretch receptor neurons during this phase of the locomotor cycle (see figure 6.2A). Thus, efferent control of the stretch receptor neurons is well designed to maintain their excitability at an optimal level during the different phases of the movement; this is similar to the role of the alpha-gamma linkage in mammals. The phasic modulatory input to the intraspinal stretch receptor neurons is primarily of segmental origin, with glutamatergic excitation alternating with glycinergic, chloride-mediated inhibition (Vinay et al., 1996). In addition, the stretch receptor neurons are subject to a tonic inhibition exerted by GABAergic (and possibly somatostatin) neurons (Vinay et al., 1996). Such a tonic control of the excitability of the stretch receptor neurons could set the gain of the stretch reflex, thereby keeping it well adapted to the ongoing movement.

Sensory Feedback Control of Fin Movements during Swimming

Sensory Input to Fin Motoneurons

The dorsal fin musculature of the lamprey is innervated by a separate class of motoneurons with a morphology distinct from that of myotomal motoneurons (Shupliakov et al., 1992). In contrast to myotomal motoneurons, which do not send dendrites into the dorsal column, fin motoneurons frequently do so (Wallén et al., 1985; Shupliakov et al., 1992). Electron microscopic (EM) studies have shown that most of the close appositions between fin motoneuron dendrites and dorsal column axons represent synaptic contacts (Shupliakov et al., 1992). Dorsal cells are primary mechanosensory neurons that have their cell bodies in the spinal cord and their axons in the dorsal column; intracellular stimulation of these cells produce monosynaptic excitatory postsynaptic potentials (EPSPs) in fin motoneurons (see figure 6.2C; El Manira et al., 1996). No such connections have been found between dorsal cells and myotomal motoneurons (Teräväinen and Rovainen, 1971). In a recent study, dorsal cells innervating the dorsal fin and fin motoneurons were retrogradely labelled from the dorsal fin, demonstrating that dorsal cells that innervate the skin of the dorsal fin indeed form close appositions with fin motoneurons (El Manira et al., 1996). Thus, a separate monosynaptic reflex loop appears to be subserving the dorsal fin, a reflex loop distinct from the one involving the intraspinal stretch receptor neurons and the myotomal motoneurons. Again, this arrangement is similar to the monosynaptic stretch reflex of higher vertebrates.

Movement of the Dorsal Fin during Swimming

During fictive locomotion, fin motoneurons are active in antiphase with respect to the main locomotor burst produced by the myotomal motoneurons (see figure 6.1B; Buchanan and Cohen, 1982; Shupliakov et al., 1992). This arrangement corresponds to the mechanical situation during actual swimming, as depicted schematically in figure 6.2D (cf., El Manira et al., 1996). When, for instance, the myotomal musculature on the right side of

the body contracts, the body segment moves toward the left due to the curvature formed. Without activation of the dorsal fin musculature—or with activation of its right side portion—the fin would bend, as shown by the dashed outline in figure 6.1D, thereby reducing the body-surface area that acts against the water to produce the thrust for propulsion. Instead, the contralateral side of the fin musculature contracts, resulting in a stiffening of the fin and thereby maintaining a maximal surface area for the thrust.

Such a different movement pattern of the dorsal fin obviously cannot rely on feedback from intraspinal stretch receptor neurons for sensory control, but instead must require a separate control circuit. The direct connections between the sensory dorsal cells that innervate the fin, presumably very efficiently signalling any deviation from an upright position, and the fin motoneurons form the basis for this newly described sensory feedback mechanism (see figure 6.2E; El Manira et al., 1996).

Concluding Remarks

A comparison of the description of lamprey swimming in this chapter to the description of *Xenopus* embryo swimming in chapter 7 (Roberts et al., this volume) reveals several organizational features common to both systems: fast excitation mediated by glutamate as well as fast reciprocal inhibition mediated by glycine (see also Kiehn et al., chapter 4 this volume). Some characteristics may differ, due, in part, to the rapid developmental changes in the *Xenopus* embryo nervous system. Nevertheless, both systems together constitute a platform for a detailed analysis of the cellular basis for rhythmogenesis during locomotion in vertebrates.

In the lamprey, the cellular mechanisms underlying the sensory feedback control during swimming have been analyzed in considerable detail. Two different sensory feedback networks have been described (see figure 6.2E). The first involves movement feedback from intraspinal stretch receptor neurons that assist in the control of trunk undulatory movements; the second serves to control dorsal fin movements during swimming. The different requirements for the two sensory feedback systems during locomotion are reflected in the separate solutions revealed for the two cases.

Acknowledgments

Thanks are due to G. N. Orlovsky and D. Parker for valuable manuscript comments. The work reviewed was supported by the Swedish Medical Research Council (proj. no. 3026), the Karolinska Institute, and the European Commission (contract no. SCI*-CT92-0832).

References

Anadon R, Molist P, Pombal MA, Rodriguez-Moldes I, Rodicio MC (1995) Marginal cells in the spinal cord of four elasmobranchs (*Torpedo marmorata, T. torpedo, Raja undulata* and *Scyliorhinus canicula*): Evidence for homology with lamprey intraspinal stretch receptor neurons. *Eur J Neurosci* 7:934–943.

Andersson O, Forssberg H, Grillner S, Wallén P (1981) Peripheral feedback mechanisms acting on the central pattern generators for locomotion in fish and cat. *Can J Physiol Pharmacol* 59:713–726.

Bacskai BJ, Wallén P, Lev-Ram V, Grillner S, Tsien RY (1995) Activity-related calcium dynamics in lamprey motoneurons as revealed by video-rate confocal microscopy. *Neuron* 14:19–28.

Barthe J-Y, Vinay L, Matsushima T, Tegnér J, Grillner S (1992) GABA$_B$-ergic modulation of the spinal locomotor network in lamprey. III. Modulation of intraspinal stretch receptor neurons and of rebound excitation. *Suppl Eur J Neurosci* 5:134.

Brodin L, Grillner S, Rovainen CM (1985) N-Methyl-D-aspartate (NMDA), kainate, and quisqualate receptors and the generation of fictive locomotion in the lamprey spinal cord. *Brain Res* 325:302–306.

Buchanan JT, Cohen AH (1982) Activities of identified interneurons, motoneurons, and muscle fibers during fictive swimming in the lamprey and effects of reticulospinal and dorsal cell stimulation. *J Neurophysiol* 47:948–960.

Buchanan JT, Grillner S (1987) Newly identified "glutamate interneurons" and their role in locomotion in the lamprey spinal cord. *Science* 236:312–314.

El Manira A, Shupliakov O, Fagerstedt P, Grillner S (1996) Monosynaptic input from cutaneous sensory afferents to fin motoneurons in lamprey. *J Comp Neurol* 369:533–542.

Grillner S, Deliagina T, Ekeberg Ö, El Manira A, Hill RH, Lansner A, Orlovsky GN, Wallén P (1995) Neural networks coordinating locomotion and body orientation in lamprey. *Trends Neurosci* 18:270–279.

Grillner S, Matsushima T, Wadden T, Tegnér J, El Manira A, Wallén P (1993) The neurophysiological bases of undulatory locomotion in vertebrates. *Sem Neurosci* 5:17–27.

Grillner S, McClellan A, Perret C (1981a) Entrainment of the spinal pattern generators for swimming by mechanosensitive elements in the lamprey spinal cord in vitro. *Brain Res* 217:380–386.

Grillner S, McClellan A, Sigvardt A, Wallén P, Wilén M (1981b) Activation of NMDA receptors elicits "fictive locomotion" in lamprey spinal cord in vitro. *Acta Physiol Scand* 113:549–551.

Grillner S, Wallén P, Brodin L, Lansner A (1991) Neuronal network generating locomotor behavior in lamprey: Circuitry, transmitters, membrane properties, and simulation. *Ann Rev Neurosci* 14:169–199.

Grillner S, Williams TL, Lagerbäck P (1984) The edge cell, a possible intraspinal mechanoreceptor. *Science* 223:500–503.

Matsushima T, Tegnér J, Hill RH, Grillner S (1993) GABA$_B$-ergic modulation of the spinal locomotor network in the lamprey: Suppression of HVA Ca^{2+}-currents, postinhibitory rebound and post-spike afterhyperpolarization in lamprey neurons. *J Neurophysiol* 70:2606–2619.

Ohta Y, Grillner S (1989) Monosynaptic excitatory amino acid transmission from the posterior rhombencephalic reticular nucleus to spinal neurons involved in the control of locomotion in lamprey. *J Neurophysiol* 62:1079–1089.

Schroeder DM (1986) An ultrastructural study of the marginal nucleus, the intrinsic mechanoreceptor of the snake's spinal cord. *Somatosensory Res* 4:127–140.

Schroeder DM, Egar MW (1990) Marginal neurons in the urodele spinal cord and the associated denticulate ligaments. *J Comp Neurol* 301:93–103.

Shupliakov O, Wallén P, Grillner S (1992) Two types of motoneurons supplying dorsal fin muscles in lamprey and their activity during fictive locomotion. *J Comp Neurol* 321:112–123.

Teräväinen H, Rovainen CM (1971) Electrical activity of myotomal muscle fibers, motoneurons, and sensory dorsal cells during spinal reflexes in lampreys. *J Neurophysiol* 34:999–1009.

Tråvén HGC, Brodin L, Lansner A, Ekeberg Ö, Wallén P, Grillner S (1993) Computer simulations of NMDA and non-NMDA receptor-mediated synaptic drive: Sensory and supraspinal modulation of neurons and small networks. *J Neurophysiol* 70:695–709.

Tsien RY, Bacskai BJ (1995) Video-rate confocal microscopy. In: *Handbook of Biological Confocal Microscopy* (Pawley JB, ed.), 459–478. New York: Plenum.

Viana Di Prisco G, Wallén P, Grillner S (1990) Synaptic effects of intraspinal stretch receptor neurons mediating movement-related feedback during locomotion. *Brain Res* 530:161–166.

Vinay L, Barthe J-Y, Grillner S (1996) Central modulation of stretch receptor neurons during fictive locomotion in lamprey. *J Neurophysiol* 76:1224–1235.

Wallén P, Grillner S (1987) N-Methyl-D-Aspartate receptor induced, inherent oscillatory activity in neurons active during fictive locomotion in the lamprey. *J Neurosci* 7:2745–2755.

Wallén P, Grillner S, Feldman JL, Bergelt S (1985) Dorsal and ventral myotome motoneurons and their input during fictive locomotion in lamprey. *J Neurosci* 5:654–661.

Wallén P, Lansner A (1984) Do the motoneurons constitute a part of the spinal network generating the swimming rhythm in the lamprey? *J Exp Biol* 113:493–497.

7

Spinal Networks Controlling Swimming in Hatchling *Xenopus* Tadpoles

Alan Roberts, Steve R. Soffe, and Ray Perrins

Abstract

The hatchling *Xenopus* tadpole or embryo provides one of the simplest and best understood model systems for studying the generation of locomotor motor output patterns in vertebrates. In this chapter we review the connections and functions of spinal and brainstem neurons involved in the initiation, generation, coordination, and termination of the swimming motor pattern in the *Xenopus* tadpole, which invites comparison with similar circuits in lampreys (Wallén, chapter 6, this volume).

Spinal Rhythm Generation, or What the Tadpole Can Do

The *Xenopus* tadpole is small and swims at 10 to 20 Hz in response to a brief touch to its skin. It usually continues to swim until it contacts a solid object or the surface meniscus, at which point it stops abruptly. In the immobilized tadpole, the same stimulus produces many seconds of fictive swimming in the same frequency range (reviewed by Dale et al., 1990; Roberts et al., 1986; Roberts, 1990; references to unattributed data in this account can be traced through these reviews). Even the spinal tadpole can swim for several cycles when a 1 msec current pulse excites the touch-sensitive sensory neurites in the skin. We have concluded that the spinal cord contains sufficient neurons and connections to generate a basic motor output for swimming and to sustain this output without reflexes and without applied chemical excitants. Finally, pressure stimuli to the head skin or cement gland stop both actual and fictive swimming, which means that the spinal networks can be studied during their full natural range of operation in response to the stimuli that normally start and stop swimming.

Swimming is not the only motor output that the spinal cord can produce. When attempts are made to grasp *Xenopus* tadpoles, they show strong, slow (2 to 10 Hz) bending movements with waves of bending that spread from tail to head (Kahn and Roberts, 1982). This struggling pattern of motor output can be generated by the spinal cord in response to repetitive stimulation of the same skin sensory neurons that initiate swimming

(Soffe, 1991). The pattern of motor output thus depends on the pattern of sensory input in a common sensory pathway. Soffe (1993) has presented evidence that the circuitry that generates swimming can also generate the struggling pattern. Furthermore, in swimming of the one day old larva, the motoneurons fire multiply on each cycle, and the activity becomes similar to that seen during locomotion in larger, more mature vertebrates (Sillar et al., chapter 17, this volume).

Spinal Circuitry

The spinal cord of the hatchling tadpole is very small, only 100 μm or less in diameter. It contains eight types of neuron (Roberts and Clarke, 1982) that are homologs of those described in fish embryos (Bernhardt et al., 1990). Figure 7.1A shows the six spinal neuron types that have roles in the swimming circuitry and have been studied by intracellular recording. All six neurons form continuous longitudinal columns consisting of 100 to 300 cells on each side of the CNS. The columns extend rostrally into the hindbrain to the level of the vagus, so some of the neurons lie in the brain stem. In this position, some of them have descending axons (e.g., premotor descending and commissural interneurons) and could be called reticulospinal neurons. However, because they form coherent longitudinal columns that extend without any breaks into the spinal cord, we treat the whole column as a single neuron class or population. As a result, our "spinal" neuron classes include some brain-stem neurons (discussed in Roberts and Alford, 1986). As in other vertebrates, the tadpole brain stem also contains further distinct classes of reticulospinal neurons that influence locomotion, such as the well-known Mauthner neurons and *midhindbrain reticulospinal* interneurons (mr in figure 7.1A). The functions of two spinal neuron types remain unclear: *Kolmer-Agdur* cells have cilia and microvillae in the neural canal and are probably sensory (Dale et al., 1987); *ascending* interneurons are GABAergic and active during swimming.

In the next section we outline some broad conclusions on the operation of the spinal circuitry, saving the discussion of reservations and uncertainties for later in the chapter.

Initiation of Swimming

Rohon-Beard neurons (RBs) innervate the trunk skin with free nerve endings and fire one or two impulses to touch or an electrical current pulse in their receptive field. A single impulse in a single RB neuron can initiate

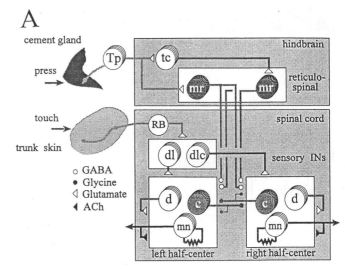

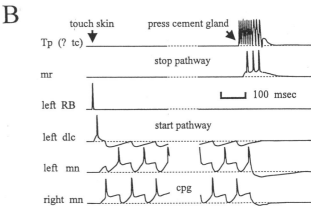

Figure 7.1

Neuronal circuitry (A) and its activity (B) during swimming in *Xenopus* tadpoles. Swimming is started by touching the trunk skin (touch arrow) to excite neurons in the sensory initiation pathway—including Rohon-Beard neurons (RBs) and neurons with decussating axons (dlcs) or ipsilateral axons (dls). The swimming motor output rhythm is generated within the spinal cord by a central pattern generator (CPG) made up of premotor descending (d) and commissural (c) interneurons and motoneurons (mn). Swimming can be stopped by pressure on the cement gland (press arrow) on the head. Trigeminal sensory neurons (Tp) then excite (partly indirectly via trigeminal commissural neurons [tc]) inhibitory reticulospinal interneurons (mr), which turn off swimming. Supraspinal swim initiation pathways not shown. More details in text.

swimming. RBs have central longitudinal axons in the dorsal spinal cord that excite sensory interneurons with decussating (dlcs) or ipsilateral (dls) axons in the tadpole equivalent of the dorsal horn. A single RB excites many sensory interneurons so that its excitation is amplified and then relayed to premotor interneurons and motoneurons on both sides of the body. Like RBs, the sensory interneurons fire only one or two spikes. They are phasically inhibited, and they gate sensory input during swimming (Wallén, chapter 6, this volume). The head

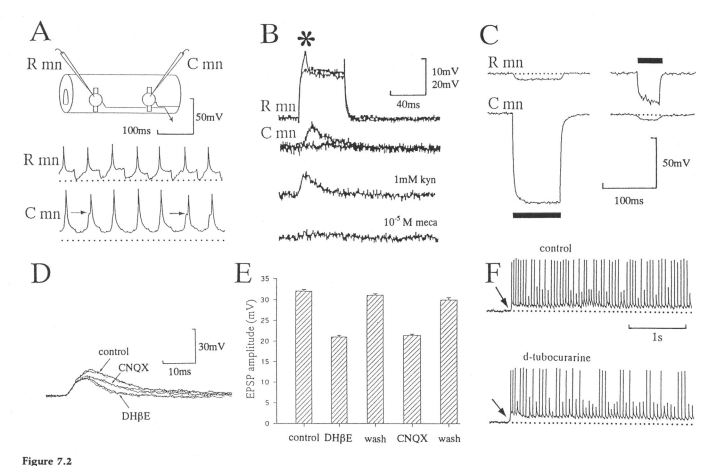

Figure 7.2

Motor neuron central synapses and cholinergic contribution to the spinal central pattern generator. (A, B, and C) Two microelectrodes were used to record from a rostral (Rmn) and caudal (Cmn) motor neuron up to 230 μm apart. During fictive swimming, the motor neurons showed typical activity (A, dots show resting potential), and in the Cmn the fast EPSPs underlying the spikes are sometimes clear (at arrows). In 50% of such pairs a current-evoked spike in the rostral neuron (*) led to a large EPSP (mean 7 mV) in the caudal neuron (B), which was blocked by nicotinic antagonists (e.g., mecamylamine) but not by glutamatergic anatagonists (e.g., kynurenate). In 5 pairs recorded 70 μm or less apart, the motoneurons were connected by electrical junctions, and current injected into either motoneuron (bar) spread to the other (C). (D, E, and F) The EPSP underlying motoneuron spikes during fictive swimming was revealed (D) when inhibition was blocked pharmacologically and spiking was prevented by negative current injection. This EPSP was reduced by local application of both nicotinic (DHβE) and glutamatergic AMPA (CNQX) antagonists (D, E). (F) Premotor interneurons do not fire reliably during swimming. Blocking their cholinergic drive with d-tubocurarine reduced the EPSP under the spike (not shown) and caused a clear decrease in the reliability of firing. Swimming was started by skin stimuli at arrows.

skin is innervated by touch-sensitive trigeminal sensory neurons, which when stimulated can also initiate swimming (not shown in figure 7.1).

Functions of Neurons Active during Swimming

Three neuron types seem sufficient to generate the basic swimming motor pattern: motoneurons, descending interneurons, and commissural interneurons (designated as mn, d, and c in figure 7.1). All three show a very similar pattern of activity during fictive swimming (see mns in figure 7.1B). They fire a single spike on each cycle, partly driven by phasic synaptic excitation; are tonically excited; and receive mid-cycle inhibition. The evidence for their function comes from paired intracellular recordings, dye injections, pharmacology, and immunocytochemistry.

Commissural interneurons (c) project to the opposite side of the cord where the axon branches to ascend and descend. They show glycine-like immunoreactivity, produce strychnine-sensitive inhibition of rhythmically active motoneurons and premotor interneurons on the opposite side, and are therefore responsible for mid-cycle reciprocal inhibition. Some commissural interneurons also have an ipsilateral axon, which may be responsible for recurrent on-cycle inhibition of sensory decussating interneurons and some rhythmically active neurons (commissural, descending, and motoneurons).

Descending interneurons (d) project caudally on the same side of the cord. We have concluded that they are the premotor excitatory interneurons that produce dual-component AMPA and NMDA receptor-mediated excitation of motoneurons, commissural interneurons, and other descending interneurons in their own side of the spinal cord or half-center (see c and d in figure 7.1A). Descending interneurons therefore provide a fast AMPA excitation that assists more caudal neurons to reach firing threshold and a slow NMDA excitation that sustains the next cycle of activity on the same side of the spinal cord. Because we conclude that descending interneurons both provide and receive the excitation, we regard it as a form of positive feedback within each half-center.

Motoneuron (mn) peripheral axons excite the segmentally organized swimming muscles, but they also have descending longitudinal axons in the spinal cord that make central synapses with other neurons. Recent paired recordings have shown directly that these synapses produce cholinergic excitation of other more caudal motoneurons (see figures 7.2A and 7.2B). In addition to this excitation mediated by nicotinic acetylcholine receptors, motoneurons within one segment also make electrical connections with each other (figure 7.2C). Are these central motoneuron synapses important during swimming? Very local microapplications of nicotinic, AMPA, and other receptor antagonists were made to spinal motoneurons and interneurons during fictive swimming to assess the different components of the excitation underlying firing. These experiments emphasized the importance of the electrical component of excitation to motoneurons and showed that both motoneurons and premotor interneurons receive a significant amount of nicotinic excitation that sums with the glutamatergic excitation from descending interneurons (see figures 7.2D and 7.2E; Perrins and Roberts, 1995a, 1995b, 1995c). Because nicotinic antagonists can reduce the reliability of premotor interneuron firing (figure 7.2F) and lead to a drop in the frequency of swimming, cholinergic excitation is fundamental to spinal rhythm production. The simplest explanation for these results is that the nicotinic excitation to interneurons, which is another form of positive feedback, also comes from spinal motoneurons.

Mechanisms of Rhythm Generation

Spinal neurons fire only once per cycle during swimming. Most spinal motoneurons recorded with sharp microelectrodes fire repetitively when depolarized only

if caesium is used in the microelectrode, suggesting a role for K^+ channels in limiting repetitive firing (Dale, 1991; Soffe, 1989; Dale, chapter 8, this volume). If tonically depolarized from a resting voltage, motor neurons can fire on rebound from hyperpolarization caused by an inhibitory postsynaptic potential (IPSP) or an injected current. When tonically depolarized during swimming, neurons will respond to reciprocal inhibition from the commissural interneurons on the other side of the spinal cord and should similarly fire on rebound. The two sides of the spinal cord can therefore operate as reciprocally inhibitory half-centers (Brown, 1914; Stein and Smith, chapter 5, this volume), where firing in each occurs as reciprocal inhibition wanes.

We have concluded that tonic drive is generated within the spinal rhythm generator by the cycle-by-cycle feedback of long-duration, NMDA receptor–mediated excitatory postsynaptic potentials (EPSPs) from glutamatergic descending interneurons. Because the rhythmically active spinal neuron classes extend into the brain stem, we expect that the positive feedback tonic drive mechanism also extends into the brain stem. This proposal is rather different from Brown's hypothesis, which suggested a separate tonic drive mechanism in the brain. The plausibility of our proposal has been demonstrated by realistic simulations of the spinal circuitry based on current clamp measurements of neuron properties and paired intracellular recordings to determine synaptic interactions (Roberts and Tunstall, 1990). The voltage dependent properties of the NMDA receptor–gated channels in the presence of Mg^{2+} are not necessary for fictive swimming but appear to increase the stability of rhythm generation (Soffe and Roberts, 1989). Simulations suggest that the increase in stability is achieved by an enhancement of postinhibitory rebound (Roberts et al., 1995). In addition, recent evidence shows that cholinergic excitation from motor neurons contributes to the feedback excitation that controls frequency and sustains activity in the swimming rhythm generator (Perrins and Roberts, 1995c).

Rebound from reciprocal inhibition cannot be the only mechanism contributing to rhythm generation because a single, surgically isolated side of the spinal cord (half-center) can still generate a rhythm. The rhythm generation may depend on rebound from recurrent inhibition provided within each half-center by the ipsilateral axons of some commissural interneurons (figure 7.1A). The half spinal cord can also produce some rhythm without glycinergic inhibition (Soffe, 1989), suggesting an underlying cellular rhythmicity. However, oscillations seen elsewhere in NMDA and TTX (Kiehn et al, chapter 4,

Roberts, Soffe, and Perrins

this volume) appear absent in embryonic neurons, even in the presence of 5HT, which permits oscillations in older larval neurons (Sillar et al., chapter 17, this volume). Furthermore, such oscillations are usually too slow (around 1 Hz) to provide the basis for tadpole swimming at 10 to 20 Hz.

Based on current evidence, we conclude that: (1) Rhythm is sustained within each side of the spinal cord by positive feedback excitation from glutamatergic premotor descending interneurons activating NMDA receptors and cholinergic motoneurons activating nicotinic receptors. (2) Rhythmicity involves overlapping mechanisms: (a) Within an isolated half-center in which inhibition has been blocked, rhythmic activity may require feedback excitation to synchronize firing and intrinsic membrane properties—particularly K^+ conductances—to limit or "tune" rhythmic firing to the appropriate frequencies for swimming (see Dale, chapter 8, this volume). (b) Also within a half-center, recurrent inhibition can facilitate rhythm generation by spacing firing and by producing a hyperpolarization that closes voltage-dependent K^+ channels, reactivates inactivated Na^+ channels, and closes voltage-dependent NMDA channels. As inhibition wanes, residual NMDA and cholinergic synaptic conductances, additional glutamatergic and cholinergic input from more rostral neurons (plus electrical input to motoneurons), and depolarization-dependent enhancement of NMDA conductances produce depolarization. Firing on rebound will finally depend on the opening of voltage-gated Na^+ channels. (c) In the intact spinal cord, a powerful glycinergic reciprocal inhibition is also at work. Like recurrent inhibition but more strongly, this glycinergic inhibition will produce delayed rebound firing and organize the alternation of the two half-centers.

Control of Frequency during Swimming

After the initiation of swimming, the frequency of swimming usually drops slowly. Many ionic, cellular and synaptic functions may contribute to this (Dale, chapter 8, this volume). In our research, we have asked what network mechanisms contribute to the drop and to the rise in frequency that follows brief stimulation to the skin during swimming. We have observed that, as frequency falls, motoneurons spiked reliably on every cycle, but premotor interneurons fire less and less, and might stop entirely (cf. figures 7.2A and 7.2F). If the skin was stimulated during swimming, the frequency increased, and premotor interneurons were recruited to fire again for a short period. Those results led us to propose that frequency can be controlled by determining the number of active premotor interneurons (Sillar and Roberts, 1993). We have used computer simulations of spinal networks to demonstrate that swimming frequency can depend on the number of active premotor interneurons in the population (Wolf and Roberts, 1995).

Longitudinal Coordination during Swimming

During swimming, waves of bending pass from the head to the tail to drive the tadpole forward and usually away from the source of stimulation (Boothby and Roberts, 1995). In fictive swimming, a corresponding small rostrocaudal delay occurs in the motor output along the body. In 1991 we proposed that this delay might result from a head-to-tail gradient in the synaptic drive to the neurons generating motor output. Pharmacological manipulations designed to increase or decrease such a gradient led to the expected changes in the rostrocaudal delays (Tunstall and Roberts, 1991). A head-to-tail gradient in the excitation and inhibition of spinal motoneurons was demonstrated by recording intracellularly from motoneurons at different longitudinal positions during fictive swimming (Tunstall and Roberts, 1994). Simulations of a chain of coupled segmental rhythm generators suggest that the gradient might provide a sufficient explanation for the head-to-tail sequencing of motor output (Tunstall and Roberts, in preparation).

Stopping Swimming

Swimming usually stops when the head of the tadpole bumps into the water surface or the side of the dish and becomes attached by mucus secreted from the cement gland (located near where the mouth will form). Fictive swimming can be stopped by pressure on the cement gland, which excites *trigeminal pressure receptors* (Tp in figure 7.1) projecting into the hindbrain. The pressure excites some reticulospinal hindbrain neurons and leads to GABAergic IPSPs in spinal motoneurons (Boothby and Roberts, 1992). Because immunocytochemistry has revealed GABAergic midhindbrain reticulospinal neurons (mr in figure 7.1) in the same location, with bilateral projections to the spinal cord, we have concluded that the trigeminal sensory neurons excite the midhindbrain reticulospinal neurons directly, and indirectly via *trigeminal commissural* neurons (tc in figure 7.1), to inhibit spinal rhythm generation and to stop swimming (see figure

7.1). GABAergic reticulospinal neurons with direct inhibitory connections to spinal motoneurons have also been found in the rat (Holstege, 1991).

Discussion and Conclusions

Characterization of the stopping pathway means that we can provide a framework for the circuitry that controls all major aspects of the swimming behavior of the hatchling frog tadpole (figure 7.1). It also gives us a clear role for four major synaptic transmitters: glutamate, acetylcholine, glycine, and GABA. The *Xenopus* tadpole preparation has many great advantages. First, it allows investigation of a range of fictive behavior that very closely matches actual behavior and does not require external chemical excitants for its expression. Second, the structure of the tadpole's nervous system, especially its spinal cord, is extremely simple. One disadvantage in using the tadpole is that intracellular recording and dye injection are very difficult, so we still lack direct evidence for some neuronal connections (for example, d to other d interneurons, mn to d or c interneurons). However, the simplicity of the neuroanatomy gives us confidence in our conclusions (e.g., midhindbrain reticulospinal neurons are the only GABAergic hindbrain neurons that project to the spinal cord; decussating sensory interneurons are the only spinal neurons with commissural axons that do not show glycine immunoreactivity; trigeminal commissural neurons have been shown by backfilling, though their function has been inferred only from lesion experiments).

We have provided a brief review of the current evidence for the mechanisms that initiate, generate, and terminate tadpole swimming. There remain some important gaps in our understanding of each of these mechanisms. The pathway by which a stimulus initiates activity in rhythmic neurons on the same side is yet to be demonstrated. Our conclusions on rhythm generation are based on properties of motoneurons; the situation in premotor interneurons may or may not be the same but, like the degree of heterogeneity within each neuron class, remains largely unknown. No role can yet be assigned to the ascending interneurons, though they are rhythmically active during swimming. We know little about the connections that organize longitudinal coordination. More generally, we do not know how the swimming circuitry is modified to produce the very different pattern that underlies struggling behavior. However, the relative simplicity of the *Xenopus* preparation gives us confidence that these and other gaps in our knowledge can be filled.

Acknowledgments

We would like to thank the Wellcome Trust, the Wolfson Trust, the MRC, and the SERC (United Kingdom) for their support of the work reviewed here.

References

Arshavsky Y, Orlovsky GN, Panchin YV, Roberts A, Soffe SR (1993) Neuronal control of swimming locomotion: Analysis of the pteropod mollusc *Clione* and embryos of the amphibian *Xenopus*. *Trends Neurosci* 16:227–233.

Bernhardt RR, Chitnis AB, Lindamer L, and Kuwada JY (1990) Identification of spinal neurons in the embryonic zebrafish. *J Comp Neurol* 302:603-616.

Boothby KM, Roberts A (1992) The stopping response of *Xenopus laevis* embryos: Pharmacology and intracellular physiology of rhythmic spinal neurons and hindbrain neurons. *J Exp Biol* 169:65–86.

Boothby KM, Roberts A (1995) Effects of site and strength of tactile stimulation on the swimming responses of *Xenopus laevis* embryos. *J Zool* 235:113–125.

Brown TG (1914) On the nature of the fundamental activity of the nervous centres. *J Physiol* (Lond) 48:18–46.

Dale N (1991) The isolation and identification of spinal neurons that control movement in the *Xenopus* embryo. *Europ J Neurosci* 3:1025–1035.

Dale N, Roberts A, Ottersen OP, Storm-Mathisen J (1987) The morphology and distribution of 'Kolmer-Agduhr cells', a class of cerebrospinal-fluid-contacting neurons revealed in the frog embryo spinal cord by GABA immunocytochemistry. *Proc R Soc Lond B Biol Sci* 232:193–203.

Dale N, Roberts A, Soffe SR (1990) The anatomy, development, physiology, and role of glycinergic neurons in the *Xenopus* embryo spinal cord. In: *Glycine Neurotransmission* (Ottersen OP, Storm-Mathisen J, eds.), 329–353. Chichester, UK: Wiley & Sons.

Holstege JC (1991) Ultrastructural evidence for GABAergic brainstem projections to spinal motoneurones in the rat. *J Neurosci* 11:159–167.

Kahn JA, Roberts A (1982) The neuromuscular basis of rhythmic struggling movements in embryos of *Xenopus laevis*. *J Exp Biol* 99:197–205.

Perrins R, Roberts A (1995a) Cholinergic and electrical synapses between synergistic spinal motoneurons in the *Xenopus laevis* embryo. *J Physiol* 485:135–144.

Perrins R, Roberts A (1995b) Cholinergic and electrical motoneuron-to-motoneuron synapses contribute to on-cycle excitation during swimming in *Xenopus* embryos. *J Neurophysiol* 73:1013–1019.

Perrins R, Roberts A (1995c) Cholinergic contribution to excitation in a spinal locomotor central pattern generator in *Xenopus* embryos. *J Neurophysiol* 73:1005–1012.

Roberts A (1990) How does a nervous system produce behaviour? A case study in neurobiology. *Sci Progress* (Oxford) 74:31–51.

Roberts A, Alford ST (1986) Descending projections and excitation during fictive swimming in *Xenopus* embryos: Neuroanatomy and lesion experiments. *J Comp Neurol* 250:253–261.

Roberts A, Clarke JDW (1982) The neuroanatomy of an amphibian embryo spinal cord. *Phil Trans Roy Soc B* 296:195–212.

Roberts A, Dale N, Soffe SR (1986) Spinal interneurones and swimming in frog embryos. In: *Neurobiology of Vertebrate Locomotion* (Grillner S, Stein PSG, Stuart DG, Forssberg H, Herman RM, eds.), 279–306. London: Macmillan.

Roberts A, Tunstall MJ (1990) Mutual re-excitation with post-inhibitory rebound: A simulation study on the mechanisms for locomotor rhythm generation in the spinal cord of *Xenopus* embryos. *Europ J Neurosci* 2:11–23.

Roberts A, Tunstall MJ, Wolf EW (1995) Properties of networks controlling locomotion in a simple vertebrate and significance of voltage-dependency of NMDA channels: A simulation study of rhythm generation sustained by positive feedback. *J Neurophysiol* 73:485–496.

Sillar KT, Roberts A (1993) Control of frequency during swimming in *Xenopus* embryos: A study on interneuronal recruitment in a spinal rhythm generator. *J Physiol* 472:557–572.

Soffe SR (1989) Roles of glycinergic inhibition and N-methyl-D-aspartate receptor-mediated excitation in the locomotor rhythmicity of one half of the *Xenopus* embryo CNS. *Europ J Neurosci* 1:561–571.

Soffe SR (1990) Active and passive membrane properties of spinal cord neurons which are rhythmically active during swimming in *Xenopus* embryos. *Europ J Neurosci* 2:1–10.

Soffe SR (1991) Triggering and gating of motor responses by sensory stimulation: Behavioural selection in *Xenopus* embryos. *Proc R Soc B* 246:197–203.

Soffe SR (1993) Two distinct rhythmic motor patterns are driven by common premotor and motor neurons in a simple vertebrate spinal cord. *J Neurosci* 13:4456–4469.

Soffe SR, Roberts A (1989) The influence of magnesium ions on the NMDA mediated responses of ventral rhythmic neurons in the spinal cord of *Xenopus* embryos. *Europ J Neurosci* 1:507–515.

Tunstall MJ, Roberts A (1991) Longitudinal coordination of motor output during swimming in *Xenopus* embryos. *Proc R Soc Lond B* 244:27–32.

Tunstall MJ, Roberts A (1994) A longitudinal gradient of synaptic drive in the spinal cord of *Xenopus* embryos and its role in coordination of swimming. *J Physiol* (Lond) 474:393–405.

Wolf EW, Roberts A (1995) The influence of premotor interneurone populations on the frequency of the spinal pattern generator for swimming in *Xenopus* embryos: A simulation study. *Europ J Neurosci* 4:671–678.

8

Role of Ionic Currents in the Operation of Motor Circuits in the *Xenopus* Embryo

Nicholas Dale

Abstract

Xenopus embryo spinal neurons possess at least six classes of ion channel: a fast Na^+ channel; a mix of kinetically similar Ca^{2+} channels; a fast K^+ channel; a slow K^+ channel; a Na^+-dependent K^+ channel; and a slowly activating Ca^{2+}-dependent K^+ channel. The roles of the voltage-gated currents in determining neuronal firing properties and operation of the locomotor circuitry have been examined both pharmacologically and in realistic computer simulations.

Model neurons fire repetitively in response to current injection. The Ca^{2+} current seems essential for repetitive firing. The fast K^+ current appears mainly to control spike width, whereas the slow K^+ current exerts a powerful influence on repetitive firing. The spinal locomotor circuitry appears to tolerate a wide variation in the relative strengths of the component synapses but is very sensitive to the magnitudes of the voltage-gated currents. Feedback mechanisms may therefore be present to maintain the correct balance of ionic currents—a role possibly performed by the Na^+-dependent K^+ current.

Like many other rhythmic motor patterns, swimming in the *Xenopus* embryo is episodic: it undergoes rundown and self-termination even in the absence of sensory inputs. The Ca^{2+}-dependent K^+ current appears to play an important role in the self-termination of swimming.

Understanding the central generation of motor patterns necessitates bringing together three types of information: identification of the involved neurons and their synaptic connectivity; characterization of the voltage-gated currents possessed by the component neurons; and description of the properties of the interconnecting synapses (Selverston, 1980).

This dauntingly comprehensive catalogue of information has not yet been fully achieved for any motor system. Even with partial descriptions, however, it becomes interesting to evaluate the possible contributions of the circuit components at different levels, including the roles of whole neurons, as well as those of individual ionic currents and synapses. Two approaches are presently available. First, pharmacological agents can be used to manipulate the individual components in a selective manner while studying their effects on neuronal properties and circuit function (El Manira et al., 1994; Tierney and Harris-Warrick, 1992; Wall and Dale, 1994a, 1995). Second, physiologically based computer models that incorporate accurate descriptions of the known components can be used to explore how they may contribute to overall circuit function (Getting, 1989; Traub et al., 1991; McCormick and Huguenard, 1992). Because pharmacological agents often have poor specificity, they may affect several components of the circuit at the same time, making it difficult to interpret the role of any single component. Computer models allow modification of individual components in highly specific ways and can potentially offer a fundamental understanding of how, for example, ion channels contribute to circuit function. For computer models to be valuable in this way, though, they must be based upon experimentally obtained descriptions of ionic currents and synapses.

The stage 37/38 *Xenopus* embryo is an advantageous model for studying the control of locomotion in vertebrates (see also Roberts et al., chapter 7, this volume). Its nervous system is very simple, containing only eight anatomical classes of neuron in the spinal cord (Roberts and Clarke, 1982). Furthermore, the neurons have very limited dendritic arborizations, thus allowing them to be modelled as a single compartment. The neural circuit and transmitters underlying the control of swimming have been at least partly elucidated (Dale, 1985; Dale and Roberts, 1985; Perrins and Roberts, 1995). "First-generation" computer simulations of this neural circuit have been attempted (Roberts and Tunstall, 1990; Wall and Dale, 1994a; Roberts et al., 1995), but they were made prior to the description of the ion channels of *Xenopus* neurons.

In this chapter I describe the progress that Mark Wall and I have made in characterizing the ionic currents of *Xenopus* spinal neurons. We have used both pharmacological experiments and computer simulations that incorporate the latest physiological information to explore the roles of these currents.

Ionic Currents of *Xenopus* Embryo Spinal Neurons

To study the ionic currents of the *Xenopus* embryo, I devised methods for acutely isolating *Xenopus* embryo spinal neurons so that patch clamp techniques could be used (Dale, 1991). The properties of the isolated neurons remained substantially unchanged by the dissociation procedure, and certain anatomical categories of neuron could be identified after isolation (Dale, 1991).

Compared to the neurons of many adult vertebrates, or indeed of invertebrates, the neurons of the *Xenopus* embryo have rather simple electrical properties. For example, they do not display the plateau potentials seen in neurons of many motor systems. Their complement of

ion channels is thus somewhat restricted. So far, the currents that I describe in the sections below have been seen in all types of acutely dissociated *Xenopus* spinal neurons, including "commissural-like neurons"—90% of which are glycinergic interneurons—and "multipolar neurons," a mixture of motoneurons and excitatory interneurons (Dale, 1991).

Inward Currents

The embryo spinal neurons possess a very fast TTX-sensitive, Na^+ current (I_{Na}), which undergoes very fast inactivation. The activation time constants range from 0.1 msec at 40 mV to 0.25 msec at -60 mV, whereas those for inactivation range from 0.3 msec to 8 msec over physiological voltages (Dale, 1995a).

A mixture of Ca^{2+} currents is also present. Two currents can be blocked by ω-conotoxin GVIA (ω-CgTX), one reversibly and the other irreversibly (Wall and Dale, 1994b). The remaining 40% of the Ca^{2+} current is resistant to both ω-CgTX and dihydropyridines. Although at least three different Ca^{2+} channels are thus indicated by pharmacological experiments, they are sufficiently similar kinetically to be modeled by a single current (I_{Ca}) over the physiological range of voltage (Dale, 1995a). The Ca^{2+} currents activate with time constants of 0.3 msec at -40 mV to 0.8 msec at -30 mV and are thus slower than I_{Na}. The Ca^{2+} currents undergo slow inactivation at rather positive potentials (≥ 20 mV). Although this inactivation has not been completely analyzed, it has time constants that are three orders of magnitude slower than the inactivation of I_{Na}.

Outward Currents

Xenopus embryo neurons possess several K^+ currents that are hard to separate either through voltage protocols or pharmacological methods. However, two components of the delayed rectifier have very distinct kinetics (Dale, 1995a): the fast and slow K^+ currents ($I_{K(f)}$ and $I_{K(s)}$, respectively). Although $I_{K(f)}$ activates with time constants ranging from 0.5 msec at 30 mV to 2 msec at -40 mV, $I_{K(s)}$ is much slower, with time constants of 5 msec at 30 mV and 25 msec at -30 mV. The activation of $I_{K(f)}$ is comparable to, but slightly slower than, the Ca^{2+} currents, but $I_{K(s)}$ activates some 2 orders of magnitude more slowly. We know that both $I_{K(f)}$ and $I_{K(s)}$ inactivate slowly, with time constants greater than 100 msec, but further characterization of this inactivation has not yet been possible.

A fast-activating, voltage- and Na^+-dependent K^+ current ($I_{K(Na)}$) is also present in *Xenopus* neurons (Dale,

1993). This current resembles a delayed rectifier that depends not only on voltage, but also on the levels of internal Na^+ that comes primarily from a steady inward leak through a nonselective cation channel (Dale, 1993). Na^+ will also enter during action potentials; however, this source becomes significant only during sustained repetitive firing. Another major source of intracellular Na^+ during neural activity is the activation of excitatory synaptic channels (Dale, 1993, 1995b).

Finally, *Xenopus* neurons also possess a Ca^{2+}-dependent K^+ current ($I_{K(Ca)}$; Wall and Dale, 1995). This current activates very slowly with a time constant of 437 msec at 0 mV: some four orders of magnitude slower than the fast-activating, voltage-gated currents. Such slow kinetics must obviously place constraints on its function. $I_{K(Ca)}$ is selectively and potently blocked by apamin, which enables the use of apamin to explore the roles of $I_{K(Ca)}$ in the motor behaviour of the whole embryo (Wall and Dale, 1995).

To summarize, six main currents appear to be possessed by the spinal neurons of the *Xenopus* embryo. The currents have the following order in speeds of activation: $I_{Na} > I_{Ca} > I_{K(f)} = I_{K(Na)} \gg I_{K(s)} \gg I_{K(Ca)}$. Such a wide range in activation speed suggests that the different currents may play quite distinct roles in controlling neuronal properties and the operation of spinal motor circuits.

Roles of the Voltage-Gated Ionic Currents

Because specific blockers have not yet been found for many of the channels present in *Xenopus* embryo neurons, much of the investigation of the roles that these channels may play in determining the control of motor behavior depends upon the use of computer simulations (Dale, 1995b). In discussing the channels' roles, I mention corroborative pharmacological experiments where they exist.

Firing Properties of Neurons

When computer simulations of *Xenopus* embryo neurons are performed by incorporating the six described currents into model neurons at realistic densities, the model neurons exhibit an outwardly rectifying membrane. They fire repetitively at progressively higher frequencies as more current is injected. Although I_{Ca} is small in magnitude when compared to I_{Na}, its inactivation is much slower than that of I_{Na}. Relatively more of the current will remain unaffected by inactivation at physiological voltages. Thus, I_{Ca} plays an important role in spike initiation and repetitive firing of the model neurons. This

conclusion is supported by the effect of ω-CgTX, which can block spike initiation in real spinal neurons (Wall and Dale, 1994b).

An interesting division of labor exists between $I_{K(f)}$ and $I_{K(s)}$ in the model neurons (Dale, 1995b). $I_{K(f)}$ has a powerful effect on both spike width and threshold without affecting the frequency of repetitive firing. In contrast, $I_{K(s)}$ has little effect on spike width and a modest effect on the threshold, but a very powerful effect on repetitive firing. Owing to its slow kinetics of activation and deactivation, $I_{K(s)}$ appears to slow the rate of repetitive firing and to space out action potentials. With realistic levels of $I_{K(s)}$ present, if model neurons are given unpatterned synaptic excitation alone (similar in magnitude to that which occurs during swimming), they exhibit a rate of firing about twice that seen during swimming.

The model neurons have rather different properties from those previously reported for *Xenopus* embryo spinal neurons (Soffe, 1990). Earlier reports were based upon experiments using sharp microelectrodes to record from spinal neurons and suggested that *Xenopus* neurons showed strong membrane accommodation. I have investigated this discrepancy and have found that if the model neurons are given input resistances typical of those measured with sharp microelectrode recordings, then they too fail to fire repetitively (Dale, 1995b). Thus, previous reports of strong membrane accommodation in these small neurons may be partly artifactual: a result of damage during intracellular recording.

Generation of Swimming Motor Pattern

Several years ago, Mark Wall and I examined how K^+ currents might be important in motor pattern generation in *Xenopus*. By applying nonspecific K^+ channel blockers (TEA and 3,4-DAP) to the spinal cord, we found that the swimming motor pattern was surprisingly sensitive to these blockers. If as little as 20% of the outward current was blocked, several types of abnormalities in the motor pattern could be seen that were characterized by an increased tendency of neurons to fire at the midpoint of the cycle, when they are normally silent (Wall and Dale, 1994a). We were able to replicate some of the actions of these K^+ channel blockers with first-generation computer models. Using the latest computer simulations, I examined the roles of the two K^+ currents in motor pattern generation (Dale, 1995b) and have come to four broad conclusions:

1. The circuit is relatively insensitive to reductions in $I_{K(f)}$ alone.

2. The circuit ceases to function if $I_{K(s)}$ is removed altogether, although it can be made to work in the absence of $I_{K(s)}$ if the other K^+ currents are raised to unrealistic levels.

3. All three effects of the non-specific K^+ channel blockers can be reproduced, but only if *both* $I_{K(f)}$ *and* $I_{K(s)}$ are reduced.

4. The circuit is very sensitive to the balance between the inward (I_{Na} and I_{Ca}) and outward ($I_{K(f)}$, $I_{K(s)}$, and $I_{K(Na)}$) currents. If the outward currents are reduced, subsequent weakening of the inward currents can restore correct circuit operation.

Clearly, I_{Ks} plays an important role in generation of the motor pattern for swimming in *Xenopus*. It seems to endow the spinal neurons with an intrinsic firing rate about twice that of the swimming motor pattern. If two populations of neurons possessing this intrinsic firing rate are coupled together by reciprocal inhibition, alternating activity will result at about half the rate of each cell's intrinsic firing frequency. Each population is inhibited at about the time at which its cells would naturally fire a spike. For this hypothesis, the slow K^+ current—largely responsible for setting the intrinsic firing rate—is vital for the production of the swimming motor pattern. It could thus be considered as the "pacemaker current" for swimming.

In many rhythmic systems, some neurons are either (1) *endogenous bursters* that exhibit pacemaker-like activity in the absence of any input—for example, the AB neuron of the stomatogastric ganglion (Marder and Meyrand, 1989); or (2) *conditional bursters* that exhibit pacemaker-like activity only in the presence of neuromodulators or transmitters—e.g., lamprey spinal neurons during activation of NMDA receptors (Wallén and Grillner, 1987). So far, the *Xenopus* embryo has appeared to lack either an endogenous or a conditional burster in its pattern-generating circuit. At later stages of development, 5HT combined with NMDA can activate conditional oscillations. My hypothesis—that $I_{K(s)}$ endows the neurons with a characteristic firing rate in the presence of unpatterned excitation—makes the *Xenopus* circuit somewhat akin to a conditional burster. In this case, the excitation from the network would allow the neurons to exhibit their own characteristic firing pattern (single spikes rather than bursts of discharge).

Implications for the Development of Spinal Motor Circuits and a Possible Role for $I_{K(Na)}$

Both the real and the simulated circuit are very sensitive to the balance of currents expressed in individual neu-

rons. During development of the central pattern generator for swimming, if correct motor pattern generation is to occur, there must be mechanisms that rather precisely regulate the relative levels of expression of several different channels (see Lindsell and Moody, 1994). Without compensatory feedback mechanisms, however, the operation of such a precisely determined circuit would be very inflexible. For example, temperature may differentially affect the balance of currents, and swimming speed may differentially alter the temporal summation of channel activation and inactivation. Real motor circuits, therefore, require not only precise regulation of ion channel expression but also feedback mechanisms to adjust the balance of inward and outward currents.

$I_{K(Na)}$ might mediate such corrective feedback. If, for example, the circuit became too excitable, and too many midcycle spikes were generated, the level of intracellular Na^+ would rise, and the magnitude of $I_{K(Na)}$ would also increase. Simulation studies suggest that $I_{K(Na)}$ can partly compensate for the absence of $I_{K(s)}$ (Dale, 1995b). Similarly, a decrease in excitability might be at least partly offset by the resulting decrease in intracellular Na^+ and $I_{K(Na)}$. My modelling studies suggest that intracellular Na^+ does indeed change within the ranges in which $I_{K(Na)}$ is sensitive (5–20 mM; Dale 1993, 1995b). This mechanism remains speculative, however, until the magnitudes of the changes in $I_{K(Na)}$ and intracellular Na^+ can be measured directly.

Roles of Synaptic Connections

I have also used computer simulations to investigate the roles of synaptic connectivity within the circuit—in particular, to test whether classes of synaptic input might influence the frequency of motor output. I arrived at three predictions based on this work (Dale, 1995b):

1. The absolute magnitude and the ratio of the inhibitory to excitatory conductances is *relatively* unimportant for generation of the correct motor pattern for swimming. An alternating pattern can be produced when the ratio of feedback excitation to reciprocal inhibition varies from 0.63 to 200.

2. As feedback excitation increases, the frequency of the motor pattern increases.

3. As reciprocal inhibition decreases, the frequency of the motor pattern increases.

I have experimentally tested the third prediction by blocking the glycinergic reciprocal inhibition in the real circuit. Strychnine is a potent glycine receptor antagonist (K_D = 14 nM) and, at nanomolar levels, is quite selective for the glycine receptor. By applying strychnine at doses from 1 to 100 nM, I have shown that the frequency of swimming increases as the magnitude of reciprocal inhibition is reduced. The dependence of swimming on the magnitude of inhibition is very similar to that predicted by my model (Dale, 1995b).

In the real animal, neurons within the spinal network receive inputs from several convergent inhibitory and excitatory interneurons (Dale and Roberts, 1985; Wall and Dale, 1993; Sillar and Roberts, 1993). The number of presynaptic interneurons that converge on a single neuron is an important determinant of the strength of the inhibitory and excitatory synaptic drive received by that neuron. The ability of the model circuit to generate an alternating pattern over a wide range of strengths of synaptic inputs suggests that the real circuit may also be able to tolerate considerable variation in the number of convergent synaptic inputs per neuron, while still preserving the capacity for motor pattern generation. This ability to tolerate variation contrasts with the rather critical balance needed in the voltage-gated currents for correct operation of the circuit.

Motor Patterns Rundown

Real rhythmic motor behaviors are not invariant from cycle to cycle. Instead, they are rather like a clockwork toy and exhibit a steady rundown in frequency that leads to spontaneous termination. Many motor behaviors shown this rundown—including swimming (McClellan and Grillner, 1983), walking (Iwahara et al., 1991), scratching (Robertson et al., 1985), fictive sexual climax (McKenna et al., 1991), and micturition (Shefchyk, 1989).

Although the mechanisms of rhythm generation have been extensively studied, those underlying a rundown of motor patterns have received relatively little attention. Swimming in the *Xenopus* embryo runs down: it starts at a frequency of around 20 Hz, which gradually decreases to around 10 Hz before the embryo spontaneously stops swimming (Kahn and Roberts, 1982; Wall and Dale, 1995). I have begun to examine the nature of this "clockwork spring" in the *Xenopus* embryo.

The $I_{K(Ca)}$ current contributes to the spontaneous termination of swimming in the *Xenopus* embryo. It activates very slowly, with a time constant several times longer than a single cycle of swimming, therefore clearly playing little role in the generation of a single cycle of swimming (Wall and Dale, 1995). The role of this current can be contrasted with an apamin-sensitive Ca^{2+}-dependent K^+ current in the lamprey, which may contribute to generation of the rhythmic motor pattern itself (El Manira et al., 1994). If intracellular Ca^{2+} in spinal neurons were to increase slowly during swimming, activation of $I_{K(Ca)}$ would progressively increase, which might plausibly contribute to the rundown and termination of swimming. Possible sources of a Ca^{2+} influx during swimming include I_{Ca} as well as NMDA receptors that are activated in a sustained manner. Mark Wall and I tested this hypothesis by using apamin to block $I_{K(Ca)}$ selectively. We found that 10 nM apamin extended the length of swimming episodes by 40%: enough time for several hundred extra cycles of swimming (Wall and Dale, 1995). However, apamin did not affect the rundown of swimming. In the control state, the final cycle period for swimming (just before cessation) is around 176% of the initial starting cycle period. Apamin did not change the initial starting cycle period of swimming but did increase the final cycle period to 194% of the initial cycle period, thus allowing the circuit to continue to produce activity with longer cycle periods than normal: it blocked the spontaneous termination of swimming. Even when $I_{K(Ca)}$ is blocked, swimming in the *Xenopus* embryo still runs down and terminates (albeit after a longer period). Other mechanisms must therefore contribute to rundown of the motor pattern generator—for example, purinergic transmitters (Dale and Gilday, 1996).

Why should rundown be such an omnipresent feature of central pattern generators? Two reasons are plausible. First, it may be an inbuilt mechanism to prevent automaton-like activity in the absence of a specific terminating signal. Second, by ensuring that stereotyped motor patterns have an inherent tendency to stop, it may protect against a build-up of muscle fatigue under conditions in which motor activity is neither needed nor desirable, thus preserving the system at a peak of readiness for those circumstances in which maximal motor output is necessary.

Acknowledgments

I thank the Royal Society and the BBSRC for their generous support and Fred Kuenzi for reading an earlier version of this chapter.

References

Dale N (1985) Reciprocal inhibitory interneurons in the *Xenopus* embryo spinal cord. *J Physiol* 363:61–70.

Dale N (1991) The isolation and identification of spinal neurons that control movement in the *Xenopus* embryo. *Eur J Neurosci* 3:1025–1035.

Dale N (1993) A large, sustained Na⁺- and voltage-dependent K⁺ current in spinal neurons of the frog embryo. *J Physiol* 462:349–372.

Dale N (1995a) Kinetic characterization of the voltage-gated currents possessed by frog embryo spinal neurons. *J Physiol* 489:473–488.

Dale N (1995b) Experimentally derived model for the locomotor pattern generator in the *Xenopus* embryo. *J Physiol* 489:489–510.

Dale N, Gilday D (1996) Regulation of rhythmic movements by purinergic neurotransmitters in frog embryos. *Nature* 383:259–263.

Dale N, Roberts A (1985) Dual-component amino-acid-mediated synaptic potentials: Excitatory drive for swimming in *Xenopus* embryos. *J Physiol* 363:35–59.

El Manira A, Tegnér J, Grillner S (1994) Calcium-dependent potassium channels play a critical role for burst termination in the locomotor network in lamprey. *J Neurophysiol* 72:1852–1861.

Getting PA (1989) Reconstruction of small neural networks. In: *Methods in Neuronal Modelling: From Synapses to Networks* (Koch C, Segev I, eds.), 171–194. Cambridge, Mass.: MIT Press.

Iwahara T, Atsuta Y, Garcia-Rill E, Skinner RD (1991) Locomotion induced by spinal cord stimulation in the neonate rat in vitro. *Somatosensory Motor Res* 8:281–287.

Kahn JA, Roberts A (1982) The central nervous origin of the swimming motor pattern in embryos of *Xenopus laevis*. *J Exp Biol* 99:185–196.

Lindsell P, Moody WJ (1994) Na⁺ channel mis-expression accelerates K⁺ channel development in embryonic *Xenopus laevis* muscle. *J Physiol* 480:405–410.

Marder E, Meyrand P (1989) Chemical modulation of an oscillatory neural circuit. In: *Neuronal and Cellular Oscillators* (Jacklet JW, ed.), 317–338. New York: Marcel Dekker.

McClellan AD, Grillner S (1983) Initiation and sensory gating of "fictive" swimming and withdrawal responses in an in vitro preparation of the lamprey spinal cord. *Brain Res* 269:237–250.

McCormick DA, Huguenard JR (1992) A model of the electrophysiological properties of thalamocortical relay neurons. *J Neurophysiol* 68:1384–1400.

McKenna KE, Chung SK, McVary KT (1991) A model for the study of sexual function in anaesthetised male and female rats. *Am J Physiol* 261:R1276–R1285.

Perrins RJ, Roberts A (1995) Cholinergic contribution to excitation in a spinal locomotor central pattern generator in *Xenopus* embryos. *J Neurophysiol* 73:1013–1019.

Roberts A, Clarke JDW (1982) The neuroanatomy of an amphibian embryo spinal cord. *Phil Trans Roy Soc B* 296:195–212.

Roberts A, Tunstall MJ (1990) Mutual re-excitation with post inhibitory rebound: A simulation study on the mechanisms for locomotor generation in the spinal cord of *Xenopus* embryos. *Eur J Neurosci* 2:11–23.

Roberts A, Tunstall MJ, Wolf E (1995) Properties of networks controlling locomotion in a simple vertebrate and significance of voltage-dependency of NMDA channels: A simulation study of rhythm generation sustained by positive feedback. *J Neurophysiol* 73:485–495.

Robertson GA, Mortin LI, Keifer J, Stein PSG (1985) Three forms of the scratch reflex in the spinal turtle: Central generation of motor patterns. *J Neurophysiol* 53:1517–1534.

Selverston AI (1980) Are central pattern generators understandable? *Behav Brain Sci* 3:535–571.

Shefchyk SJ (1989) The effects of lumbrosacral deafferentation on pontine micturition centre-evoked voiding in the decerebrate cat. *Neurosci Lett* 99:175–180.

Sillar KT, Roberts A (1993) Control of frequency during swimming in *Xenopus* embryos: A study on interneuronal recruitment in a spinal rhythm generator. *J Physiol* 472:557–572.

Soffe SR (1990) Active and passive membrane properties of spinal cord neurones that are rhythmically active during swimming in *Xenopus* embryos. *Eur J Neurosci* 2:1–10.

Tierney AJ, Harris-Warrick RM (1992) Physiological role of the transient potassium current in the pyloric circuit of the lobster stomatogastric ganglion. *J Neurophysiol* 67:599–209.

Traub RD, Wong RKS, Miles R, Michelson H (1991) A model of a CA3 hippocampal pyramidal neuron incorporating voltage-clamp data on intrinsic conductances. *J Neurophysiol* 66:635–650.

Wall MJ, Dale N (1993) GABA-B receptors modulate glycinergic inhibition and spike threshold *Xenopus* spinal neurons. *J Physiol* 469:275–290.

Wall MJ, Dale N (1994a) A role for potassium currents in the generation of the swimming motor pattern of *Xenopus* embryos. *J Neurophysiol* 72:337–348.

Wall MJ, Dale N (1994b) GABA_B receptors modulate an ω-conotoxin sensitive calcium current which is required for synaptic transmission in the *Xenopus* embryo spinal cord. *J Neurosci* 14:6248–6255.

Wall MJ, Dale N (1995) A slowly activating Ca²⁺-dependent K⁺ current that plays a role in termination of swimming in *Xenopus* embryos. *J Physiol* 487:557–572.

Wallén P, Grillner S (1987) N-Methyl-D-aspartate receptor-induced, inherent oscillatory activity in neurons active during fictive locomotion in the lamprey. *J Neurosci* 7:2745–2755.

9

Integration of Cellular and Network Mechanisms in Mammalian Oscillatory Motor Circuits: Insights from the Respiratory Oscillator

Jeffrey C. Smith

Abstract

Recent studies with in vitro systems have produced new mechanistic models of respiratory rhythm and pattern generation in mammals. This chapter summarizes these models and outlines a set of principles regarding the operation of the pattern generation networks in the lower brain stem. The respiratory networks are postulated to consist of two basic interacting elements at the interneuronal level: an oscillator that produces the breathing rhythm and a pattern formation network. The oscillator is modeled as a hybrid pacemaker-network, in which oscillatory bursting properties of coupled, conditional pacemaker-like neurons—in conjunction with synaptic interactions—generate and control the rhythm. The main locus of pacemaker neurons is proposed to be in the pre-Bötzinger complex, the region of the ventrolateral medulla shown to contain the neuronal kernel for rhythm generation. The oscillator is embedded in and drives the larger pattern formation network that produces the three phases of neural activity during the respiratory cycle. The pattern formation network consists of excitatory interneurons, which generate the excitatory drive to (pre)motoneurons, and populations of inhibitory interneurons, which generate at least three waves of synaptic inhibition. The inhibitory interactions, together with intrinsic cellular properties, regulate the transitions and durations of the cycle phases, as well as shape neuronal bursting patterns. A major recent hypothesis states that rhythm and pattern generation mechanisms can undergo transformation between different functional states. The network structure and cellular properties are such that multiple modes of rhythm generation may exist; the mechanisms of rhythmogenesis in particular may transform between pacemaker-driven and more network-based mechanisms. These principles, derived from studies of the respiratory system, may serve as a paradigm for the analysis of other oscillatory motor networks in the mammalian central nervous system.

Breathing in mammals is a complex motor act generated by a neuronal network in the lower brain stem that is designed to produce appropriately coordinated activity of spinal and cranial motoneurons during inspiration and expiration—the two main behavioral phases of breathing (see also Calabrese and Feldman, chapter 11, this volume). The underlying rhythmic pattern of neural activity consists of three phases: inspiratory, post-inspiratory (also termed stage-1 expiratory), and stage-2 expiratory. The pattern results from spatial and temporal interactions of cellular and network processes that are not yet fully understood. The difficulty of probing cellular mechanisms in the mammalian central nervous system (CNS) in vivo has led to the development of in vitro model systems that provide conditions for concurrently investigating processes at cellular and network levels. Data from the model systems have resulted in new hypotheses and models, which I discuss and synthesize with models derived from in vivo studies. This chapter focuses on the principles of organization and operation of the respiratory network, with particular emphasis on how cellular and network mechanisms are integrated for rhythm and pattern generation. (For an overview and background, see recent reviews: Richter et al., 1992; Bianchi et al., 1995; Feldman and Smith, 1995; Smith et al., 1995; Richter, 1996; see also Calabrese and Feldman, chapter 11, this volume).

The In Vitro Model Systems

The respiratory pattern can be generated by the CNS in the absence of movement-related afferent signals. Several isolated in vitro systems have been developed with functional respiratory networks: the en bloc brainstem-spinal cord preparations from neonatal rodents (rats and mice; see Smith et al., 1990), and the more reduced transverse medullary slice preparations from neonatal and juvenile rodents. The slice preparations, originally developed by Smith and others (1991), isolate the critical elements for rhythm and inspiratory burst pattern generation. They have accordingly become important for the analysis of rhythm generation mechanisms, including developmental studies (Funk et al., 1993, 1994; Ramirez et al., 1996). The main hypothesis in formulating models based on these highly reduced preparations asserts that mechanisms operating in vitro represent fundamental substrates for rhythm and pattern generation (Smith et al., 1990, 1995; Feldman and Smith, 1995). These mechanisms are, however, assumed to undergo some transformation when embedded in the intact CNS and possibly during development. Important aspects of the models, therefore, explain the transformations in the mechanisms that are expressed in different preparations (e.g., in vitro vs. in vivo) and at different stages of development.

Organization of Pattern Generation Network

The respiratory network structurally consists of two bilaterally distributed, interconnected columns of interneurons in the ventrolateral reticular formation of the medulla. The network is organized for two processes: rhythm generation and spatiotemporal pattern formation.

Specific, interacting network components—a rhythm generator (oscillator) and a pattern formation network—are postulated to be dedicated to these two processes (see Feldman et al., 1990). The main classes of inspiratory (I) and expiratory (E) interneurons, as well as their postulated synaptic connections, are illustrated in figure 9.1. The excitatory interneurons that form the kernel of the oscillator are embedded in the larger and more spatially distributed pattern formation network, which consists of interacting populations of excitatory and inhibitory interneurons driven in parallel by the oscillator and synaptically organized to generate the three phases of neuronal activity during the respiratory cycle. The excitatory interneurons generate synaptic drive in parallel transmission pathways to cranial and spinal (pre)motoneurons, whereas the highly interconnected inhibitory interneurons generate a temporal pattern of synaptic inhibition that operates on the excitatory interneurons to produce the appropriate three-phase pattern of excitatory drive. Feedback inhibitory connections from the network to the oscillator are critical for the control of rhythm generation. The main hypotheses about the operation of the oscillator and pattern formation network are considered in the two main sections below. "Realistic" computational models (Smith et al., 1995; Smith, 1995) have been used to test the plausibility of many of the principles outlined, and this chapter considers the results from the modeling.

The Oscillator

Locus of the Oscillator

The critical populations of oscillator interneurons must be located to identify the mechanisms of rhythmogenesis. Implicit in earlier models (e.g., Richter et al., 1986; Bianchi et al., 1995) has been the concept of a spatially distributed oscillator involving network interactions throughout the ventrolateral columns of medullary respiratory cells. More recent in vitro studies have shown, however, that a critical locus of interneurons is segregated in a functionally specialized subregion called the pre-Bötzinger complex (Smith et al., 1991). This region is postulated to contain the kernel of the oscillator and is presumed to be the site where convergent inputs, including those from modulatory afferent circuits, interact with the kernel for regulation of rhythm. Although the supporting evidence for this hypothesis from both in vitro and in vivo studies is compelling (reviewed in Smith et al., 1995), it remains an important problem to establish causality between the activity of oscillatory neurons found in the

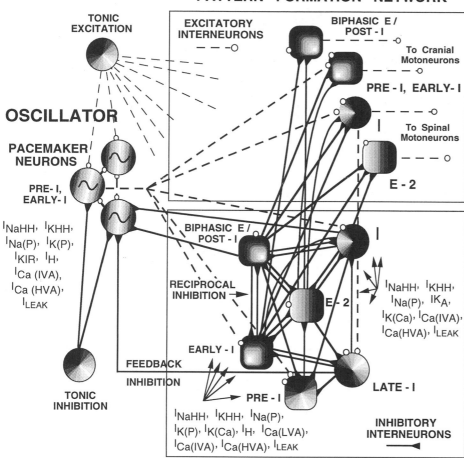

PATTERN FORMATION NETWORK

Figure 9.1

Postulated configuration of respiratory rhythm and pattern formation network in ventrolateral medulla. Classification of interneurons is based on spiking patterns in relation to inspiratory (I) and expiratory (E) phases of the respiratory cycle. In each class, subpopulations of excitatory and inhibitory neurons are hypothesized. Each neuron type is distributed bilaterally in the medulla. Connections are postulated from patterns of spike discharge and synaptic activation in vitro (see Smith et al., 1990; Onimaru et al., 1996) and in vivo (see Richter, 1996; Bianchi et al., 1995), where homologous cell classes have been identified. Hypothesized conductances in each cell class are indicated; excitatory and inhibitory subpopulations are postulated to have similar currents. The model represents the kernel for rhythm and pattern generation; afferent circuits active in vivo not included in the model would operate on the kernel for control of breathing in the intact mammal. Conductance abbreviations: I_{NaHH}, fast Na^+; $I_{Na(P)}$, persistent Na^+; I_{KHH}, delayed rectifier K^+; I_{KIR}, inwardly rectifying K^+; $I_{K(P)}$, slowly activating, persistent K^+; I_{KA}, hyperpolarization-activated K^+; $I_{K(Ca)}$, Ca^{2+}-dependent K^+; $I_{Ca(LVA)}$, low-voltage-activated Ca^{2+}; $I_{Ca(HVA)}$, high-voltage-activated Ca^{2+}; $I_{Ca(IVA)}$, intermediate-voltage-activated Ca^{2+}; I_H, hyperpolarization-activated, mixed cation conductance.

pre-Bötzinger complex (Smith et al., 1991; Schwarzacher et al., 1995) and the actual production of the rhythm.

Cellular and Synaptic Mechanisms: The Hybrid Pacemaker-Network Model

The central issue regarding the oscillator has been whether it is (1) a network oscillator in which rhythmogenesis is an emergent property of synaptic interactions among functionally distinct populations of inhibitory neurons; (2) a pacemaker-driven oscillator consisting of neurons with endogenous bursting properties and in

which rhythmogenesis is explicable in terms of intrinsic membrane conductance mechanisms; or (3) some combination of both types of mechanisms (see also Selverston et al., Calabrese and Feldman; Harris-Warrick et al., chapters 10, 11, and 19, this volume). The evidence obtained from in vitro preparations strongly indicates that the oscillator must, in general, be modeled as a hybrid of pacemaker and network properties (Smith et al., 1995), as depicted in figure 9.1, which shows a complex oscillator. Pacemaker-driven and network-based modes of oscillation exist only in principle for now, but we postulate that the mechanisms of rhythm generation can transform from a pacemaker-driven mode to an inhibitory network-based mode. In the in vitro preparations, synaptic inhibition is not essential for rhythm generation, so the oscillator operates mainly in a pacemaker-driven mode (see Smith et al., 1995; Feldman and Smith, 1995). The network-based modes are postulated to exist primarily under certain conditions in vivo. The hybrid model thus provides a unified explanation of rhythm generation mechanisms in these different states.

The Pacemaker-Driven Oscillator

A population of synaptically coupled, conditional bursting, pacemaker-like neurons (figure 9.1) are hypothesized to generate excitatory drive during the inspiratory phase. These pacemaker-like neurons are assumed to be bilaterally distributed in the pre-Bötzinger complex, where there is a concentration of neurons with intrinsic oscillatory bursting properties (Smith et al, 1991; Johnson et al., 1994). Synaptic inputs are proposed to converge on these cells from beating (tonic-spiking) excitatory and inhibitory neurons, as well as from bursting (phasic) inhibitory neurons in the pattern formation network. The major operating principles of the oscillator include:

Voltage-dependent bursting behavior of pacemaker neurons
The candidate pre-Bötzinger complex pacemaker neurons exhibit voltage-dependent oscillatory bursting in which the burst frequency increases as the baseline membrane potential is depolarized (Smith et al., 1991). The voltage-dependence of bursting is assumed to be a major mechanism for control of the rhythm, which results from a set of intrinsic membrane conductances that produce a subthreshold current-voltage (I-V) relationship with a negative slope region. At more depolarized levels, the neurons undergo a transition to a stable beating mode of action potential generation (Smith et al., 1995). At hyperpolarized levels, the neurons are quiescent. Because the neurons exhibit several functional states, the oscillatory bursting is assumed to be "conditional" (i.e., depolarizing synaptic inputs and/or activation of particular membrane conductances is required to establish bursting). The membrane currents producing the voltage-dependent behavior have not been identified. From models that mimic this behavior, we postulate a complex set of subthreshold voltage-dependent conductances (Smith et al., 1995; see also figure 9.1) that include a subthreshold activating, slowly inactivating (persistent) Na$^+$ conductance ($I_{Na(P)}$) as the main inward current that produces bursting and the negative slope region of the I-V relationship, as well as a more slowly activating, persistent K$^+$ conductance ($I_{K(P)}$) critical for burst termination.

Synaptic interactions regulating oscillatory behavior
Tonic inputs Excitatory amino acid (EAA)—mediated, as well as inhibitory (GABAergic and glycinergic) inputs from beating neurons (figure 9.1) are postulated to control baseline membrane potential and thus regulate oscillatory frequency as well as determine the pacemaker neurons' functional state (quiescence, bursting, beating). The pacemaker and beating cells therefore form rudimentary substrates for the control of rhythm. In addition, synaptic inputs mediated by modulatory neurotransmitters that affect subthreshold conductances, including by second messenger—linked processes, would also be important mechanisms for controlling rhythm (see Smith et al., 1995). Neuromodulator effects on the activation and inactivation properties of conductances that shift membrane potential and voltage-dependent behavior might cause transitions between functional states.

Dynamic regulation by phasic inhibition Feedback inhibition from neurons active in the inspiratory phase (I and Late-I neurons; see figure 9.1) and the post-inspiratory phase (Biphasic E/Post-I neurons) is postulated to terminate bursting and to reset the pacemaker neuron oscillation for each cycle. Modeling has shown that resetting dynamically regulates bursting and produces stable network oscillations (Smith et al., 1995; below).

Synchronization of pacemaker neurons Bursting must be synchronized within the bilaterally distributed pacemaker cell population, presumably by excitatory amino acid (non-NMDA receptor)—mediated interconnections. The candidate pre-Bötzinger complex pacemaker neurons receive phasic excitatory synaptic input (Smith et al., 1991). Many of the cells within the population are assumed to be relatively hyperpolarized, therefore requiring the excitatory input to activate the voltage-dependent inward currents that produce bursting. Synaptic interactions are presumed to be due to both local and bilateral axon collaterals. Imperfect synchronization can be expected due to nonuniform properties and synaptic coupling, and we can predict a dispersion of spiking onset times before and during the inspiratory phase, with some neurons bursting early (Pre-I and Early-I neurons). Such Pre-I bursting neurons have been identified in the pre-Bötzinger complex; in some cases, spiking occurs several hundred milliseconds before inspiratory motor discharge (Smith et al., 1990; Johnson et al., 1994; Schwarzacher et al., 1995).

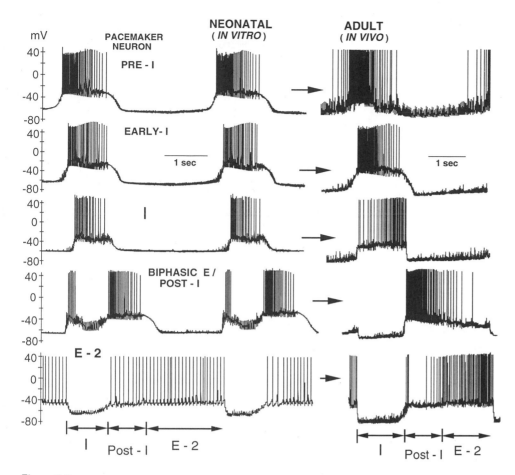

Figure 9.2

Discharge patterns and membrane potential trajectories of several main classes of respiratory interneurons. Shown are simulations with recent versions of computational model (Smith, 1995) that incorporates the different neuron types and conductances (see figure 9.1) described by Hodgkin-Huxley-like equations. Simulations mimic general features of neuronal behavior in the neonatal (rat) medulla in vitro (left; e.g., Smith et al., 1990; Onimaru et al., 1996) and in the adult mammal in vivo (right; e.g., Richter, 1996; Bianchi et al., 1995). Respiratory cycle phases are indicated. Simulated bursting patterns and membrane potential excursions are transformed from those characteristic of neonatal neurons in vitro to those more characteristic of the adult mammal in vivo when synaptic inhibition and tonic excitation in the network is increased. Under these simulated conditions, the mechanism of rhythm generation is transformed from the pacemaker-driven mode operating in vitro to a more network-based mode in vivo, requiring phasic inhibition to terminate pacemaker neuron bursting (see text for full explanation).

Multiple Modes of Oscillation and Transformation

The transformation of pacemaker neurons from bursting to beating or quiescent states can cause the rhythmogenesis mechanism to transform to other oscillatory modes inherent in the network.

Network oscillator with feedback inhibition   In their depolarized beating state (e.g., under conditions of elevated tonic excitation), pacemaker neurons continue to provide excitatory drive for inspiratory phase initiation. In this state, however, feedback inhibition from I, Late-I, and Post-I neurons becomes necessary for resetting pacemaker neuron bursting and inspiratory phase termination. The burst-generating inward currents are reset, allowing current deinactivation or reactivation and subsequent bursting, which initiates the next inspiratory phase as the inhibition declines. Rhythm is thus controlled by the dynamic interaction among ongoing tonic excitation, phasic inhibition, and voltage-dependent conductances. Simulations show that stable network oscillations can occur under these conditions (e.g., Smith et al., 1995; figure 9.2).

Network oscillator with reciprocal inhibitory interactions   Under conditions in which pacemaker cells are quiescent and there is sufficient tonic excitatory drive to the pattern formation network, reciprocal inhibitory interactions (see figure 9.1)—mainly between Early-I, Post-I, and stage-2 expiratory (E-2) neurons—might generate three-phase oscillations, as originally proposed by Richter and colleagues (1986). The reciprocal inhibition would operate cooperatively with membrane conductances that produce postinhibitory rebound bursting and burst adaptation to promote phase transitions and stable oscillations (Richter et al., 1992).

Synopsis

Several stable modes of oscillation may be inherent in the network, and it remains to be established which mode predominates under different conditions, particularly in vivo. Models for rhythm generation in vivo assume a network mode in which the reciprocal inhibitory interactions between Early-I and Post-I neurons constitute the primary oscillator (Richter et al., 1992; Richter, 1996; Bianchi et al., 1995). Such models, however, do not account for the phasic excitation that occurs in the network early in the inspiratory phase in vivo or in vitro, and they cannot account for the oscillations in vitro after experimental block of synaptic inhibition (Smith et al., 1995; Feldman and Smith, 1995). The multistate, hybrid pacemaker-network model provides a more unified explanation because it incorporates excitatory drive from pre-Bötzinger complex bursting neurons as a fundamental mechanism controlling the timing of inspiratory burst generation. The excitation mainly sets the rhythm in the highly reduced system in vitro, in which network inhibitory interactions appear reduced and the intrinsic bursting properties of the oscillator kernel are strongly expressed. We postulate that with elevated tonic excitation and synaptic inhibition in vivo, transformation to a network-based mode (e.g., a network oscillator with feedback inhibition) can occur; simulations with these conditions mimic neuronal activity in vivo (see figure 9.2). Direct evidence for such transformations in vivo is required, however, and the mechanisms that control mode switching need to be more fully understood.

Pattern Formation Network: Principles of Operation

Functions of Excitatory and Inhibitory Neurons

Separate populations of excitatory interneurons are active during each cycle phase; each population generates the rhythmic drive in specific transmission pathways to spinal or cranial inspiratory and expiratory motoneurons (see figure 9.1). Current evidence suggests that excitatory transmission of rhythmic drive in the network is mediated by excitatory amino acids (primarily non-

NMDA receptors), including at the site of premotoneuron to motoneuron synapses (reviewed in Smith et al., 1995; see also Calabrese and Feldman, chapter 11, this volume).

The inhibitory interneurons serve several functions. First, they generate a pattern of synaptic inhibition that shapes the spiking profiles and burst patterns of individual neuron populations. Second, they produce the three cycle phases and the appropriate temporal sequences of neuron bursting within a phase. Reciprocal inhibitory interactions between Early-I, Post-I, and E-2 neurons (figure 9.1) are the basic substrate for generating the three phases. Third, they produce stable phase transitions; and fourth, they control cycle frequency by interacting with pacemaker neurons and by controlling phase durations. The four functions are best illustrated by outlining cellular and synaptic events postulated to generate individual phases.

Generation of Inspiratory Phase Pattern

The inspiratory phase is started by phasic excitation from pacemaker neurons, which initiates depolarization and bursting in Pre-I, Early-I, and I neurons (figure 9.2). The excitation from pacemaker neurons operates cooperatively with ongoing tonic excitation and with the intrinsic bursting properties of the driven neurons to start and maintain inspiratory phase activity. The bursting of Pre-I and Early-I inhibitory neurons generates an early inhibiting wave that delays the spiking of I and Late-I neurons, and inhibits all expiratory neurons. Early inhibition is required to produce the appropriate sequence of activation of cranial and spinal (pre)motoneurons with the activation of cranial cells that are driven by Pre-I and Early-I excitatory interneurons (figure 9.1), undergoing depolarization, and spiking up to several hundred milliseconds prior to the spiking of spinal inspiratory motoneurons, which are driven by the I interneurons. Late-I inhibitory neurons receive excitation from I neurons and produce a second inhibitory wave, which begins termination of bursting in all inspiratory neurons, including pacemaker neurons. Inspiratory phase termination results from the decline in pacemaker neuron bursting, from the late-I inhibition, and from the next wave of inhibition produced by bursting of Biphasic E/Post-I inhibitory cells.

Generation of Expiratory Phase Pattern

The bursting of Biphasic E/Post-I neurons (figure 9.2), which initiates the expiratory phase, is assumed to result from post-inhibitory rebound depolarization potentiated by intrinsic bursting properties and tonic excitation. The bursting of excitatory Biphasic E/Post-I cells provides the excitatory drive to cranial (laryngeal) expiratory motoneurons. The bursting of inhibitory Biphasic E/Post-I neurons, besides inhibiting inspiratory neurons, delays the discharge of stage-2 expiratory (E-2) neurons, thus allowing development of the post-inspiratory phase. Stage-2 of expiration (figure 9.2) develops with the decline of Post-I discharge. The discharge of E-2 neurons is presumed to result from tonic excitation (figure 9.1) and intrinsic conductances that maintain these cells in a depolarized state. E-2 activity is poorly developed in vitro (figure 9.2), where the reciprocal inhibitory interactions between Post-I and E-2 neurons are postulated to be weak. In the adult, in vivo, E-2 discharge is robust, and the interactions are typically strong. The inhibitory wave terminating the expiratory phase occurs with the bursting of Pre-I and Early-I inhibitory neurons driven by pacemaker neurons. We postulate that pacemaker neurons do not receive inhibition or are only weakly inhibited during E-2, thus allowing the development of preinspiratory excitatory drive.

Cellular Properties Involved in Pattern Formation

Intrinsic currents have not been extensively measured in pattern formation network neurons in vitro or in vivo, but we assume a heterogeneous set of voltage-dependent Na^+, K^+, Ca^{2+}, and mixed cationic conductances in different cell types (see figure 9.1; Richter et al., 1992; Richter, 1996; Onimaru et al., 1996; see also Calabrese and Feldman, chapter 11, this volume). The intrinsic currents would dynamically interact with synaptic drive to promote bursting and shape discharge patterns. Conductances that promote postinhibitory rebound depolarization (e.g., I_H, $I_{Ca(LVA)}$), support bursting ($I_{Na(P)}$, $I_{Ca(IVA)}$), $I_{Ca(HVA)}$), and facilitate burst termination and repolarization ($I_{K(P)}$, $I_{K(Ca)}$) are assumed to be important, particularly in Pre-I, Early-I, and Biphasic E/Post-I neurons. The cationic currents that support bursting also promote depolarization in response to excitatory synaptic drive and are therefore considered important for facilitating excitatory drive transmission in many of the pattern-forming neurons; bursting behavior has been documented in several types of respiratory neurons, particularly I neurons, in vitro (Johnson et al., 1994).

Developmental Transformations

Rhythm and pattern generation mechanisms are assumed to undergo some postnatal developmental elaboration (e.g., Funk et al., 1994; Ramirez et al., 1996), but the developmental properties of interneurons (figure 9.1) have not been studied. Two hypotheses dominate our current analysis: (1) Pre-Bötzinger complex neurons remain the kernel for rhythm generation throughout development (e.g., Schwarzacher et al., 1995; Ramirez et al., 1996); and (2) network inhibitory interactions become more important in the production and control of individual cycle phases with development. Adult neurons in vivo exhibit more prominent inhibitory hyperpolarization, which may reflect developmental shifts in Cl^- equilibrium potentials as well as changes in the expression and properties of GABA and glycine receptors. Simulations indicate that inhibitory currents must be increased to transform neuronal discharge patterns and membrane potential trajectories from those characteristic of the neonatal rodent in vitro to those more characteristic of the anesthetized adult in vivo (Smith, 1995; see also figure 9.2). As inhibitory potentials increase, hyperpolarization activated or deinactivated conductances (e.g., I_H, $I_{Ca(LVA)}$) may become more important in burst pattern formation and rhythm control. A fundamental question is whether developmental changes occur in neuronal pacemaker properties, or in the control of these cells, so that inhibitory network modes of rhythm generation predominate in mature mammals, as some studies speculate (e.g., Richter et al., 1992). Developmental analysis of cellular and network properties in the pre-Bötzinger complex in vivo and in vitro should resolve this issue.

References

Bianchi AL, Denavit-Saubie M, Champagnat J (1995) Central control of breathing in mammals: Neuronal circuitry, membrane properties, and neurotransmitters. *Physiol Rev* 75:1–45.

Feldman JL, Smith JC (1995) Neural control of respiratory pattern in mammals: An overview. In: *Regulation of Breathing* (Dempsey JA, Pack AI, eds), 39–69. New York: Dekker.

Feldman JL, Smith JC, Ellenberger HH, Connelly CA, Liu G, Greer JJ, Lindsay AD, Otto MR (1990) Neurogenesis of respiratory rhythm and pattern: Emerging concepts. *Amer J Physiol* 259:R879–R886.

Funk GD, Smith JC, Feldman JL (1993) Generation and transmission of respiratory oscillations in medullary slices: Role of excitatory amino acids. *J Neurophysiol* 70:1497–1515.

Funk GD, Smith JC, Feldman JL (1994) Development of thyrotropin-releasing hormone and norepinephrine potentiation of inspiratory-related hypoglossal motoneuron discharge in neonatal and juvenile mice in vitro. *J Neurophysiol* 72:2538–2541.

Johnson SM, Smith JC, Funk GD, Feldman JL (1994) Pacemaker behavior of respiratory neurons in medullary slices from neonatal rat. *J Neurophysiol* 72:2598–2608.

Onimaru H, Ballanyi K, Richter DW (1996) Calcium-dependent responses in neurons of the isolated respiratory network of newborn rats. *J Physiol* 491(3):677–695.

Ramirez JM, Quellmalz UJA, Richter DW (1996) Postnatal changes in the mammalian respiratory network as revealed by the transverse brainstem slice of mice. *J Physiol* 491:799–812.

Richter DW (1996) Neural regulation of respiration: Rhythmogenesis and afferent control. In: *Comprehensive Human Physiology*, vol. 2 (Greger R, Windhorst U, eds), 2079–2095. Heidelberg: Springer.

Richter DW, Ballantyne D, Remmers JE (1986) Respiratory rhythm generation: A model. *News in Physiol Sci* 1:109–112.

Richter DW, Ballanyi K, Schwarzacher S (1992) Mechanisms of respiratory rhythm generation. *Curr Opin Neurobiol* 2:788–793.

Schwarzacher SW, Smith JC, Richter DW (1995) Pre–Bötzinger complex in the cat. *J Neurophysiol* 73:1452–1461.

Smith JC (1995) New computational models of the respiratory oscillator in mammals. In: *Modeling and Control of Ventilation* (Semple S, Guz A, Adams L, eds), 7–13, New York: Plenum.

Smith JC, Ellenberger HH, Ballanyi K, Richter DW, Feldman JL (1991) Pre-Bötzinger complex: A brainstem region that may generate respiratory rhythm in mammals. *Science* 254:726–729.

Smith JC, Funk GD, Johnson SM, Feldman JL (1995) Cellular and synaptic mechanisms generating respiratory rhythm: Insights from in vitro and computational studies. In: *Ventral Brainstem Mechanisms and Control of Respiration and Blood Pressure* (Trouth CO, Millis RM, Kiwull-Schöne H, Schlafke ME, eds), 463–496. New York: Dekker.

Smith JC, Greer JJ, Liu G, Feldman JL (1990) Neural mechanisms generating respiratory pattern in mammalian brain stem–spinal cord in vitro. I. Spatiotemporal patterns of motor and medullary neuron activity. *J Neurophysiol* 64:1149–1169.

10

Shared Features of Invertebrate Central Pattern Generators

Allen I. Selverston, Yuri V. Panchin, Yuri I. Arshavsky, and Grigori N. Orlovsky

Abstract

The organization of invertebrate central pattern generators and their role in motor control systems are described. This review emphasizes some general principles of motor control common to both invertebrates and vertebrates. The spatiotemporal organization of motor outputs produced by central pattern generators is determined by endogenous properties of generator neurons and their interactions with each other and with output neurons. Cellular properties and intercellular connections are under the control of different command (modulatory) neurons and hormonal influences, which makes the central pattern generators into flexible, multifunctional systems capable of generating various motor outputs that depend on ongoing conditions. The central pattern generators send signals of their activity to higher centers. Here, we discuss the contribution these signals make to motor behavior.

How the central nervous system (CNS) copes with the complexity of the external and internal world is one of the central problems of neurophysiology. Concerning the problem of motor control, the main objective of motor coordination is to overcome the redundant number of degrees of freedom of the motor apparatus (Bernstein, 1967). According to the concept of hierarchical control, complex nervous systems include relatively autonomus subsystems, each dedicated to a particular function. Higher levels of the system that have all the information concerning a solved task do not control each element at lower levels. They instead send a general command to those various subsystems. Motor outputs produced by subsystems are thus determined not by detailed higher order commands, but by subsystem organization. The central pattern generators (CPGs) underlying "automatic" movements (locomotion, respiration, swallowing, defense reactions, etc.) are examples of such subsystems.

At the present time, the problem of understanding the basis for the operation of CPGs at the *cellular* level can *only* be solved in animals with "simpler" nervous systems, such as invertebrates and lower vertebrates. Invertebrate CPGs have been of interest for many years because they offer the possibility of studying rhythmic behaviors in terms of the interactions between identifiable neurons in defined circuits. In principle, the neural

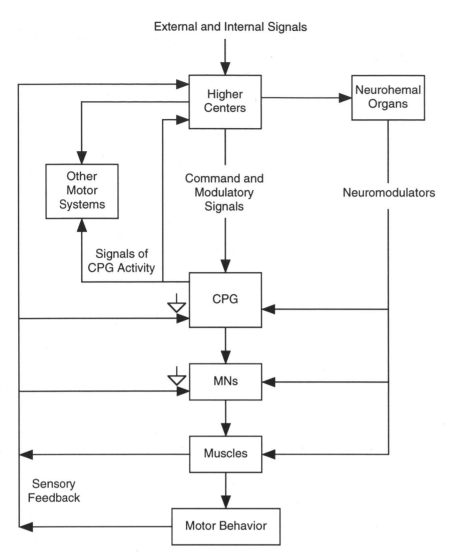

Figure 10.1
Overall scheme for the role of CPGs in the formation of motor programs. White arrows show that sensory feedback acting on the basis of a motor behavior can be "explained" from the cellular to the system level. Work on many invertebrate systems has not only identified neural circuits unique to individual animals, but also suggested entirely new mechanisms for the production of spatiotemporal patterns in general. Here, we summarize the main achievements obtained by studying invertebrate CPGs and their role in motor control (figure 10.1). We describe not only the basic mechanisms of how patterns are generated, but also how they are controlled and modulated.

Neural Organization of CPGs

The most detailed analysis of CPG organization has been carried out for rhythmical movements. The CPG and motoneurons (MNs) are under control of higher centers and neuromodulators.

concept is an operational one. The CPG is usually defined as the ensemble of neural elements necessary and sufficient for the production of a coordinated motor pattern in response to short or tonic inputs. Sensory feedback, however, is *not* necessary for the production of the motor pattern. Of course, CPGs are in reality integrated into the rest of the CNS and are influenced to various degrees by sensory feedback as well as by other factors. It is often possible, however, to examine a CPG in an isolated condition so that fundamental questions can be asked about the formation of the motor pattern. In order to answer the major question, "How do the CPGs that control rhythmical movements operate?" we have to ask the following questions:

1. What are the sources of the rhythmical activity within CPG networks?

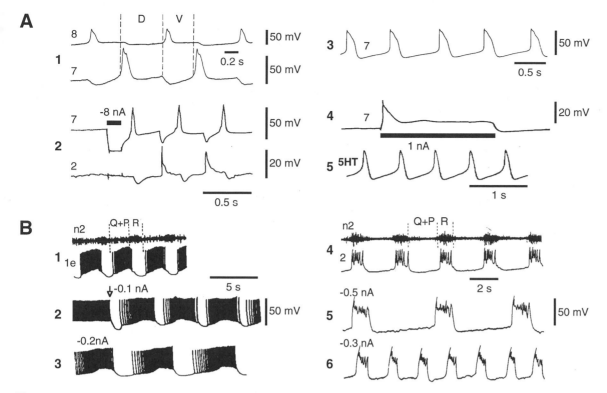

Figure 10.2
Characteristics of generator neurons in mollusks. (A) The swimming CPG in *Clione limacina*. (1) Alternating activity of group 7 and 8 interneurons (see figure 10.4A) in isolated pedal ganglia; D and V are the phases of the cycle corresponding to dorsal and ventral wing flexions. (2) Simultaneous recording of antagonistic neurons 7 and 2; in the absence of rhythm generation, injection of a pulse of hyperpolarizing current into the interneuron (period of current injection is marked by a solid line) produced a bout of swimming activity consisting of three cycles (modified from Arshavsky et al., 1985). (3) Endogenous activity of the isolated interneuron 7 (modified from Arshavsky et al., 1991). (4, 5) Isolated interneuron 7 generated no rhythmical activity, sponta-

neously or in response to depolarizing current injection (4); the rhythmical activity was triggered by serotonin (5×10^{-7} M) application (5) (modified from Panchin et al., 1996). (B) The feeding CPG in the snail *Planorbis corneus*. (1, 4) Buccal interneurons 1e and 2 were recorded together with electroneurogram in buccal nerve (n2); quiescent (Q), protraction (P), and retraction (R) phases of the cycle are indicated. (2, 3, 5, 6) The same interneurons were recorded after extraction from the ganglia at different levels of the membrane potential; in (2) the beginning of hyperpolarizing current injection is marked by an arrow (modified from Arshavsky et al., 1991).

2. What mechanisms determine the frequency of the motor output and the duration of the cycle phases?

3. What mechanisms shape the pattern of the motor output—that is, determine the number of phases in the cycle and the transition from one phase to another?

The above questions can be answered for only a few favorable preparations. All or most of the cells constituting the CPGs as well as the synaptic connections between cells have been identified for these preparations, so the mechanisms by which the CPGs operate in terms of neuron-to-neuron interactions can be reasonably well understood.

Sources of Rhythmicity

Rhythm generation in the overwhelming majority of the CPGs that have been studied to date is mainly based on the endogenous pacemaker properties of generator

neurons. This has been demonstrated in the heartbeat CPG of crustacea (Tazaki and Cooke, 1990), the swimming CPG in the mollusk *Clione limacina* (Arshavsky et al., 1991), the pyloric and gastric CPGs of the crustacean stomatogastric system (Selverston and Moulins, 1987; Harris-Warrick et al., 1992; Panchin et al., 1993), the feeding CPG in mollusks (Arshavsky et al., 1989, 1991), and the flight CPG in the locust (Ramirez and Pearson, 1991). The decisive role of endogenous bursting for rhythm generation has also been shown in vertebrate CPGs (Wallén, chapter 6, this volume, and Smith, chapter 9, this volume). The most conclusive evidence for endogenous properties has been obtained in experiments involving the physical or functional isolation of single neurons (figures 10.2 and 10.3). After isolation, generator neurons exhibited rhythmical activity similar to the activity they generated before isolation.

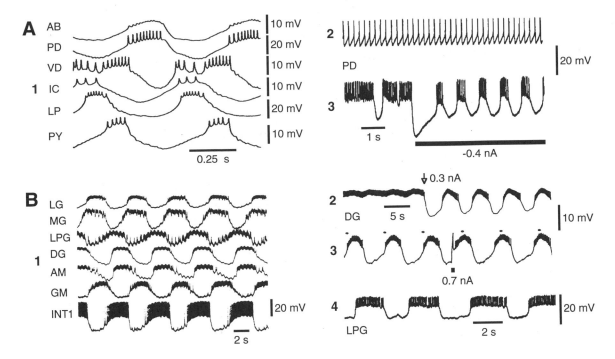

Figure 10.3

Characteristics of generator neurons in the crustacean stomatogastric system. (A) The pyloric CPG from the crustacean stomatogastric system. (1) Simultaneous recordings of neurons constituting the pyloric CPGs (modified from Selverston and Moulins, 1987). (2, 3) PD neuron isolated with an axon and neuropilar processes after two days in culture. (2) Initial activity. (3) After pilocarpine (5×10^{-5} M) application, the neuron generated a pyloric rhythm when hyperpolarized (modified from Panchin et al., 1993). (B) The gastric CPG from the crustacean stomatogastric system. (1) Simultaneous recordings of neurons constituting the gastric CPG (modified from Selverston and Moulins,

1987). (2, 3) A functionally isolated DG neuron generated the gastric rhythm under influence of pilocarpine at a definite level of the membrane potential; the beginning of hyperpolarizing current injection is marked by an arrow. (3) Resetting of the rhythm by injection of a depolarizing pulse; dots show expected times of burst initiation (modified from Elson and Selverston, 1992). (4) LPG neuron isolated with an axon and neuropilar processes after two days in culture; the neuron generated a gastric rhythm after pilocarpine application (modified from Panchin et al., 1993).

Potentials produced by neurons from different CPGs display various forms. They can be prolonged (approximately 100 msec) action potentials (e.g., interneurons of groups 7 and 8 from *Clione's* swimming CPG, figure 10.2A); slow waves of depolarization (bursting potentials) that underlie bursts of spike discharges (interneurons of group 1 from the snail feeding CPG, figure 10.2B, 1–3; generator neurons from the pyloric and gastric CPGs, figure 10.3); rectangular-shaped waves of depolarization (interneurons of group 2 from the snail feeding CPG, figure 10.2B, 4–6). In all cases, periodic cell discharges are preceded by a ramp depolarization (pacemaker potential). Depolarizing pulses reset the rhythmic discharges of isolated cells (figure 10.3B, 3), as is characteristic of pacemakers. In some cases, generator neurons are constitutive bursters: they exhibit spontaneous rhythmical activity after isolation (figures 10.2A, 3, and 10.2B). In most cases, however, generator neurons are conditional bursters: they exhibit rhythmical activity only under the influence of command neurons, their

transmitters, or neuromodulatory substances carried in the blood (figures 10.2A, 4 and 5, 10.3A, and 10.3B).

The endogenous rhythmical activity of generator neurons is produced by different membrane currents interacting with one another. Most generator neurons exhibit endogenous activity at a definite level of membrane potential (figures 10.2B, 10.3A, and 10.3B) because of activation and inactivation of currents participating in rhythm generation. The ionic requirements for bursting activity have been investigated in the electrically coupled group of PD-AB stomatogastric neurons that play a kernel role in pyloric rhythm generation (Gola and Selverston, 1981). It has been suggested that the pacemaker potential is determined by a decrease of K^+ conductance because the interburst ramp depolarization is accompanied by an increase in the membrane resistance. This suggestion was supported by the fact that, in the isolated AB neuron, rhythmical activity was induced by reducing the K^+ current (Harris-Warrick and Johnson, 1987). When the pacemaker potential reaches a threshold level, Na^+ and Ca^{2+} channels open, and the inward current caused by the entrance of these ions results in the generation of a slow depolarizing wave. At the same time, a small outward K^+ current is activated that reduces the slow wave amplitude. This current is a candidate mechanism for modulating the burst discharge. A progressive intracellular accumulation of Ca^{2+} activates the Ca^{2+}-dependent K^+ current, which, in cooperation with voltage-sensitive outward currents, terminates the depolarizing wave. Thus, the temporal characteristics of the slow waves are determined by the dynamics of the Ca^{2+} current and the activation of the Ca^{2+}-dependent K^+ current. Such a mechanism can be observed in many systems. For example, the dynamics of the Ca^{2+} current and the Ca^{2+}-dependent K^+ current determine the timing of the driver potentials in neurons from the crustacean cardiac CPG (Tazaki and Cooke, 1990).

It may be the case that reciprocal inhibitory coupled neurons assist in burst formation, as has been shown directly in pyloric neurons of the stomatogastric system (Miller and Selverston, 1982). A necessary condition for rhythm generation in such a system is the existence of time-dependent mechanisms (such as a Ca^{2+}-dependent K^+ current), which ensure burst termination. Another factor that assists in reinforcing rhythmicity in systems of reciprocal inhibitory coupled neurons is postinhibitory rebound, a property typical of generator neurons (Perkel and Mulloney, 1974; Arshavsky et al., 1985; Harris-Warrick et al., 1992). In preparations of *Clione*'s pedal ganglia that do not exhibit endogenous activity, injection of a short pulse of hyperpolarizing current into a generator interneuron resulted in a bout of rhythmical activity consisting of several cycles (see figure 10.2A, 2). In this case, postinhibitory rebound is of crucial importance for the rhythm generation. Thus, the endogenous activity of generator neurons and network properties *do not exclude*, but *add* to each other, ensuring reliable rhythm generation. Postinhibitory rebound, however, is not the main source of the rhythmical activity. Activity based solely on postinhibitory rebound is noise sensitive, and any accidental failure will stop rhythm generation. Furthermore, networks heavily dependent on postinhibitory rebound lose the flexibility necessary to make changes in the spatiotemporal pattern of a motor output.

An exception to the rule of rhythmic motor patterns being driven by pacemaker neurons has been described in the swimming CPG of the marine snail *Tritonia* (Getting, 1989; Frost et al., chapter 16, this volume). For this preparation, it has been concluded that the rhythmic pattern is a result of synaptic interactions only. The swimming rhythm in *Tritonia* lasts for only a few cycles, and Getting has suggested that such short-lived behavior may depend less on the need for pacemaker neurons than do systems that cycle for long periods of time.

Mechanisms Determining the Frequency of a Motor Output and the Duration of the Cycle Phases

Like the generation of the rhythmical activity, the temporal pattern of the motor output produced by the CPGs is to a great extent determined by intrinsic properties of generator neurons. These properties are due to the combination of ion channels contained in the neurons that make up the CPG. As shown in figures 10.2 and 10.3, the frequency of the rhythmical activity produced by isolated generator neurons is within the range of frequencies typical of a given CPG. In a system consisting of a number of coupled oscillator neurons, the frequency of the rhythmical activity is determined by the fastest element(s). This is true not only for systems with excitatory interconnections (as in the cardiac ganglion of the crustacea), but also for systems with inhibitory connections between neurons. For example, the pyloric CPG consists of 14 neurons, all of which are conditional bursters with different intrinsic frequencies. Although pyloric neurons interact via inhibitory connections (figure 10.4D), the CPG's rhythmical activity is determined by the neuron with the highest intrinsic activity, the AB neuron (Bal et al., 1988; Harris-Warrick et al., 1992). Correspondingly, command signals for switching on the pyloric CPG and for controlling its frequency are addressed primarily to the AB neuron (Marder and Meyrand, 1989). After inactivation of the AB neuron, the leading role in rhythm generation is played by the PD neurons, whose intrinsic frequency is closest to that of the AB (Bal et al., 1988).

Intrinsic properties of generator neurons play an important role in determining the temporal organization of single cycles. The duration of action potentials or of bursting discharges in generator neurons (and therefore the duration of the postsynaptic potentials they produce onto target neurons) is comparable with the duration of cycle phases (see figures 10.2 and 10.3).

Membrane properties of generator neurons determine the temporal patterns of motor outputs not only in the CPGs underlying rhythmical movements but also in the CPGs underlying single movements, as demonstrated in a study of the neural mechanisms of a defense reaction in *Planorbis*. Interneurons that constitute the CPG for the defense reaction produce prolonged action potentials (up to 2 seconds). The duration of the action potentials is

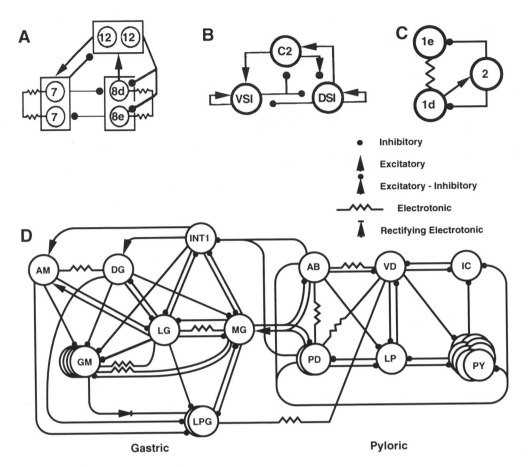

Figure 10.4

Examples of network organization of CPGs in invertebrates. (A) The swimming CPG in *Clione*; thin lines show connections functioning during "weak" and "intense" modes of operation; thick lines show connections functioning during "intense" mode of CPG operation only (modified from Arshavsky et al., 1985). (B) The swimming CPG in *Tri-*

tonia (modified from Getting, 1989). (C) The feeding CPG in *Planorbis* (modified from Arshavsky et al., 1991). (D) The pyloric and gastric CPGs in crustacea; some connections shown are not monosynaptic, but functional (modified from Selverston and Moulins, 1987). Types of neurons are indicated inside large circles.

comparable with the duration of the defense reaction itself (Arshavsky et al., 1991).

In addition to the membrane properties of generator neurons, intercellular interactions also make important contributions to the organization of the temporal pattern of rhythmical movements. For example, although intrinsic mechanisms exist for termination of bursting discharges in the isolated group 1 interneurons from the feeding CPG in *Planorbis* (see figures 10.2B, 2, and 10.2B, 3), during normal CPG functioning, burst termination in these neurons is caused by inhibitory inputs from the group 2 interneurons (figure 10.4C). A similar situation can be observed in the stomatogastric pyloric and gastric CPGs.

Shaping the Pattern of the Motor Output

The shaping of motor output in terms of burst sequences is mainly determined by the interactions of generator neurons with each other and with output neurons. The organization of the circuits appears to be quite distinct for different CPGs, although all circuits have variations of the same fundamental synaptic connections. The differences in circuit organization may exist because of differences in the mechanical properties of the peripheral motor apparatus: the simpler a movement is, the simpler is the organization of intercellular connections. In CPGs that produce monophasic activity (e.g., the crustacean cardiac CPG), there are only excitatory intercellular connections that determine the synchronous activity of the whole system. In contrast, the pattern of biphasic swimming movements in mollusks *Clione* and *Tritonia* is mainly determined both by excitatory connections between synergistic neurons and by inhibitory interconnections between antagonistic neurons (see figures 10.4A and 10.4B). Even within the CPGs that underlie biphasic movements, however, additional mechanisms contribute to reliable alternation between the two phases of the cycle.

One mechanism that contributes to reliable alteration is delayed excitation of antagonistic neurons that exist in parallel with inhibitory interconnections. Excitatory connections between antagonistic neurons were found in the swimming CPGs of *Clione* and *Tritonia* (figures 10.4A and 10.4B). In *Clione*, a simple CPG organization (two groups of antagonistic interneurons, 7 and 8e, inhibiting each other) is realized only during "weak" swimming (figure 10.4A). During "intense" swimming, an additional mechanism that includes the high-threshold group 8d interneurons and plateau-generating group 12 interneurons comes into operation (Arshavsky et al., 1985). The interneurons 12 inhibit the group 8 interneurons and activate the group 7 interneurons (figure 10.4A). Consequently, they contribute to the termination of the ventral (V) phase and to the onset of the next dorsal (D) phase. In *Tritonia*, an alternation of the dorsal and ventral flexions is determined by reciprocal inhibition between the dorsal swim interneurons (DSIs) and the ventral swim interneurons (VSIs) (figure 10.4B). In parallel with inhibitory interconnections, an excitatory connection from the DSI to VSI neurons is realized through the interneurons C2, which form multicomponent (excitatory-inhibitory) synapses on the DSIs and excitatory synapses on the VSIs (Getting, 1989; Frost et al., chapter 16, this volume). When starting to fire, the C2s initially contribute to excitation of the DSIs; they then inhibit the DSI activity and promote an excitation of the antagonistic VSI neurons. Thus, in *Clione* and *Tritonia*, although specific mechanisms for the delayed excitation between antagonistic neurons are different, their functional role is the same.

The other mechanism that contributes to reliable transitioning from one cycle phase to another is postinhibitory rebound (see also Calabrese and Feldman, chapter 11, this volume). The excitation of generator neurons active in a given phase of the cycle is facilitated after termination of the inhibitory postsynaptic potential (IPSP) produced by antagonistic interneurons active in the previous phase. The kinetics of the voltage trajectory during postinhibitory rebound plays an important role in determining the onset of the next burst. The rebound phenomenon also contributes to maintaining stable rhythm generation. Thus, mechanisms that determine the rhythmicity of a system and the pattern of the rhythmical activity are tightly interconnected, and their division is rather arbitrary.

The three-phase pattern typical of the feeding motor output in pulmonate mollusks (Arshavsky et al., 1991) is determined by interactions of interneurons of groups 1e, 1d, and 2 (figure 10.4C). In contrast to the swimming CPGs, which have mutual inhibitory connections between antagonistic generator neurons, the feeding CPG essentially has asymmetrical connections between interneurons active in opposite phases of the cycle. Group 1 interneurons exert an excitatory action on group 2 interneurons, whereas the latter inhibit group 1 interneurons. Multiphasic patterns of activity underlying rhythmic movements of the foregut in the crustacea are determined by complex electrical, inhibitory, and excitatory connections between neurons of the pyloric and gastric CPGs (figure 10.4D). In some invertebrate circuits, the motor pattern is formed by nonspiking (graded) interactions between neurons (Raper, 1979; Selverston and Moulins, 1987; Harris-Warrick et al., 1992).

Although isolated CPGs are able to produce the basic spatiotemporal patterns underlying automatic movements, during actual behavior the final motor outputs are strongly influenced by sensory feedback from the peripheral motor apparatus. Due to sensory feedback, motor outputs produced by CPGs adapt to environmental variations (Pearson, 1993; Pearson and Ramirez, chapter 21, this volume). The more variable are the conditions for executing a given movement, the greater the role played by sensory mechanisms in forming the motor output. Feedback signal efficiencies are not constant; instead, they are regulated by higher centers in relation to the motor task. In addition, CPGs themselves regulate feedback efficiency depending on the cycle phase due to presynaptic inhibition of primary afferents (Cattaert et al., 1992; Nusbaum et al., chapter 22, this volume). Sensory feedback may also have a modulatory function by acting for longer periods on metabotropic receptors located on generator neurons in the CPG (Harris-Warrick et al., chapter 19, this volume).

Reliability

Descriptions of CPG organization demonstrate that CPGs are highly reliable systems. Everything that is crucial for stable rhythm generation (e.g., origin of rhythmicity, factors determining the duration of cycle phases, and transition from one phase to another) is determined by not one but several complementary factors acting in concert. The redundancy within the CPGs guarantees their high reliability and adaptability to different conditions as well as their resistance to accidental local damage. For example, the pyloric and gastric CPGs from the crustacean stomatogastric system continue to produce rhythmical activity and a recognizable pattern even after the elimination of some neurons or connections that seem to be important for CPG operation (Miller and Selverston, 1982; Harris-Warrick et al., 1992). In *Clione*, the alternating activity of antagonistic neurons is preserved even after blockading the inhibitory connection from group 8 to group 7 interneurons—one of the kernel connections within the swimming CPG (Panchin et al., 1995).

Command Neurons

Because basic patterns of motor output produced by CPGs are determined by their internal organization, CPGs can be switched into the active state by a simple unpatterned command. We use the term *command neuron* to designate higher level neurons, excitation of which activates or suppresses a CPG. In some cases, command neurons act by changing the membrane potential of CPG neurons. More commonly, command neurons act by changing membrane properties of generator neurons. They transform conditional bursters that constitute a CPG from a passive to a rhythm-generating state. In addition, command neurons affect intercellular connections within a CPG. Thus, command neurons can be regarded as types of modulatory neurons (Harris-Warrick et al., chapter 19, this volume). Command neurons are activated by external signals (e.g., danger) or by a change of internal state (e.g., motivational state) of the organism. The effects of command neuron activation are not fixed but depend on the state of the motor system. For example, stimulation of the same command neuron in the cockroach triggers either the running or the flying CPG depending on whether or not the legs are in contact with the substrate (Ritzmann et al., 1980).

CPGs Controlled by a Number of Command Neurons Using Different Neurotransmitters

The multiplicity of command neurons has been shown in studies of the crustacean stomatogastric system (Nagy and Dickinson, 1983; Nusbaum and Marder, 1989; Harris-Warrick et al., 1992 and chapter 19, this volume). The pyloric and gastric CPGs located in the stomatogastric ganglion produce rhythmical activity only if the ganglion is connected with anterior centers located in the commissural ganglia. Therefore, rhythmical activity in the CPGs is triggered and maintained by inputs from command neurons located in the commissural ganglia. Several command neurons that trigger the pyloric and gastric rhythms were identified: a cholinergic neuron, a proctolinergic neuron, and several neurons with unknown transmitters. In addition, cholecystokinin (CCK)-containing

fibers were identified in the stomatogastric nerve. Correspondingly, generation of the pyloric and gastric rhythms in the isolated stomatogastric ganglion can be triggered or altered by applying different neurotransmitters.

Multiple command neurons seem to be a common phenomenon. In mollusks, different neurons that initiate the feeding CPG have been identified (Croll et al., 1985). Correspondingly, the feeding CPG can be switched on by serotonergic (Gillette and Davis, 1977) and GABAergic mechanisms (Arshavsky et al., 1993a). In *Clione*, the swimming CPG is activated by both serotonergic and nonserotonergic cerebropedal neurons (Arshavsky et al., 1985, 1993b; Panchin et al., 1996).

Command Neurons and Chemical Signaling

Based on results obtained with invertebrates, Horridge (1961) suggested the existence of two types of signaling in the CNS: anatomically addressed and chemically addressed (paracrine transmission) signaling. In the latter case, presynaptic fibers do not form synapses on target cells but release a transmitter into some area of the neuropile, affecting all neurons in the immediate area that are susceptible to the transmitter. Chemical signaling seems to be used by modulatory neurons, including command neurons, that affect the whole population of neurons forming a CPG and that do not require exact (point-to-point) addressing. Indirect support for this hypothesis was obtained in *Clione* (Arshavsky et al, 1988). In the isolated CNS, the swimming CPG often works irregularly when bouts of the rhythmical activity alternate with periods of "silence." The bouts of rhythmical activity are caused by spontaneous excitation of command neurons. It was shown that the activity of pedal neurons, which were physically isolated and then manually reinserted into the ganglion, changed in relation to "locomotor bouts," suggesting that command neurons release transmitters in concentrations sufficient to affect target neurons in the absence of synaptic contacts. These transmitters may thus operate to produce a specific behavior by selecting the appropriate neurons and modifying their cellular and synaptic properties.

Integrative Role of Command Neurons

In many cases, the effect of command neurons is not restricted to one CPG system but can influence other systems as well. The simplest example of such influence has been obtained in studying the neural mechanisms of swimming in *Clione*. Serotonergic command neurons that activate the swimming CPG simultaneously activate the heart-exciting neuron (Arshavsky et al., 1992), which ensures coordination of the locomotor and circulatory systems. Command neurons with more complex integrative functions have been found in molluskan feeding behavior. In *Aplysia*, the command neurons from the cerebral ganglia initiate the feeding CPG and simultaneously affect neurons involved in the control of feeding posture (Teyke et al., 1990; Kupfermann et al., chapter 20, this volume). In *Clione*, the "cerebral hunting interneuron" exerts a widespread action on different systems involved in hunting behavior (Arshavsky et al., 1993b): in addition to activating the swimming CPG, it excites tentacle muscle motoneurons and affects statocyst receptors, thus ensuring changes in spatial orientation during hunting.

Inhibitory Command Neurons

In addition to excitatory command neurons that initiate activity of CPGs, there are also *inhibitory command neurons* in many invertebrates. Activation of inhibitory command neurons results in prompt termination of CPG activities. Although the function of these neurons is as important as that of excitatory command neurons, they have not been studied in as much detail. In some cases, inhibitory command neurons produce short-term effects due to hyperpolarization of generator neurons (Arshavsky et al., 1992). In other cases, inhibitory neurons act in a long-lasting manner, their effects resulting from the suppression of the ability of generator neurons to produce an endogenous rhythm (Cazalets et al., 1987). These inhibitory command neurons can thus also be regarded as types of modulatory neurons.

CPGs Send Signals of Their Activity to Higher Centers

Higher centers involved in motor control receive input signals not only from proprioceptors, but also from elements within the CPGs. These network properties were initially described in cats (Arshavsky et al., 1986). During fictive locomotion and scratching in immobilized cats, ascending signals that carry information about the activity of the spinal CPGs produce rhythmical oscillations in cerebellar and descending tract neurons. Similar phenomena have subsequently been described in many other preparations, including invertebrates (Weiss et al., 1978; Croll et al., 1985; Harris-Warrick et al., 1992). When operating, the CPGs drive rhythmical activity in neurons of anterior ganglia. The rhythmical signals coming from CPGs are involved in different aspects of motor control. In the simplest cases, those signals contribute to

coordination of the activity in different motor centers. For example, in *Clione*, signals from the feeding CPG produce the rhythmical activity of tentacle muscle motoneurons (Arshavsky et al., 1993a), which ensures coordinated movements of the buccal apparatus and tentacles.

In many cases, signals sent by a CPG produce rhythmical activity in neurons that project back to the CPG. Thus, a closed loop emerges between the CPG and neurons of higher centers. During CPG operation, rhythmical signals circulate within the loop. Some researchers have proposed that rhythmically active neurons at higher levels should be regarded as a part of a CPG because they can reset the ongoing rhythm. Rhythmically active neurons of higher centers may participate in stabilizing the CPG, although we do not think that rhythmically active neurons at higher levels should be regarded as CPG neurons. It has been shown that tonic descending inputs are sufficient for driving the CPG (Selverston and Miller, 1980). Arshavsky and colleagues (1986) advanced a hypothesis for the role of rhythmical activity in descending tract neurons based on their studies of motor control in cats. The highest motor centers can influence the spinal CPGs only via descending tracts. Due to the rhythmical oscillation of activity in descending tracts, signals from the highest centers are transmitted to the spinal cord only in definite phases of the cycle. Thus, CPGs regulate a temporal pattern of signals they receive from the highest centers—a "gate mechanism." As a result, the highest centers affect spinal mechanisms without disturbing the basic motor pattern. One can suggest that, in invertebrates, rhythmical oscillations of activity in higher neurons, exerting short-term influences on CPGs, play a similar gating function.

It is more surprising that signals from CPGs can produce rhythmical oscillations of the activity in descending modulatory neurons—for example, in the molluskan giant serotonergic neurons (Weiss et al., 1978) and in modulatory neurons from the crustacean stomatogastric system (Harris-Warrick et al., 1992)—because modulatory neurons trigger a long-lasting cascade of events that overlap the duration of a single cycle. We can hypothesize that neuromodulators are more effective when released in a pulsatile manner rather than continuously.

CPGs as Multifunctional Systems

Currently, it is a truism to say that CPGs are not hardwired circuits, but flexible multifunctional systems capable of producing different motor outputs. Understanding this, to a great extent, came from studies on invertebrates. Modifications in CPG operation can display a wide range of variation within a given "theme" or can totally change a "theme." Three main sources of modification in CPG operation are often interconnected: afferent signals, command and modulatory neurons, and hormonal influences (Pearson, 1993).

In simpler cases, modifications in CPG operation are determined by strengthening the input signals that recruit new network elements. As mentioned previously, a transition from a "weak" to an "intense" mode of operation in *Clione*'s swimming CPG is based on the involvement of two groups of interneurons. In *Tritonia*, a neural network controlling defense reaction includes the low-threshold I neurons that react to a weak stimulus; they produce local withdrawal and simultaneously inhibit interneurons that participate in swimming rhythm generation (Getting, 1989). With stronger stimulation, the C2 neurons begin to fire. They inhibit the I neurons and thus release the network for swimming rhythm generation.

More commonly, different modes of CPG operation are determined by different modulatory influences that modify both cellular properties and intercellular connections. CPGs are usually controlled by a set of command neurons that use different neurotransmitters. As a result, each command neuron produces a specific mode of CPG operation. The system that best illustrates the multifunctionality of CPGs is the crustacean stomatogastric system (Selverston and Moulins, 1987; Harris-Warrick et al., 1992; Harris-Warrick et al., chapter 19, this volume). The pyloric and gastric CPGs can be triggered by identified cholinergic and proctolinergic command neurons as well as by elevated blood levels of CCK. Each input produces a different motor output. Similar results were obtained in other preparations. In mollusks, excitation of different command neurons produces different modes of operation of the feeding CPG, including switching from an ingestion to a rejection pattern (Croll et al., 1985). The CPG controlling ventilation in the crab produces two motor programs that ensure different directions of water flow during gill perfusion. Switching of CPG operation from one mode to another is determined by central command signals (DiCaprio, 1990). The cardiac CPG in the leech produces excitation of heart motoneurons in a rear-to-front progression on one side and synchronous excitation of motoneurons on the other side. This right-left coordination of CPG operation switches every 20–40 cycles, the switch from one to the other mode of operation being controlled by special interneurons (Gramoll et al., 1994). One can

suggest that, in all these examples, as in the crustacean stomatogastric system, command neurons modify membrane properties and synaptic connections of generator neurons, thus producing dramatic changes in CPG operation.

Work on the stomatogastric system has also demonstrated that neuromodulatory substances not only reconfigure specific circuits, but also elicit interactions between functionally diverse circuits in many different ways (Harris-Warrick et al., 1992). It has been shown that neurons do not remain restricted to one CPG but can switch from one to another. For example, the VD neuron (figure 10.4D) can switch from the pyloric to the cardiac sac rhythm when a modulatory neuron is stimulated (Hooper and Moulins, 1989). The peptide, red pigment–concentrating hormone, fuses the gastric mill and cardiac sac pattern into a novel blended pattern (Dickinson et al., 1990). When a modulatory neuron—the pyloric suppressor—is stimulated, neurons from the esophageal, pyloric, and gastric network are combined into an entirely de novo circuit that has been termed a "swallowing" network (Meyrand et al., 1991).

These results have broad implications for our understanding of CPGs and rhythmic motor behavior because they constrain our definition of a CPG. It is now impossible to regard a CPG as separate from its chemical environment. The chemical environment and its action on cellular and synaptic properties is as important in understanding the mechanisms of CPG action as the actual neural circuit.

Conclusion

Box 10.1 summarizes the main conclusions on the functional organization and the role of CPGs in motor control. During the last 20 years, our notions concerning the functioning of CPGs have changed radically, largely due to results obtained on invertebrates. Originally, the dominant point of view was that CPGs were hardwired networks formed by uniform, "digital" elements; the source of the rhythmical activity was an interaction between the elements, which by themselves were not capable of rhythmical activity. It is now evident that CPGs are formed by complex elements capable of generating prolonged action potentials, bursting potentials, plateau potentials, and so on. What is especially important is that some generator neurons are constitutive or conditional pacemakers whose endogenous activity underlies rhythm generation. Spatiotemporal organiza-

Box 10.1
Invertebrate Contributions to CPG Systems

Functional CPG Neural Circuits   It has been possible to describe the formation of rhythmic motor patterns in terms of the interactions between the identified neurons.

Mechanism of Pattern Formation   Rhythmic motor patterns are a form of spatiotemporal activity that is derived from a combination of oscillator cells and synaptic interactions. The former is due to the presence of constitutive or conditional pacemaker potentials, and the latter to the unique combination of synaptic and electrical connections between neurons in the circuit. In some invertebrate circuits, the principal characteristics of the motor pattern are formed by nonspiking interactions between CPG neurons—that is, by *graded release* of neurotransmitters.

Diversity and Uniformity   Although invertebrate neural circuits have different arrangements of their connections, all circuits use variations of the same fundamental cellular and synaptic properties. Reciprocal inhibition and reciprocal excitation-inhibition are usually the most common connections described. Postinhibitory rebound following inhibition contributes to rhythm generation and to transitions from one phase of the cycle to another.

Redundancy   Everything that is crucial for CPG activity (origin of rhythmicity, factors determining duration of cycle phases and transition from one phase to another, etc.) is based on several mechanisms acting in concert. Some neurons or connections can be removed from circuits without major degradation of the pattern.

Circuit Anatomy   The anatomical connections between neurons in CPG circuits *constrain* the total range of motor patterns observed. Changes in the functional properties of the neurons and synapses, however, permit a wide range of motor patterns within the boundaries set by the anatomical connections and mechanical properties of the peripheral motor apparatus.

Sensory Feedback   Sensory receptors activated by rhythmic movements affect CPG neurons on a cycle-by-cycle basis and therefore determine the final output pattern. The effectiveness of feedback signals is regulated (presynaptic inhibition) by a CPG depending on the cycle phase. In addition, sensory signals are controlled by higher centers. Sensory inputs may also modulate the CPG over a longer period by acting on metabotropic receptors located on CPG neurons (modulatory function).

"Command" Neurons   Command neurons initiate CPG rhythmical activity by changing the membrane potential of constitutive bursters or transforming membrane properties of conditional bursters. Furthermore, they change synaptic interconnections between CPG neurons. Usually the CPGs are under the control of several command neurons that use different transmitters and thus determine different modes of CPG operation. In addition to excitatory command neurons, there are *inhibitory* command neurons that produce prompt termination of the CPG activity. In some cases, command neurons are modulated presynaptically by the same neurons that they are affecting.

Signaling to Higher Centers   CPG timing signals are usually sent to higher control centers, where they rhythmically entrain descending inputs back to CPG neurons. Thus, CPGs control a temporal pattern of signals that they receive from higher centers ("gating mechanism").

Neuromodulatory Control   Neuromodulatory substances, discharged onto CPG circuits either by specific neurons acting in paracrine fashion or released into the bloodstream, alter CPG circuits. These substances usually act on second messenger systems in CPG neurons. By changing cellular and synaptic properties, they produce *functionally* different circuits and therefore different motor output patterns (multifunctional circuits). Not only are specific circuits reconfigured, but neurons can be transposed between one circuit and another to form "blended" circuits or be selected to form entirely de novo circuits.

tion of motor output is determined both by endogenous properties of generator neurons and by their interaction with each other and with output neurons. Thus, the old question of whether CPGs are cell-driven or network-driven oscillators is not topical; network and cellular properties do not exclude but add to each other in generating proper motor output. Cellular properties and intercellular connections are under the control of different command and modulatory neurons as well as hormonal neuromodulators. As a result, the CPGs are flexible systems capable of generating various motor outputs depending on descending signals and local environment. The CPGs send a copy of their activity to higher centers, which contributes to the integration of motor behavior. As described in this and many other chapters of this volume, in spite of great differences in the complexity of nervous systems, some general principles of motor control are common for both invertebrates and vertebrates. Therefore, lessons from the study of invertebrate CPGs are likely to be important in understanding CPGs of vertebrates.

Acknowledgments

This work was supported by NIH grants NS 09322 and NS 25916, by National Science Foundation grant IBN-9222029, by ISF grants MRO 000 and MRO 300, and by the Royal Swedish Academy of Sciences (research grant for Swedish-Russian scientific cooperation).

References

Arshavsky YI, Beloozerova IN, Orlovsky GN, Panchin YV, Pavlova GA (1985) Control of locomotion in marine mollusc *Clione limacina*. 1–4. *Exp Brain Res* 58:255–293.

Arshavsky YI, Deliagina TG, Gamkrelidze GN, Orlovsky GN, Panchin YV, Popova LB, Shupliakov OV (1993a) Pharmacologically induced elements of the hunting and feeding behavior in pteropod mollusk *Clione limacina*. 1. Effect of GABA. *J Neurophysiol* 69:512–521.

Arshavsky YI, Deliagina TG, Gamkrelidze GN, Orlovsky GN, Panchin YV, Popova LB (1993b) Pharmacologically induced elements of the hunting and feeding behavior in pteropod mollusk *Clione limacina*. 2. Effect of physostigmine. *J Neurophysiol* 69:522–532.

Arshavsky YI, Deliagina TG, Gelfand IM, Orlovsky GN, Panchin YV, Pavlova GA, Popova LB (1988) Non-synaptic interaction between neurons in molluscs. *Comp Biochem Physiol* 91C:199–203.

Arshavsky YI, Deliagina TG, Orlovsky GN, Panchin YV (1989) Control of feeding movements in pteropod mollusc *Clione limacina*. *Exp Brain Res* 78:387–397.

Arshavsky YI, Deliagina TG, Orlovsky GN, Panchin YV, Popova LB (1992) Interneurons mediating the escape reaction of the marine mollusc *Clione limacina*. *J Exp Biol* 164:307–314.

Arshavsky YI, Gelfand IM, Orlovsky GN (1986) *Cerebellum and Rhythmical Movements*. Berlin: Springer.

Arshavsky YI, Grillner S, Orlovsky GN, Panchin YV (1991) Central generators and the spatiotemporal pattern of movements. In: *The Development of Timing Control* (Fagard J, Wolff PH, eds.), 93–115. Amsterdam: Elsevier.

Bal T, Nagy F, Moulins M (1988) The pyloric central pattern generator in Crustacea: A set of conditional neuronal oscillators. *J Comp. Physiol* 163:715–727.

Bernstein N (1967) *The Coordination and Regulation of Movements*. Oxford: Pergamon.

Cattaert D, El Manira A, Clarac F (1992) Direct evidence for presynaptic inhibition in crayfish sensory afferents. *J Neurophysiol* 67:610–624.

Cazalets JR, Nagy F, Moulins M (1987) Suppressive control of a rhythmic central pattern generator by an identified modulatory neuron in crustacea. *Neurosci Lett* 81:267–272.

Croll LP, Kovak MP, Davis WJ, Matera EM (1985) Neural mechanisms of motor program switching in the mollusc *Pleurobranchaea*. *J Neurosci* 5:64–71.

DiCaprio RA (1990) An interneurone mediating motor programme switching in the ventilatory system of the crab. *J Exp Biol* 154:517–535.

Dickinson PS, Mecsas C, Marder E (1990) Neuropeptide fusion of two motor pattern generator circuits. *Nature* 344:155–158.

Elson RC, Selverston A (1992) Mechanisms of gastric rhythm generation in the isolated stomatogastric ganglion of spiny lobsters. *J Neurophysiol* 68:890–907.

Getting PA (1989) Emerging principles governing the operation of neural networks. *Ann Rev Neurosci* 12:185–204.

Gillette R, Davis WJ (1977) The role of the metacerebral giant neuron in the feeding behavior of *Pleurobranchaea*. *J Comp Physiol (A)* 116:129–159.

Gola M, Selverston A (1981) Ionic requirements for bursting activity in lobster stomatogastric neurons. *J Comp Physiol* 145:191–207.

Gramoll S, Schmidt J, Calabrese RL (1994) Switching in the activity state of an interneuron that controls coordination of the hearts in the medicinal leech. *J Exp Biol* 186:157–171.

Harris-Warrick RM., Johnson BR (1987) Potassium channel blockade induces rhythmic activity in a conditional burster neuron. *Brain Res* 416:381–386.

Harris-Warrick RM, Marder E, Selverston AI, Moulins M, eds. (1992) *The Stomatogastric Nervous System*. Cambridge, Mass.: MIT Press.

Hooper SL, Moulins M (1989) Switching of a neuron from one network to another by sensory induced changes in membrane properties. *Science* 244:1587–1589.

Horridge GA (1961) The organization of the primitive central nervous system as suggested by the examples of inhibition and the structure of neuropile. In: *Nervous Inhibition* (Florey E, ed.), 395–409. Oxford: Pergamon.

Marder E, Meyrand P (1989) Chemical modulation of an oscillatory neural circuit. In: *Neuronal and Cellular Oscillators* (Jacklet JW, ed.), 317–338. New York: Dekker.

Meyrand P, Simmers J, Moulins M (1991) Construction of a pattern-generating circuit with neurons of different networks. *Nature* 351:60–63.

Miller JP, Selverston AI (1982) Mechanisms underlying pattern generation in lobster stomatogastric ganglion as determined by selective inactivation of identified neurons. 4. Network properties of pyloric neurons. *J Neurophysiol* 48:1416–1432.

Nagy F, Dickinson PS (1983) Control of a central pattern generator by an identified modulatory interneurone in crustacea. I. Modulation of the pyloric motor output. *J Exp Biol* 105:33–58.

Nusbaum MP, Marder E (1989) A modulatory proctolin-containing neuron (MPN). II. State-dependent modulation of rhythmic motor activity. *J Neurosci* 9:1600–1607.

Panchin YV, Arshavsky YI, Deliagina TG, Orlovsky GN, Popova LB, Selverston A (1996) Control of locomotion in marine mollusk *Clione limacina*. 11. Effect of serotonin. *Exp Brain Res* 109:361–365.

Panchin YV, Arshavsky YI, Selverston A, Cleland TA (1993) Lobster stomatogastric neurons in primary culture. *J Neurophysiol* 69:1967–1992.

Panchin YV, Sadreev RI, Arshavsky YI (1995) Control of locomotion in marine mollusk *Clione limacina*. 10. Effects of acetylcholine antagonists. *Exp Brain Res* 106:135–144.

Pearson KG (1993) Common principles of motor control in vertebrates and invertebrates. *Annu Rev Neurosci* 16:265–297.

Perkel DH, Mulloney B (1974) Motor pattern production in reciprocally inhibitory neurons exhibiting postinhibitory rebound. *Science* 185:181–183.

Ramirez JM, Pearson KG (1991) Octopominergic modulation of interneurons in flight system of the locust. *J Neurophysiol* 66:1522–1537.

Raper JA (1979) Nonimpulse-mediated synaptic transmission during the generation of a cyclic motor program. *Science* 205:304–306.

Ritzmann RE, Tobias ML, Fourtner CR (1980) Flight activity initiated via giant interneurons of the cockroach: Evidence for bifunctional trigger interneurons. *Science* 210:443–445.

Selverston AI, Miller JP (1980) Mechanisms underlying pattern generation in lobster stomatogastric ganglion as determined by selective inactivation of identified neurons. 1. Pyloric system. *J Neurophysiol* 44:1102–1121.

Selverston AI, Moulins M, eds. (1987) *The Crustacean Stomatogastric System*. Berlin: Springer.

Tazaki K, Cooke IM (1990) Characterization of Ca current underlying burst formation in lobster cardiac ganglion motorneurons. *J Neurophysiol* 63:370–384.

Teyke T, Weiss KR, Kupfermann I (1990) An identified neuron (CPR) evokes neuronal responses reflecting food arousal in *Aplysia*. *Science* 247:85–87.

Weiss KR, Cohen JL, Kupfermann I (1978) Modulatory control of buccal musculature by a serotonergic neuron (metacerebral cell) in *Aplysia*. *J Neurophysiol* 41:181–203.

11

Intrinsic Membrane Properties and Synaptic Mechanisms in Motor Rhythm Generators

Ronald L. Calabrese and
Jack L. Feldman

Abstract

Our research has focused on the cellular, synaptic, and network mechanisms of rhythmic motor pattern formation and its modulations for the automatic functions of heartbeat in leeches and respiration in mammals. The rhythmic activity that drives these patterns is generated by a network of interneurons, then elaborated into a functional motor pattern through the interaction of the neural oscillators with premotor interneurons and motoneurons. The intrinsic membrane properties and synaptic interactions of the component neurons of leech heartbeat and mammalian respiratory neural oscillators are widely applicable to the oscillators found in other motor pattern-generating networks. The first part of this review focuses on the intrinsic membrane properties that promote oscillation in all motor pattern generators with special reference to examples from neurons that program leech heartbeat. Although the mechanisms by which rhythmic activity is translated into a functional motor pattern are not well understood in any system, considerable progress is being made in the mammalian respiratory system. The second part of the review focuses on how oscillatory activity is elaborated into a precise motor pattern in the mammalian respiratory system by synaptic mechanisms that control the synaptic drive to and the excitability of motoneurons.

Intrinsic Membrane Properties

Some neurons are capable of producing rhythmic bursts of impulses that can drive oscillation in neuronal networks. The best characterized motor pattern generator possessing such neurons is the pyloric network of the crustacean stomatogastric ganglion (Harris-Warrick et al., 1992, and chapter 19, this volume; Harris-Warrick, 1993; Selverston et al., chapter 10, this volume). According to the modulatory state of the ganglion, each pyloric neuron may burst endogenously, although one or more of an electrically coupled group of three neurons usually act as bursting pacemakers. The pacemaker neurons are imbedded in a network of inhibitory synaptic connections with other pyloric neurons that are themselves bursters or have complex intrinsic membrane properties, including the ability to produce plateau potentials. The interactions of the pacemaker neurons with the other neurons strongly influence the final pyloric pattern that is produced, in terms of both period and phase relations among the participating neurons. Thus, network interactions play a defining role even in a system that has been considered to be dominated by bursting pacemakers. Recent experimental and modeling studies have emphasized the dynamic regulation of bursting properties in this system (Siegel et al., 1994; Turrigiano et al., 1995; Marder et al., chapter 13, this volume). Crab stomatogastric ganglion neurons in primary cell culture undergo a progressive change from being relatively inexcitable, to producing large action potentials upon depolarization with injected current, to spontaneous (or inducible with current injection) bursting over the course of four days. Several ionic currents were identified in these neurons using a two-electrode voltage-clamp technique. The assumption of the bursting phenotype is associated with an increase in inward current densities and a decrease in outward current densities; modeling studies indicate that such changes in current densities are sufficient to explain the changes in cellular properties. These results indicate that ionic conductances are dynamically regulated in neurons and that the regulation may be associated with the activity state of neurons in situ.

Rhythmically active interneurons (Arshavsky et al., 1993; Selverston et al., chapter 10, this volume) are found in the nearly continuously active swim pattern generator of the pelagic mollusk *Clione*, and such activity is gated by sensory input in the spinal interneurons that pace the swimming motor pattern in early stage tadpoles of *Xenopus* (Arshavsky et al., 1993; Roberts et al., chapter 7, this volume). Rhythmic activity is elicited in nonspiking interneurons in the lamprey spinal cord by NMDA, which also gates the swimming motor pattern (Grillner et al., 1991; Wallén, chapter 6, this volume). In these systems, reciprocally inhibitory connections among interneurons are thought to predominate in pacing rhythmic activity. For example, in *Clione*, dorsal- and ventral-phase swim interneurons form reciprocally inhibitory synapses; neurons from each population are capable of producing endogenous rhythmic activity when isolated from the nervous system. If inhibitory transmission from the ventral-phase swim interneurons to the dorsal-phase interneurons in the intact isolated nervous system is blocked (Panchin et al., 1995), both populations continue to alternate, albeit at a somewhat lower frequency, which has been interpreted to indicate that endogenous pacemaking by the interneurons is the dominant mechanism for rhythm generation. Although these experiments reveal endogenous pacemaking capabilities, the period change associated with blockade of one half of the reciprocal inhibitory interaction suggests that the synaptic interactions are crucial in pacing the

rhythm. In the leech heartbeat pattern generator, two reciprocally inhibitory pairs of rhythmically active interneurons pace the heartbeat fictive motor program. Blockade of the inhibitory synapses between the neurons with bicuculline leads to tonic firing (Schmidt and Calabrese, 1992, see also figure 11.3A), thus indicating that in this system reciprocal inhibition is necessary for oscillation.

Both endogenous membrane properties intrinsic to individual neurons and synaptic interactions contribute to the generation of motor rhythms. It is important, therefore, to understand in detail all of the basic membrane properties that contribute to rhythmicity. Such widespread membrane phenomena as endogenous bursts, plateau potentials, and sag potentials are important contributors (Getting, 1989; Marder, 1991; Pearson and Ramirez, 1992; Wang and Rinzel, 1995). In the context of neuronal networks with reciprocally inhibitory neurons, postinhibitory rebound is also often considered a basic membrane characteristic that promotes oscillation (Roberts and Tunstall, 1990; Friesen, 1994; Selverston et al., chapter 10, this volume).

Membrane Bistability, Plateau Potentials, and Action Potentials

If neurons possess voltage-gated inward currents that do not inactivate, they can have a bistable membrane potential: one level situated below the activation level for the inward current and one level situated where the inward current is activated. Transition between the two can be brought about from the lower level by transient depolarization and from the upper level by transient hyperpolarization. The expression of membrane bistability depends on the maximal conductance, steady-state activation properties, kinetics, and reversal potential of *both* the inward current and the available voltage-gated outward currents. In some neurons, such bistability is expressed only when outward currents are blocked.

Plateau potentials are regenerative depolarizations. Plateau potentials, unlike action potentials, do not function in long-distance axonal conduction, but serve to regulate neuronal excitability and synaptic transmission. Most plateau potentials are relatively long-lasting (tens of milliseconds to seconds in duration) and are a special case of membrane bistability (Marder, 1991). During a plateau potential, an inward current may inactivate slowly or an outward current—e.g., a Ca^{2+}-activated K^+ current—may slowly develop. The membrane bistability is thus transient; that is, plateau potentials are terminated by inactivation and/or repolarization by outward currents. If the underlying inward current inactivates relatively rapidly, such potentials are sometimes called "spikes," even though much faster Na$^+$ spikes (action potentials) ride atop them. Action potentials, plateau potentials, and membrane bistability form a continuum with only arbitrary subdivisions. We refer to all regenerative phenomena that range from temporally stable membrane bistability to rapid Na$^+$ action potentials as *plateau potentials*. Multiple current mechanisms can contribute to plateau formation in a given neuron.

Plateau potentials are generally thought to provide the excitatory drive for burst formation during pattern generation. Intrinsic bursting can indeed be thought of as repetitive plateau formation—that is, much like intrinsic repetitive spike production in spontaneously active neurons (Wang and Rinzel, 1995). To the extent that spontaneous impulse activity is regular, with constant inter-impulse intervals, we consider the neuron a beating pacemaker; if spontaneous bursting (i.e., plateau formation) is regular, the neuron is a bursting pacemaker. The ability to produce plateau potentials does not establish that such potentials occur during normal activity, however; rather, they indicate the presence of a sustained inward current that can provide voltage-dependent excitatory drive to the system. The inward currents that mediate plateau potentials can be modulated so that plateau potentials may be produced only in the proper physiological context. NMDA-gated channels can provide sustained excitatory drive in the larval *Xenopus* (Arshavsky et al., 1993; Roberts et al., 1995, and chapter 7, this volume) and lamprey (Grillner et al., 1991; Wallén, chapter 6, this volume) swim motor pattern generators because their voltage-dependent properties endow them with the ability to produce membrane bistability or plateau potentials.

Examples from our own work illlustrate these ideas. Certain neurons in the pre–Bötzinger complex of the neonatal rat brain stem in vitro produce rhythmic plateau potentials that appear to pace the fictive respiratory motor pattern (Smith et al., 1991; Smith, chapter 9, this volume). When rapidly released from hyperpolarized membrane potentials, leech heartbeat oscillator interneurons can produce sustained plateaus that support high-frequency bursts of action potentials; the plateaus do not occur when the oscillator interneurons are depolarized from their normal (i.e., uninhibited) membrane potential (see figures 11.1B and 11.1C; Arbas and Calabrese, 1987a). The plateaus produce strong graded inhibition of the opposite neuron; in addition, they support high-frequency spiking and, in turn, strong spike-mediated inhibition of the opposite cell (see figure 11.1C; Arbas and Calabrese, 1987b). Low-threshold, relatively slowly

inactivating Ca^{2+} currents, which are substantially inactivated at rest, produce the plateaus and the graded synaptic inhibition (Angstadt and Calabrese, 1991). Within the context of normal rhythmic activity, this inactivation is partially removed by inhibition. Low-threshold Ca^{2+} currents are thus available to help sustain burst formation and graded synaptic inhibition, although regenerative plateaus are not produced during each cycle (see figure 11.1C, 2). The oscillator heart interneurons also possess a persistent Na$^+$ current, whose regenerative properties are revealed when outward currents are blocked by internal TEA injection. Under these conditions, the neurons produced sustained plateaus that reach such depolarized levels that no spikes are produced (Opdyke and Calabrese, 1994). The plateaus are mediated by the persistent Na$^+$ current because they also occur when Ca^{2+} currents are blocked with Co^{2+}. With large doses of TEA, the membrane becomes bistable. The normal function of the persistent Na$^+$ current appears to sustain spiking in the absence of excitatory drive, not in plateau formation per se.

Sag Potentials

A sag potential is a slowly developing relaxation in membrane potential following hyperpolarization. It is generated by the hyperpolarization-activated inward current, I$_h$, that paces the vertebrate cardiac rhythm (DiFrancesco and Noble, 1989). I$_h$ is slow to activate and also relatively slow to deactivate. Neurons with a strong I$_h$ can escape from sustained inhibition and return to firing level. Because of its slow deactivation, I$_h$ persists long enough after the resumption of the depolarized level to provide some extra excitatory drive. Thus, in neurons of motor pattern generators as well as in cardiac muscle cells, I$_h$ can act as a rhythmic pacemaker. Our own work illustrates these points. Leech heartbeat oscillator neurons produce pronounced sag potentials; I$_h$ appears to play an important role in producing oscillation of the reciprocally inhibitory interneurons (Angstadt and Calabrese, 1989). Blocking the I$_h$ current and its associated sag potential with external Cs$^+$ disrupts oscillation and thus produces tonic firing or sporadic bursting.

Plateau potentials and I$_h$ can interact to generate oscillations. For example, thalamocortical neurons produce sleep-state dependent oscillations in mammals (Steriade et al., 1993; Sejnowski et al., 1995) because they possess inactivating, low-threshold (T-like) Ca^{2+} currents that produce plateau potentials when they are released from hyperpolarized levels and also have a well-developed I$_h$. Exposure to sleep-state dependent transmitters hyperpolarizes the neurons by activating a K$^+$ leak current so

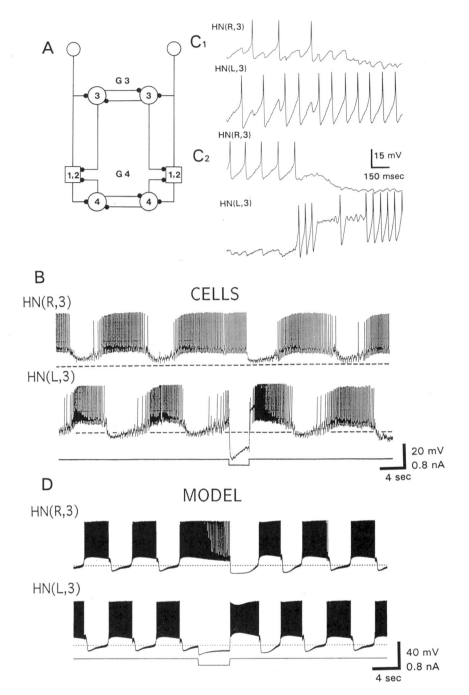

Figure 11.1

(A) Circuit diagram showing inhibitory connections among heart (HN) interneurons that pace fictive heartbeat in the leech. Cells are indexed by ganglion number and body side in this and in figures 11.2 and 11.3. The HN cells of the third and fourth segmental ganglia make reciprocal inhibitory connections across the ganglionic midline, and each pair constitutes an independent neural oscillator. The oscillators are coordinated through their connections with the HN(1) and HN(2) interneurons, which are here lumped together because they are functionally equivalent. (B) Typical alternate bursting activity of a pair of oscillator interneurons in an isolated ganglion in normal saline. The HN(L,3) cell

responds to a hyperpolarizing current pulse with a pronounced sag potential; it has a robust plateau and intense impulse burst upon release from the current pulse. The plateau is so intense that spikes are inactivated for a brief period, and associated with the plateau is strong graded inhibition of the opposite HN(R,3) neuron. (C) The transition to a burst in the HN(L,3) cells and the corresponding synaptic inhibition in the opposite HN(R,3) neurons during normal oscillation and following a hyperpolarizing pulse. (D) Model of HN oscillator neurons displays similar activity and responses to hyperpolarizing pulses as the real HN oscillator neurons. Dashed lines indicate −50 mV.

that they are brought into a range where inactivation is removed from the low-threshold Ca^{2+} current and I_h is activated. I_h rapidly depolarizes the neuron to a level at which a Ca^{2+} plateau is generated, producing a burst of spikes. The plateau deactivates I_h, but it also relatively quickly inactivates; the membrane potential is again driven to the hyperpolarized levels that reinitiate the oscillatory cycle by the K^+ leak current. In this system, the hyperpolarizing drive necessary to activate I_h (so that is acts as a pacemaker current and inactivation is removed from low-threshold Ca^{2+} currents) is provided by the K^+ leak current. In contrast, in reciprocally inhibitory networks, the hyperpolarizing drive is provided by synaptic inhibition. In the appropriate sleep state, the thalamocortical neurons can indeed be considered bursting pacemakers.

Postinhibitory Rebound

Postinhibitory rebound is a tendency of neurons to show increased excitability following inhibitory input (Friesen, 1994). Attempts to define it more precisely are fraught with difficulty because many mechanisms can contribute to it. One possible mechanism is that inhibitory hyperpolarization deinactivates an inward current so that release from inhibition produces a regenerative depolarization (action potential or plateau potential), which eventually subsides (due to inactivation), and the neuron returns to rest (see figure 11.2A). Another possible mechanism involves I_h. Here, the hyperpolarization associated with inhibition activates I_h, and, upon termination of the inhibition, the lingering effects of I_h increase excitability (see figure 11.2C). Other mechanisms for producing postinhibitory rebound are possible—e.g., deactivation of a slow outward current by hyperpolarization.

Experiments in many laboratories have been performed in which hyperpolarizing current pulses are injected into a neuron, for example, the heartbeat oscillator interneurons in the leech illustrated in figure 11.2. Upon termination of the pulses, the neuron responds by producing a plateau potential or action potential(s), which is taken as evidence for postinhibitory rebound. According to this criterion, the leech heartbeat oscillator interneurons show strong postinhibitory rebound. Such experiments can be misleading in terms of the normal activity of rhythmically active neurons, however, because inhibition may not act like a hyperpolarizing current pulse. If inhibition is not strongly hyperpolarizing or wanes slowly (as it does in the leech heartbeat oscillator interneurons), then its ability to remove inactivation from inward currents, to deactivate outward currents, or to

activate I_h will be compromised (see figure 11.1). These points are illustrated by the experimental analysis and recent modeling studies of leech heartbeat oscillator interneurons.

Several ionic currents have been identified in leech heartbeat oscillator interneurons using a single-electrode voltage-clamp technique. In addition to the fast Na^+ current that mediates spikes, these currents include two low-threshold Ca^{2+} currents—one rapidly inactivating (I_{CaF}) and one slowly inactivating (I_{CaS}) (Angstadt and Calabrese, 1991); three outward currents—a fast transient K^+ current (I_A) and two delayed rectifier-like K^+ currents, one inactivating (I_{K1}) and one persistent (I_{K2}) (Simon et al., 1992); a hyperpolarization-activated inward current—a mixed Na^+/K^+ current, $E_{rev} = -20$ mV (I_h) (Angstadt and Calabrese, 1989); a low-threshold persistent Na^+ current (I_p) (Opdyke and Calabrese, 1994); and a leakage current—$E_{rev} = -52$ mV (I_L) (Nadim et al., 1995). The inhibition between oscillator interneurons consists of a graded component associated with the low-threshold Ca^{2+} currents (Angstadt and Calabrese, 1991) and a spike-mediated component that appears to be mediated by an uncharacterized high-threshold Ca^{2+} current (Simon et al., 1994). Spike-mediated transmission is sustained even at the high spike frequency observed during normal bursting, whereas graded transmission wanes during a burst owing to the inactivation of low-threshold Ca^{2+} currents. As mentioned above, blockade of synaptic transmission with bicuculline leads to tonic activity in oscillator heart interneurons (Schmidt and Calabrese, 1992); Cs^+, which specifically blocks I_h, leads to tonic activity or sporadic bursting (Angstadt and Calabrese, 1989).

A model based on these data has been recently formulated by Nadim, Olsen, and colleagues (Nadim et al., 1995; Olsen et al., 1995). Each model neuron consists of a single electrical compartment, and each voltage-gated current is represented using standard Hodgkin-Huxley equations (Hodgkin and Huxley, 1952). Spike-mediated and graded synaptic interactions are conductance based. Each presynaptic spike elicits a conductance increase in the postsynaptic cell with a double exponential time course. For graded synaptic transfer, postsynaptic conductance is a function of presynaptic Ca^{2+} build-up and decline, via low-threshold Ca^{2+} currents and a Ca^{2+} removal mechanism respectively (De Schutter et al., 1993). Free parameters in the model are the maximal conductance for each current (voltage-gated or synaptic). The maximal conductances were adjusted to be close to the average observed experimentally. The reversal potential

Intrinsic Membrane Properties and Synaptic Mechanisms

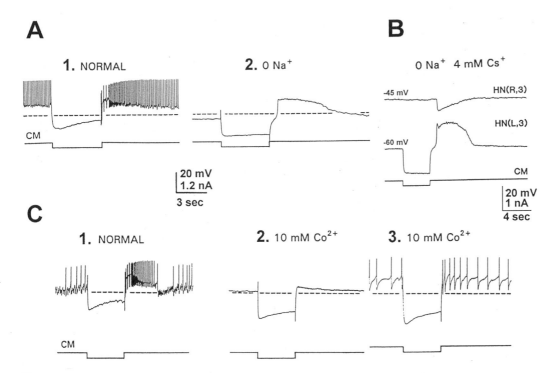

Figure 11.2

Independence of plateau and sag potentials, and plateau-mediated graded inhibition in heart (HN) interneurons. Sag and plateau potentials were evoked with hyperpolarizing current pulses; plateaus cannot be evoked with depolarizing current pulses unless the HN interneuron is hyperpolarized below −50 mV. (A) In HN interneurons, sag potentials are greatly reduced in 0 Na$^+$ saline (2) compared to normal saline (1) but plateau potentials are not. (B) In HN interneurons, sag potentials are completely blocked in 0 Na$^+$ 4 mM Cs$^+$ saline but robust plateau potentials can still be evoked that produce strong graded inhibition of the opposite HN oscillator interneuron. (C) In HN interneurons, Co^{2+} blocks plateau potential formation, regardless of whether the cell is held at rest (2) or above action potential threshold (3), but has no effect on sag potentials (1, response of the HN neuron in normal saline). A small residual depolarization associated with the sag potential is visible at the end of the current pulses in 2. This depolarization results in an increased spike frequency at the end of the current pulse in 3. The Na$^+$-mediated plateaus mentioned in the text can be evoked in 10 mM Co^{2+} saline only if outward currents are blocked with intracellular TEA injection. Dashed lines indicate −50 mV.

for each current was also determined experimentally and considered fixed. Even with these constraints on parameters, the model has myriad realizations, all of which produce stable oscillations. For the purpose of model analysis, it was necessary to settle on a canonical set of parameters, which produced oscillations that appeared most closely to approximate the biological system. Final selection of parameters to form the canonical model was dictated by model behavior under control conditions, passive response of the model to hyperpolarizing current pulses, and reaction of the model to current perturbations (see figure 11.1D). The model cells were also required to fire tonically when all inhibition between them was blocked (see figure 11.3A) because the real neurons fire tonically in bicuculline (Schmidt and Calabrese, 1992).

The canonical model generates activity that closely approximates the activity observed for a reciprocally inhibitory pair of oscillator interneurons (see figure 11.1D).

Analysis of current flows during this activity indicates that graded transmission occurs only at the beginning of the inhibitory period, which acts to turn off the opposite neuron. Sustained inhibition of the opposite neuron is all spike mediated (Olsen et al., 1995). The inward currents in the model neurons act to overcome this inhibition and to force a transition to the burst phase of oscillation. In particular, I_h is slowly activated by the hyperpolarization-associated inhibition and thus adds a delayed inward current that drives the activation of both the I_P and eventually the low-threshold Ca^{2+} currents (I_{CaS} and I_{CaF}). These inward currents support burst formation. Because it does not inactivate, I_P provides steady depolarization to sustain spiking. The low-threshold Ca^{2+} currents help force the transition to the burst phase and provide graded inhibition to silence the opposite neuron, but they inactivate as the burst proceeds. Outward currents, especially the I_{KS}, also play important roles. I_{K2}, which activates and deactivates relatively slowly and

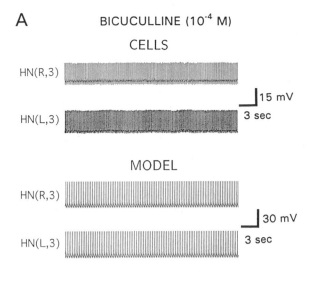

A

BICUCULLINE (10^{-4} M)

CELLS

HN(R,3)

HN(L,3)

|15 mV

3 sec

MODEL

HN(R,3)

HN(L,3)

|30 mV

3 sec

does not inactivate, regulates the depolarization that underlies the burst; whereas I_{K1}, which activates and deactivates relatively quickly and does inactivate, controls spike frequency.

Under canonical conditions, plateau formation (postinhibitory rebound) and associated graded transmission is greatly suppressed. Analysis of state variables (m and h) for low-threshold Ca^{2+} currents indicates that the removal of inactivation from these currents is not effective during the inhibitory period (Olsen et al., 1995). The membrane potential slowly rises during the period of continuous spike-mediated inhibition due primarily to I_h, thus inactivating the Ca^{2+} currents.

In the canonical model cells, as in the real cells, the potential for plateau production with its associated prolonged and intense graded transmission is revealed upon rebound from a hyperpolarizing pulse (see figure 11.1). Moreover, in the model (as in the real cells) plateau and graded transmission based oscillations occur when spikes are suppressed by reducing external Na^+ (see figure 11.3B). In the absence of sustained spike-mediated inhibition, however, recovery from inhibition (due to I_h and waning graded inhibition) is rapid enough so that Ca^{2+} currents can become regenerative, thus supporting full plateaus and strong graded inhibition.

The generation of oscillations in the leech heartbeat motor pattern generator can therefore be understood as a subtle set of interactions among voltage-gated and synaptic currents via membrane potential and intracellular messengers (e.g., Ca^{2+}). It will be important to examine other oscillatory networks with the same level of detail (see Dale, chapter 8, this volume) to elucidate generalities that may lead to a deeper understanding than conceptions based on simply recording membrane phenomena can offer.

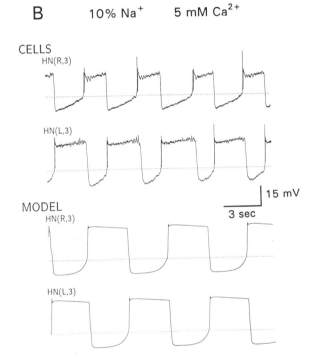

B

10% Na^+ 5 mM Ca^{2+}

CELLS

HN(R,3)

HN(L,3)

MODEL

HN(R,3)

HN(L,3)

|15 mV

3 sec

Figure 11.3

A comparison of the properties of oscillator heart (HN) interneurons of the leech and model oscillator interneurons. (A) Real and model oscillator interneurons fire tonically when the inhibitory synapses between the interneurons are blocked (10^{-4} M bicuculline). (B) Real and model oscillator interneurons produce oscillations based on plateau potentials and graded inhibition in reduced Na^+ elevated Ca^{2+} saline (10% Na^+ 5 mM Ca^{2+}). Note the sustained depolarized plateaus not observed in real or model neurons during oscillations in normal saline (see figure 11.1).

Elaboration of Motor Patterns from Oscillatory Activity: Regulation of Motoneuronal Excitability and Synaptic Drive

All movements require the nervous system to produce a precisely coordinated pattern of neuronal activity, ultimately in motoneurons. For a motoneuron, the relevant activity is the pattern and frequency of action potentials, which influence the force output of the target motor unit. For rhythmic movements, a neural oscillator generates a rhythm, which is then transformed into a regulated pattern of coordinated motoneuronal activity. The impulse activity of motoneurons is determined by their excitability (to synaptic inputs) and by the intensity and dynamics of their synaptic drive, ultimately derived from the neural oscillator. Mechanisms that control the excitability of motoneurons and modulate their synaptic drive will thus have a profound effect on motor output and, in turn, on the intensity and dynamics of movement. Understanding the regulation of rhythmic movements thus requires knowing how the excitability of motoneurons and their synaptic drive are controlled.

Breathing is continuous in mammals and is a useful model for rhythmic movement generation. For breathing movements, the end result is the exchange of metabolic gases (O_2 and CO_2) in the lung, which requires precise control of the motor pattern. Phrenic motoneurons play a key role in the generation of breathing movements; they control the diaphragm, contraction of which typically produces inspiratory air flow (or brakes expiratory air flow). Phonation and defecation are other acts requiring regulation of phrenic motoneuronal activity.

In the past decade, in vitro preparations of the mammalian brain stem and spinal cord have allowed useful studies of the specific role of identified cellular and synaptic properties in controlling neuronal excitability in mammals (Feldman et al., 1991; Funk and Feldman, 1995). An in vitro brainstem and spinal cord preparation that generates breathing rhythm offers many advantages because measurements can be made in neurons while they receive endogenous synaptic drive—in this case, rhythmic respiratory-related input. In these special preparations, spontaneously generated rhythmic membrane depolarizations (due to inward currents) and associated spiking of phrenic motoneurons occur during the inspiratory phase of the respiratory cycle (Liu et al., 1990). The envelope of the spontaneous inspiratory drive potential in a (spiking) phrenic motoneuron has a rapid onset to a peak (approximately 50 msec) followed by a plateau/declining phase that lasts 400–700 msec. The peak potential is approximately 10–20 mV above baseline potential. Superimposed on the drive's slow envelope are faster depolarizing potentials, and the initiation of action potentials occurs along with these fast potentials. When the membrane potential of a phrenic motoneuron is clamped at the end-expiratory potentials (-60 to -75 mV), the peak amplitude of the inspiratory synaptic current is typically approximately 0.8 to 2.5 nA (see figure 11.4). The excitatory postsynaptic current (EPSC) envelope has a similar shape and duration to the synaptic potential, with the basic difference that the current has a much faster rise time due to the need to charge the membrane capacitance when changing potential. Inspiratory drive current in phrenic motoneurons shows a strong voltage dependence (see figure 11.4).

Under single-electrode voltage clamp, the magnitude of the current remains relatively unchanged, with a voltage ranging from -60 to -30 mV, then shows a relatively linear dependence at more depolarized levels, which means that the magnitude of subthreshold postsynaptic potentials are relatively voltage independent. Such nonlinear behavior can have profound consequences in the transformation of synaptic input into a pattern of motoneuronal activity and thus of inspiratory movement of the diaphragm. Of interest is identification of the neurotransmitters and associated receptors that underlie not only the signaling of inspiratory drive to phrenic motoneurons, but also pre- and postsynaptic modulation of that drive.

Transmitter Identification

Glutamate mediates the transmission of inspiratory drive signals from bulbospinal inspiratory neurons onto phrenic motoneurons, thus acting on postsynaptic AMPA, KA, NMDA and metabotropic glutamate receptors (Liu et al, 1990). There is also a presynaptic AP4-sensitive metabotropic glutamate autoreceptor. Combined retrograde labeling of phrenic motoneurons and immunohistochemical detection of putative neuromessengers—for example, 5-HT, NE, substance P, thyrotropin-releasing hormone (TRH), metenkephalin, galanin, neuropeptide Y, peptide YY, vasopressin, cholecystokinin, somatostatin, neurotensin, and vasoactive intestinal polypeptide—reveal multiple neuromessengers within terminal varicosities in the phrenic nucleus (Ellenberger et al., 1992). Substance P, TRH, and metenkephalin are each colocalized with 5-HT within terminal varicosities in the phrenic nucleus and may modulate 5-HT action. The degree of terminal labeling in the phrenic nucleus varies depending on the peptide, and the coincidence of double labeling varies for each peptide colocalized with 5-HT. These results indicate that phrenic motoneuron activity is subject to modulation by many amine and peptide neuromessengers that may alter the responsiveness of phrenic motoneurons to primary excitatory (i.e., glutamate) and inhibitory inputs. This list is unlikely to be exhaustive because many other peptides and combinations of colocalized substances could also be present in the phrenic nucleus.

Why are so many putative neurotransmitters in the terminals of the phrenic nucleus, when this is a "relatively simple" relay for which glutamate is most likely the transmitter of excitatory inspiratory drive (Liu et al., 1990) and GABA is most likely the transmitter underlying inhibition during expiration? We explore below

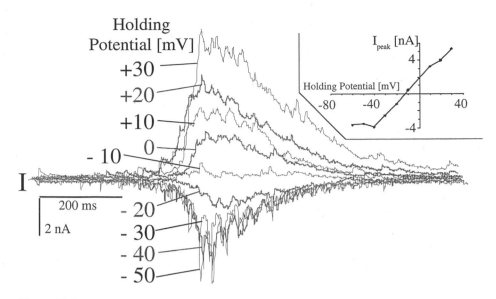

Figure 11.4

Voltage dependence of endogenous inspiratory drive currents in a phrenic motoneuron. Voltage-clamp recordings (holding potentials for each trace as indicated, −50 to +30 mV). (Inset) IV curves of peak inspiratory drive currents. (Modified from Liu and Feldman, 1992.)

some of the possible reasons for this transmitter diversity by highlighting three studies that address the modulation of the excitatory inspiratory drive to phrenic motoneurons.

Pre- and Postsynaptic Effects of Serotonin

(The information here comes from DiPasquale et al., 1992; Lindsay and Feldman, 1993; and figure 7 in Feldman and Smith, 1994.) Exogenous application of serotonin (5-HT) increases inspiratory-modulated phrenic nerve activity and produces a small amount of tonic activity during expiration. Inspiratory-modulated activity of the C4 ventral root also increases. 5-HT, in both normal and TTX-containing medium, depolarizes phrenic motoneurons and increases cell input resistance. It also increases inspiratory-modulated firing as well as the response of phrenic motoneurons to injected current. In contrast to its effect in lumbar motoneurons (Hounsgaard et al., 1988), 5-HT induces no bistable firing behavior in phrenic motoneurons. Under voltage-clamp conditions, 5-HT produces a tonic inward current of 0.1 to 0.4 nA at resting potentials. This current increases with less negative holding potentials and decreases with more negative holding potentials [−75 to −90 mV] but does not reverse. 5-HT decreases inspiratory-modulated synaptic current by approximately 25%, an attenuation unaffected by changes in holding potential. The time course for decrease in the inspiratory-modulated synaptic current is similar to the time courses for changes in tonic inward current and input resistance. Depolarization, tonic in-

ward current, and shift in the f/I relationship produced by 5-HT are antagonized by the 5-HT$_{2/1C}$ receptor antagonist ketanserin and mimicked by the 5-HT$_{2/1C}$ agonist 1(2,5dimethoxy-4-iodophenyl)2-aminopropane HC1 (DOI). However, the 5-HT-induced decrease in the inspiratory-modulated synaptic current is not reduced by ketanserin nor mimicked by DOI. The actions of 5-HT in reducing inspiratory drive appear to be mediated by a presynaptic receptor on bulbospinal inspiratory neurons. Thus, exogenously applied 5-HT simultaneously increases cell excitability and decreases inspiratory-modulated synaptic current in phrenic motoneurons via different receptors.

The combination of these effects means that 5-HT increases the excitability of phrenic motoneurons to all inputs, but decreases inspiratory inputs; this acts to stabilize inspiratory output when there are changes in 5-HT inputs. Perhaps this mechanism is valuable during sleep, when there is a dramatic drop in 5-HT release. Thus, the inspiratory throughput of phrenic motoneurons will be maintained while their excitability to all other inputs is reduced. This example may demonstrate a more general phenomenon of selective control in which the net effect of synaptic drive to motoneurons from one pathway is held constant, whereas general motoneuronal excitability is augmented (Feldman and Smith, 1995).

Pre- and Postsynaptic Effects of Adenosine

(The information here comes from Dong and Feldman, 1995.) Application of the adenosine analogue CPA in the phrenic motoneuron pool reduces whole phrenic nerve discharge and inspiratory-modulated postsynaptic currents of phrenic motoneurons in a dose-dependent manner without affecting the respiratory frequency. Application of the adenosine antagonist (IBMX) has the opposite effect of CPA; IBMX increases inspiratory discharge of the phrenic nerve and inspiratory-modulated synaptic currents of phrenic motoneurons. CPT, a selective A1 receptor antagonist, has similar effects to IBMX and also blocks the effects of CPA.

The relative pre- and postsynaptic contributions to the adenosine-induced decrease in transmission of inspiratory drive were determined by analyzing the frequency and amplitude distribution of spontaneous unitary EPSCs in phrenic motoneurons. Local application of CPA over the phrenic motoneuron pool significantly decreases the frequency of EPSCs during expiratory phase. Whether the observed effects of CPA are a consequence of a direct action on synapses onto phrenic motoneurons was investigated by applying CPA after bath application of TTX. In the presence of TTX, phrenic motoneurons exhibit miniature EPSCs (mEPSCs). CPA produces a significant reduction in mEPSC frequency, an effect consistent with the results obtained from the analysis of EPSCs during the expiratory phase.

The principal finding in these experiments is that adenosine acting at A1 receptors can modulate the synaptic transmission of inspiratory drive to phrenic motoneurons. A1 receptor antagonism increases inspiratory-modulated synaptic currents of phrenic motoneurons, suggesting that an endogenous activation of adenosine receptors reduces synaptic transmission to phrenic motoneurons. Activation of adenosine A1 receptors does not change either the steady-state membrane current or the membrane input resistance of phrenic motoneurons. Inward current induced by exogenously applied glutamate is also unaffected by adenosine receptor agonists. Furthermore, adenosine agonists produce a significant decrease in the frequency of both spontaneous EPSCs and miniature EPSCs, which are glutamatergic (Liu et al., 1990). The reduction of inspiratory drive by adenosine appears to be mediated by A1 receptors on the presynaptic terminals of bulbospinal inspiratory neurons onto phrenic motoneurons. The presynaptic modulation by adenosine may play an important role in adjusting respiratory input to phrenic motoneurons, thus regulating respiratory motor output. This regulatory mechanism may become more critical in preventing the diaphragm from becoming fatigued during high levels of ventilatory drive, such as during extreme exercise, because adenosine levels may

increase under these conditions. This activity-dependent presynaptic control may be used more generally as a governor on synaptic drive in rhythmically active motor networks (Feldman and Smith, 1995).

Role of Desensitization of AMPA Receptors in Determining Postsynaptic Inspiratory Drive

(The information here comes from Funk and Feldman, 1995.) Excitatory synaptic transmission within the vertebrate central nervous system is mediated primarily by NMDA and non-NMDA (AMPA and kainate) glutamate receptor channels. Non-NMDA receptors are primary mediators of fast excitatory transmission, and accordingly their kinetic properties have been the subject of intense study. A prominent feature of AMPA receptors is their rapid desensitization: the time-dependent decay of the current response in the presence of a constant concentration of an (exogenously applied) agonist. Desensitization may modulate the time course and efficacy of endogenous excitatory transmission. Indeed, recently discovered drugs that block desensitization increase the amplitude and, in some cases, decay time constants of AMPA receptor—mediated postsynaptic currents, a result consistent with a role of desensitization in shaping EPSCs. However, the question of whether desensitization has a physiological role in regulating signal transmission in functionally active networks in the CNS remains unanswered.

The role of desensitization in regulating activity of hypoglossal motoneurons was examined in respiratory rhythmic slices of the neonatal rat brain stem. Cyclothiazide (CYT), which reversibly blocks AMPA receptor desensitization, was used to assess the role of desensitization on inspiratory drive to hypoglossal (XII) motoneurons. To establish whether CYT could potentiate synaptic currents to XII motoneurons by acting on postsynaptic glutamate receptors at the inspiratory premotoneuron to XII motoneuron synapse, CYT was applied to the XII motor nucleus while recording (1) currents induced by exogenous application of glutamate with and without TTX, and (2) endogenous synaptic drive currents. Local application of CYT increased the inward currents produced either by spontaneous inspiratory drive (see figure 11.5) or following local application of glutamate. CYT application did not affect the input impedance in any XII motoneuron.

Individual EPSCs that comprise the inspiratory drive current cannot be resolved. However, we were able to examine the effects of CYT on the time constant, amplitude, and interval distributions of small amplitude, spon-

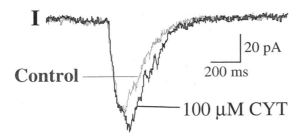

I

Control ——

20 pA

200 ms

——— 100 μM CYT

Figure 11.5
Magnitude of inspiratory drive currents in hypoglossal motoneurons is affected by AMPA receptor desensitization. Comparison under normal in vitro conditions and following removal of desensitization with application of cyclothiazide (CYT). (Modified from figure 5 in Funk and Feldman, 1995.)

taneous EPSCs recorded during the expiratory period to determine whether CYT could potentiate individual EPSCs to XII motoneurons. CYT increased the mean spontaneous EPSC peak amplitude by approximately 15%.

Transmission of respiratory drive from the rhythm-generating network to motoneurons depends on multi-quantal neurotransmitter release during relatively high-frequency bursts at all synapses in the transmission pathway. CYT-induced increases in the net change transfer of inspiratory drive current to motoneurons directly reflect an increase in the charge transfer of individual EPSCs underlying the drive current. The modulation of respiratory frequency and amplitude of motoneuron population discharge by up to 30% would have significant physiological consequences, suggesting that desensitization can have an important role in modulating signal transmission and output from this neural network. Modulation of desensitization may represent another key node for control of neuronal and network activity.

Summary

Although the research each of us performs is on widely different preparations, in both the systems on which we work, and indeed in all well-defined neuronal networks that control rhythmic movements, we can see a strong common thread. Intrinsic membrane properties and synaptic mechanisms interact to impart rhythmic activity to a neural oscillator. Thus, we saw that in the leech heartbeat system both h-current (intrinsic membrane property) and reciprocal inhibition (synaptic interaction) contribute to rhythmicity. This activity is then elaborated into a precise pattern of activity in motoneurons. Mechanisms that influence both the synaptic drive from the neural oscillator to motoneurons and the excitability of the motoneurons themselves thus have a profound influence of the motor pattern produced and ultimately on the movement. Thus, we saw that in the mammalian respiratory system both presynaptic and postsynaptic modulation in multiple forms influences the discharge patterns of motoneurons during breathing.

Acknowledgments

Our work is supported by NIH grants NS24072 (Calabrese), NS34975 (Calabrese), NS24742 (Feldman), HL37941 (Feldman), and HL40959 (Feldman).

References

Angstadt JD, Calabrese RL (1989) A hyperpolarization-activated inward current in heart interneurons of the medicinal leech. *J Neurosci* 9:2846–2857.

Angstadt JD, Calabrese RL (1991) Calcium currents and graded synaptic transmission between heart interneurons of the leech. *J Neurosci* 11:746–759.

Arbas EA, Calabrese RL (1987a) Ionic conductances underlying the activity of interneurons that control heartbeat in the medicinal leech. *J Neurosci* 7:3945–3952.

Arbas EA, Calabrese RL (1987b) Slow oscillations of membrane potential in interneurons that control heartbeat in the medicinal leech. *J Neurosci* 7:3953–3960.

Arshavsky YI, Orlovsky GN, Panchin YV, Roberts A, Soffe SR (1993) Neuronal control of swimming locomotion: Analysis of the pteropod mollusc *Clione* and embryos of the amphibian *Xenopus*. *Trends Neurosci* 16:227–233.

De Schutter E, Angstadt JD, Calabrese RL (1993) A model of graded synaptic transmission for use in dynamic network simulations. *J Neurophysiol* 69:1225–1235.

DiFrancesco D, Noble D (1989) Current I_f and its contribution to cardiac pacemaking. In: *Cellular and Neuronal Oscillators* (Jacklet JW, ed.), 31–58. New York: Dekker.

Di Pasquale E, Morin D, Monteau R, Hilaire G (1992) Serotonergic modulation of the respiratory rhythm generator at birth: An in vitro study in the rat. *Neurosci Lett* 143:91–95.

Dong, X-W, Feldman JL (1995) Modulation of inspiratory drive to phrenic motoneurons by presynaptic adenosine A1 receptors. *J Neurosci* 15:3458–3468.

Ellenberger HH, Vera PL, Feldman JL, Holets VR (1992) Multiple putative neuromessengers inputs to phrenic motoneurons in rat. *J Chem Neuroanat* 5:375–382.

Feldman JL, Smith JC (1995) Neural control of respiratory pattern in mammals: An overview. In: *Lung Biology in Health and Disease*, Vol. 79: *Regulation of Breathing* (Dempsey JA, Pack AI, eds.), 39–69. New York: Dekker.

Feldman JL, Smith JC, Liu G (1991) Respiratory pattern generation: In vitro en bloc analyses. *Curr Opin Neurobiol* 1(4):590–594.

Friesen WO (1994) Reciprocal inhibition: A mechanism underlying oscillatory animal movements. *Neurosci Biobehav Rev* 18:547–553.

Funk GD, Feldman JL (1995) Generation of respiratory rhythm and pattern in mammals: Insights from developmental studies. *Curr Opin Neurobiol* 5:778–785.

Getting PA (1989) Emerging principles governing the operation of neural networks. *Annu Rev Neurosci* 12:184–204.

Grillner S, Wallén P, Brodin L, Lasner A (1991) Neuronal network generating locomotor behavior in lamprey: Circuitry, transmitters, membrane properties, and simulation. *Annu Rev Neurosci* 14:169–199.

Harris-Warrick RM (1993) Pattern generation. *Curr Opin Neurobiol* 3:982–988.

Harris-Warrick RM, Marder E (1991) Modulation of neural networks for behavior. *Annu Rev Neurosci* 14:39–57.

Harris-Warrick RM, Marder E, Selverston AI, Moulins M, eds. (1992) *Dynamic Biological Networks: The Stomatogastric Nervous System.* Cambridge, Mass.: MIT Press.

Hodgkin AL, Huxley AF (1952) A quantitative description of membrane current and its application to conduction and excitation in nerve. *J Physiol (Lond.)* 117:500–544.

Hounsgaard J, Hultborn H, Jespersen B, Kiehn O (1988) Bistability of alpha-motor neurones in the decerebrate cat and in the acute spinal cat after intravenous 5-hydroxytryptophan. *J Physiol (Lond.)* 405:345–367.

Lindsay AD, Feldman JL (1993) Modulation of respiratory activity of neonatav rat phrenic motoneurones by serotonin. *J Physiol (Lond.)* 461:213–233.

Liu G, Feldman JL (1992) Bulbospinal transmission of respiratory drive to phrenic motoneurons. In: *Respiratory Control: Central and Peripheral Mechanisms* (Speck et al., eds.), 47–52. Lexington: University Press of Kentucky.

Liu G, Feldman JL, Smith JC (1990) Excitatory amino acid mediated transmission of inspiratory drive to phrenic motoneurons. *J Neurophysiol* 64:423–436.

Marder E (1991) Plateaus in time. *Curr Bio* 1:326–327.

Nadim F, Olsen ØH, De Schutter E, Calabrese RL (1995) Modeling the leech heartbeat elemental oscillator. I. Interactions of intrinsic and synaptic currents. *J Comput Neurosci* 2:215–235.

Olsen ØH, Nadim F, Calabrese RL (1995) Modeling the leech heartbeat elemental oscillator. II. Exploring the parameter space. *J Comput Neurosci* 2:237–257.

Opdyke CA, Calabrese RL (1994) A persistent sodium current contributes to oscillatory activity in heart interneurons of the medicinal leech. *J Comp Physiol (A)* 175:781–789.

Panchin YV, Sadreev RI, Arshavsky YI (1995) Control of locomotion in marine mollusc *Clione limacina*. X. Effects of acetylcholine antagonists. *Exp Brain Res* 106:135–144.

Pearson KG, Ramirez JM (1992) Parallels with other invertebrate and vertebrate motor systems. In: *Dynamic Biological Networks: the Stomatogastric Nervous System* (Harris-Warrick RM, Marder E, Selverston AI, Moulins M, eds.), 263–281. Cambridge, Mass.: MIT Press.

Roberts A, Tunstall MJ (1990) Mutual reexcitation with postinhibitory rebound: A simulation study on the mechanisms for locomotor rhythm generation in the spinal cord of *Xenopus* embryos. *Eur J Neurosci* 2:11–23.

Roberts A, Tunstall MJ, Wolf E (1995) Properties of networks controlling locomotion and significance of voltage dependency of NMDA channels: Simulation study of rhythm generation sustained by positive feedback. *J Neurophysiol* 73:485–495.

Schmidt J, Calabrese RL (1992) Evidence that acetylcholine is an inhibitory transmitter of heart interneurons in the leech. *J Exp Biol* 171:339–347.

Sejnowski TJ, McCormick DA, Steriade M (1995) Thalamocortical oscillations in sleep and wakefulness. In: *The Handbook of Brain Theory and Neural Networks* (Arbib MA, ed.), 976–980. Cambridge, Mass.: MIT Press.

Siegel M, Marder E, Abbott LF (1994) Activity-dependent current distributions in model neurons. *Proc Natl Acad Sci (USA)* 91:11308–11312.

Simon TW, Opdyke CA, Calabrese RL (1992) Modulatory effects of FMRFamide on outward currents and oscillatory activity in heart interneurons of the medicinal leech. *J Neurosci* 12:525–537.

Simon TW, Schmidt J, Calabrese RL (1994) Modulation of high-threshold transmission between heart interneurons of the medicinal leech by FMRF-NH2. *J Neurophysiol* 71:454–466.

Smith JC, Ellenberger HH, Ballanyi K, Richter DW, Feldman JL (1991) Pre–Bötzinger complex: A brainstem region that may generate respiratory rhythm in mammals. *Science* 254:726–729.

Steriade M, McCormick D, Sejnowski T (1993) Thalamocortical oscillations in the sleeping and aroused brain. *Science* 262:679–685.

Turrigiano G, LeMasson G, Marder E (1995) Selective regulation of current densities underlies spontaneous changes in the activity of cultured neurons. *J Neurosci* 15:3640–3652.

Wang XJ, Rinzel J (1995) Oscillatory and bursting properties of neurons. In: *The Handbook of Brain Theory and Neural Networks* (Arbib MA, ed.), 686–691. Cambridge, Mass.: MIT Press.

12

Organization of Neural Networks for the Control of Posture and Locomotion in an Insect

Malcolm Burrows

Abstract

During locomotion an insect must solve essentially the same problems as a vertebrate although it has an external, rather than an internal, skeleton. Moreover, the nervous system of an alert insect is amenable to analysis of the cellular and synaptic properties of its identified neurons and their dynamic roles in voluntary movements. The networks of neurons responsible for generating and controlling the movements of the legs are distributed; control of one pair of legs is devolved to a segmental ganglion, implying that it contains the necessary set of neurons for the expression of a coordinated leg movement. These local networks are linked by intersegmental neurons so that coordinated gaits are generated and so that postural adjustments are appropriate to movements of the other legs. It is therefore possible to analyze the properties of neurons in one ganglion and ask how they process sensory signals from receptors on a leg and convert them into a change in motor output.

The local circuits controlling locomotion and posture must generate complex but coordinated patterns of spikes (action potentials) in motor neurons so that the limbs are moved in the appropriate sequences. The circuits must also integrate commands from other parts of the central nervous system (CNS) with sensory signals generated in proprioceptors and exteroceptors by the leg movements. The cellular, synaptic, and network properties of the neurons in these circuits are all important factors in generating the underlying motor patterns, as has been revealed in vertebrates (Grillner et al., 1991), crustaceans (Selverston, 1985), insects (Burrows, 1996; Robertson, 1986), molluscs (Getting, 1989), and worms (Kristan, 1983). In this chapter I illustrate some of the general properties of the component neurons and the way they are interconnected by reference to the processing that underlies the control of insect leg movements.

The Component Neurons

Sensory Neurons

Sensory neurons provide many input channels to the CNS, in stark contrast to the few output channels provided by the motor neurons; exteroceptors on a leg, for example, outnumber leg motor neurons by almost 40 times. The majority of sensory neurons have cell bodies in the periphery close to their receptor and axonal projections that carry spikes to the CNS. The spike coding of stimuli by a leg mechanoreceptor is determined by both the mechanics of the receptor and the currents that flow across the membrane of its sensory neuron. Hairs with long, thin shafts and flexible mountings respond to air currents, whereas hairs with short, stout shafts and more rigid mountings respond only to tactile stimulation. Adaptation to a maintained stimulus is, however, caused mainly by processes that lead to the encoding of spikes, in which the slow inactivation of a Na^+ current and at least three K^+ currents are involved (French and Torkkeli, 1994). The signalling may be altered by the release of neuromodulators from neurons that may target receptors specifically.

Within the CNS, the signals of sensory neurons may be further modified by input synapses close to the output synapses on their fine branches. Many of these input synapses show GABA-like immunoreactivity associated with pleomorphic vesicles (Watson, 1992). The output synapses of the mechanosensory neurons have an excitatory action on postsynaptic neurons, probably through the release of acetylcholine. Presynaptic muscarinic receptors reduce the release of acetylcholine and consequently the amplitude of excitatory postsynaptic potentials (EPSPs). In contrast, postsynaptic muscarinic receptors increase excitability by causing a parallel, but slower depolarization to the released acetylcholine so that there are two opposing effects (Trimmer, 1994).

The central projections of the sensory neurons are highly ordered according to some feature of the signal extracted by their particular type of receptor so that their terminals are arranged as maps; this simplifies the way that signals are delivered to the appropriate postsynaptic neurons. The terminals of mechanosensitive exteroceptors, for example, form a spatial map of a leg (Newland, 1991) that corresponds to the branches of particular postsynaptic interneurons that read specific parts of that map (Burrows and Newland, 1993).

Local Interneurons

Local neurons have processes that are restricted to one segmental ganglion and are concerned with integrating signals within that segment, although they are also influenced by signals originating elsewhere. Perhaps 60% of the neurons in a segmental ganglion are spiking or nonspiking local interneurons, and within these two cat-

egories are many groups of neurons with characteristic morphologies and distinctive integrative roles.

Spiking Local Interneurons

Many spiking local interneurons have two distinct regions of branches linked by a thin process. The ventral branches are profuse with a uniform appearance, have predominantly input synapses, and occur in the most ventral and lateral regions of neuropil to which exteroceptive sensory neurons also project. The dorsal branches are sparser and varicose, have predominantly output synapses, and are in regions of neuropil in which leg motor neurons and other interneurons have branches (Siegler and Burrows, 1984; Watson and Burrows, 1985). This anatomy accords with their established synaptic connections; they receive direct synaptic inputs from sensory neurons of leg exteroceptors and make output connections with leg motor neurons and other interneurons. Interneurons in one group contain GABA, and their inhibitory actions can be blocked by drugs that block GABA (Watson and Burrows, 1987). Each interneuron synapses onto many postsynaptic neurons, but the quantal content at the different output synapses ranges from 2 to 10 because of differences in the probability of release (Laurent and Sivaramakrishnan, 1992). Thus, the effectiveness of connections of one interneuron with various postsynaptic neurons is different. The need for a spike in these interneurons must lie in some integrative action determined, at least in part, by the arrangement of the input and output synapses. The simplest scheme would have the inputs in the ventral branches initiate spikes close to the linking process, which would then channel the spikes to the output synapses in the dorsal branches.

Nonspiking Local Interneurons

Nonspiking local interneurons exert a graded control over postsynaptic neurons by the release of unknown transmitters without the intervention of spikes. Their anatomy does not immediately set them apart from spiking local interneurons; their fine neurites are profuse and of uniform appearance, and they overlap the neurites of motor neurons, other interneurons, and some sensory neurons. Input and output synapses are, however, intermingled on all the branches (Watson and Burrows, 1988) so that function might be compartmentalized, with a synaptic input activating neighboring output synapses but not more distant ones.

The membrane of nonspiking local interneurons acts nonlinearly because two voltage-sensitive K^+ channels and possibly a voltage-sensitive Ca^{2+} channel are present. Applied currents cannot depolarize the membrane by more than 10–20 mV above resting potential because of a strong outward rectification (Laurent, 1990). The whole outward current is activated at −60 mV (Laurent, 1991) and consists of a large but rapidly inactivating transient current carried by K^+ and of a later slowly inactivating current, which is also probably carried by K^+. These currents will thus be activated by the normal depolarizing synaptic inputs. The changes in membrane resistance and its time constant caused by activation of the outward K^+ currents affect the frequency response of the membranes and the time course of synaptic inputs. The integrative capacity of a nonspiking interneuron will therefore be highly dependent on its membrane potential. Fast Na^+ currents do not seem to be present, but some nonspiking interneurons produce resonant oscillations and regenerative potentials when depolarized to voltages less than −40 mV due to the activation of a voltage-dependent Ca^{2+} current (Laurent et al., 1993). This Ca^{2+} current is not responsible for regulating transmitter release, but the regenerative responses of the membrane that it causes might boost synaptic potentials in fine branches, which would counteract the shortening of the space constant caused by activation of the K^+ currents. In turn, this might enable a small input to activate nearby output synapses, or it may equalize the synaptic gain over different voltage ranges (Laurent, 1993).

The absence of spikes in these neurons means that the graded changes in membrane potential caused by synaptic inputs must affect intercellular communication. Current injection that simulates these small voltage changes alters the membrane potential of postsynaptic neurons in a continuously graded way (Burrows and Siegler, 1978), and single synaptic potentials are sometimes sufficient to cause transmitter release and to evoke synaptic potentials in postsynaptic neurons (Burrows, 1979).

Intersegmental Interneurons

Intersegmental interneurons have axons that project from one part of the CNS to another, thus providing routes for the transfer of signals between different ganglia. They typically have a cell body and an array of associated neurites in one part of the CNS and an axon that ends in a series of branches in another part, often forming side branches in the intervening ganglia through which it passes. Some have axons that project from one segment only to the neighboring one, largely collating inputs in one segment and delivering output signals to

the next one. By contrast, others have axons that project to many ganglia.

Neuromodulatory Neurons

Neurosecretory neurons release a diversity of amines and peptides, and although their total number may not be large, each can have widespread effects. One group—the so-called efferent Dorsal Unpaired Median (DUM) neurons—is known is some detail. DUM neurons have large cell bodies and bilateral axons that supply muscle and other tissue on both sides of the body. Spikes are generated in each of the two symmetrically arranged neurites that form the axons and are carried primarily by an inward Na^+ current, whereas the cell body can support spikes carried by a mixed Ca^{2+} and Na^+ current (Crossman et al., 1971; Heitler and Goodman, 1978). The fine neurites have input synapses, but only a few sites that might represent output synapses (Watson, 1984), and release sites appear to be largely restricted to the periphery. DUM neurons have not been shown to exert a central effect. They contain (Evans and O'Shea, 1978) and release octopamine (Morton and Evans, 1984), and their peripheral effects can be mimicked by octopamine. When released, octopamine acts on receptors on motor neurons, on muscle fibers, and probably on sensory neurons. Activation of one type of octopamine receptor leads to an increase in intracellular Ca^{2+} levels, whereas a second type leads to an increase in the level of cAMP (Evans, 1981). The overall effect is to change the transmitter released by motor neurons, the time course and amount of force generated by a muscle, and the response of a sensory neuron to a particular stimulus.

Each DUM neuron is activated during the motor patterns in which its target effectors are used. Thus, during the specific motor patterns that cause kicking movements of the hind legs, only those DUM neurons that supply the participating muscles are activated (Burrows and Pflüger, 1995).

Motor Neurons

Seventy motor neurons innervate the muscles of a leg. They represent only a small percentage of the overall neuronal complement of the CNS, and only a few are responsible for any particular movement.

Excitatory motor neurons innervate just one muscle, or functional group, and depolarize muscle fibers to make them contract. In contrast, inhibitory motor neurons innervate several muscles that may have antagonistic actions. They usually hyperpolarize muscle fibers to reduce their force and increase their rate of relaxation.

Most of the motor neurons can be found in one of eight groups (Siegler and Pousman, 1990). Each group is surrounded by cortical glia, and each group may be the progeny of an individual neuroblast, although the progeny of one neuroblast can occur in different groups. A few motor neurons make output synapses in the CNS from the same fine branches that receive input synapses (Watson and Burrows, 1982), but no synapses occur on the cell bodies, even though receptors for many transmitters are present.

A motor axon carries spikes that are primarily dependent on an inward Na^+ current, but the central processes do not normally support spikes; active membrane gives way to passive membrane at a zone of the primary neurite within the neuropil, and it is here that spikes are initiated (Gwilliam and Burrows, 1980). At depolarized potentials, the membrane of a cell body rectifies, probably due to the activation of a rapid transient K^+ current and a delayed rectifying K^+ current. In some neurons, an N-shaped current-voltage relationship at membrane potentials of about $+100$ mV indicates the activation of a voltage-sensitive Ca^{2+}-activated K^+ current with a reversal potential close to normal resting potential (Thomas, 1984). Certain treatments can lead to the cell body producing Na^+-dependent (Pitman et al., 1972; Pitman, 1975; Goodman and Heitler, 1979) or even Ca^{2+}-dependent spikes (Pitman, 1979). These currents are normally masked by a much larger K^+ conductance. Such channels as these may also be distributed elsewhere and may alter the responses of a motor neuron in a nonlinear way, perhaps under the action of neuromodulators. The active participation of the membrane in integration is further emphasized by its ability to produce plateau potentials associated with a large inward current, probably carried by Ca^{2+}, to an applied or a synaptically driven depolarization (Hancox and Pitman, 1991, 1993).

The Circuits

The pathways involved in generating movement that is an appropriate response to a mechanosensory stimulus are essentially the same for both proprioceptive and exteroceptive types of receptor, although for each there are important emphases of particular routes. The following conclusions can be drawn about the design of these pathways.

1. The sensory neuron to motor neuron pathways are short.

The information from a sensory neuron passes through only a few serially arranged synapses before it reaches the motor neurons. It is the general rule for proprioceptive sensory neurons to synapse directly onto motor neurons, whereas for exteroceptive sensory neurons it is the exception. Many of the interneurons process signals from both types of receptors, allowing one modality to influence another in ways relevant for locomotion.

2. There is massive convergence of sensory neurons onto interneurons.

The exteroceptive sensory neurons show massive but specific convergence onto the local interneurons—a convergence that also preserves spatial information. Each interneuron has a discrete and characteristic receptive field on a leg. In turn, the whole surface of a leg is mapped onto the interneurons as a series of overlapping receptive fields. The terminals of the proprioceptive and exteroceptive sensory neurons are segregated.

3. The processing occurs in a parallel and distributed fashion.

Each sensory neuron makes connections with several interneurons of the same class and with interneurons of different classes. A stimulus to one part of the leg is thus represented by the actions of many interneurons, so its interpretation emerges only from the interactions of interneurons with overlapping receptive fields.

4. Connections in the networks are specific.

The connections made by the sensory neurons and by the interneurons are specific. Each sensory neuron connects with only a small subset of the interneurons, and the interneurons connect with only certain other interneurons or with a particular subset of the motor neurons. Specificity of action thus results from the specificity of the connections and from the processing performed by specific interneurons.

5. Analog and digital processing operate in parallel.

Both nonspiking and spiking local interneurons dominate the processing in the networks. The reason for the use of both analog and digital coding in these networks remains as intriguing as it is obscure, but it is probably related to the morphological design and functional role of the interneurons. The graded outputs of the nonspiking interneurons might be a mechanism that provides a more precise control of the responses of its postsynaptic neurons than can be achieved by the limited range of spike coding in a few spiking interneurons. Such a mechanism may be particularly important in networks containing few neurons but in which precise movements are essential.

6. Intersegmental interneurons regulate the action of the local circuits.

Signals in intersegmental interneurons place the processing by one local circuit in the context of the processing by the local circuits of other ganglia so that a movement of one leg is always appropriate to the movements of the other legs. Local circuits can thus be considered as the local controllers for a particular limb. Coordination of the local controllers is achieved largely by the summation of the intersegmental signals with the local signals, particularly at the nonspiking interneurons. The intersegmental signals therefore modify the performance of a local response rather than initiate a new movement. The design largely devolves control of leg movements to the local controllers, upon which other signals from the brain can be superimposed to effect any desired changes.

7. Nonspiking interneurons act as gain controllers.

The nonspiking interneurons can control the expression of a local response in a graded fashion by acting as the summing points for local and intersegmental signals. Despite the parallel and distributed processing of the signals, alterations in the membrane potential of one nonspiking interneuron can alter the contribution of sets of motor neurons to a particular movement. The same input will therefore generate a different output in terms of the number of motor spikes and the force produced by the muscles.

8. The effectiveness of sensory signals is regulated by presynaptic inhibition.

The actions of a sensory neuron depend on the network of actions of other sensory neurons so that their effectiveness is reduced in a graded fashion, depending on the type and number of other sensory neurons that signal the same stimulus (Burrows and Laurent, 1993; Burrows and Matheson, 1994). This reduction is achieved by presynaptic inhibition of their terminals through the action of interneurons that are activated by yet other sensory neurons (see also Nusbaum et al., chapter 22, this volume). The result is to prevent saturation in the responses of the postsynaptic neurons when many sensory neurons are active and perhaps to extend the dynamic range of the postsynaptic neurons as well as reduce the hysteresis of their responses (Hatsopoulos et al., 1995).

The effectiveness of the sensory signals is also altered at a particular phase of the step cycle during walking (Wolf and Burrows, 1995). This presynaptic inhibition presumably matches the performance of the sensory neurons to the context of the movements of the legs.

Conclusions

Analysis of the properties of a set of neurons and the way they are connected starts to reveal some of the complex interplay between these properties when they control movements of a leg. The problems faced by an insect in controlling and coordinating the movements of its legs are similar to those faced by vertebrates, suggesting that the mechanisms revealed here may well have a wider applicability. Moreover, now that the analysis of these neurons and circuits can be performed while an alert animal is walking, it should be possible to reveal both the dynamic actions of the underlying mechanisms and how sensory feedback is integrated to shape the active performance of a movement.

References

Burrows M (1979) Synaptic potentials effect the release of transmitter from locust nonspiking interneurons. *Science* 204:81–83.

Burrows M (1996) *The Neurobiology of an Insect Brain.* Oxford, UK: Oxford University Press.

Burrows M, Laurent G (1993) Synaptic potentials in the central terminals of locust proprioceptive afferents generated by other afferents from the same sense organ. *J Neurosci* 13:808–819.

Burrows M, Matheson T (1994) A presynaptic gain control mechanism among sensory neurons of a locust leg proprioceptor. *J Neurosci* 14:272–282.

Burrows M, Newland PL (1993) Correlation between the receptive fields of locust interneurons, their dendritic morphology, and the central projections of mechanosensory neurons. *J Comp Neurol* 329:412–426.

Burrows M, Pflüger H-J (1995) Action of locust neuromodulatory neurons is coupled to specific motor patterns. *J Neurophysiol* 74:347–357.

Burrows M, Siegler MVS (1978) Graded synaptic transmission between local interneurones and motoneurones in the metathoracic ganglion of the locust. *J Physiol* 285:231–255.

Crossman AR, Kerkut GA, Pitman RM, Walker RJ (1971) Electrically excitable nerve cell bodies in the central ganglia of two insect species *Periplaneta americana* and *Schistocerca gregaria. Comp Biochem Physiol* 40A:579–594.

Evans PD (1981) Multiple receptor types for octopamine in the locust. *J Physiol* 318:99–122.

Evans PD, O'Shea M (1978) The identification of an octopaminergic neurone and the modulation of a myogenic rhythm in the locust. *J Exp Biol* 73:235–260.

French AS, Torkkeli PH (1994) The time course of sensory adaptation in the cockroach tactile spine. *Neurosci Lett* 178:147–150.

Getting PA (1989) Emerging principles governing the operation of neural networks. *Annu Rev Neurosci* 12:185–204.

Goodman CS, Heitler WJ (1979) Electrical properties of insect neurones with spiking and non-spiking somata: Normal, axotomised, and colchicine treated neurones. *J Exp Biol* 83:95–121.

Grillner S, Wallén P, Brodin L, Lansner A (1991) Neuronal network generating locomotor behavior in lamprey: Circuitry, transmitters, membrane properties, and simulation. *Annu Rev Neurosci* 14:169–199.

Gwilliam GF, Burrows M (1980) Electrical characteristics of the membrane of an identified insect motor neurone. *J Exp Biol* 86:49–61.

Hancox JC, Pitman RM (1991) Plateau potentials drive axonal impulse bursts in insect motoneurons. *Proc Roy Soc Lond B* 244:33–38.

Hancox JC, Pitman RM (1993) Plateau potentials in an insect motoneurone can be driven by synaptic stimulation. *J Exp Biol* 176:307–310.

Hatsopoulos NG, Burrows M, Laurent G (1995) Hysteresis reduction in proprioception using presynaptic shunting inhibition. *J Neurophysiol* 73:1031–1042.

Heitler WJ, Goodman CS (1978) Multiple sites of spike initiation in a bifurcating locust neurone. *J Exp Biol* 76:63–84.

Kristan WB (1983) The neurobiology of swimming in the leech. *Trends Neurosci* 6:84–88.

Laurent G (1990) Voltage-dependent nonlinearities in the membrane of locust nonspiking local interneurons, and their significance for synaptic integration. *J Neurosci* 10:2268–2280.

Laurent G (1991) Evidence for voltage-activated outward currents in the neuropilar membrane of locust nonspiking local interneurons. *J Neurosci* 11:1713–1726.

Laurent G (1993) A dendritic gain control mechanism in axonless neurons of the locust, *Schistocerca americana. J Physiol (Lond)* 470:45–54.

Laurent G, Seymour-Laurent KJ, Johnson K (1993) Dendritic excitability and a voltage-gated calcium current in locust nonspiking local interneurons. *J Neurophysiol* 69:1484–1498.

Laurent G, Sivaramakrishnan A (1992) Single local interneurons in the locust make central synapses with different properties of transmitter release on distinct postsynaptic neurons. *J Neurosci* 12:2370–2380.

Morton DB, Evans PD (1984) Octopamine release from an identified neurone in the locust. *J Exp Biol* 113:269–287.

Newland PL (1991) Morphology and somatotopic organisation of the central projections of afferents from tactile hairs on the hind leg of the locust. *J Comp Neurol* 312:493–508.

Pitman RM (1975) The ionic dependence of action potentials induced by colchicine in an insect motorneurone cell body. *J Physiol (Lond)* 247:511.

Pitman RM (1979) Intracellular citrate or externally applied TEA ions produce Ca^{++} dependent action potentials in an insect motorneurone cell body. *J Physiol (Lond)* 291:327–337.

Pitman RM, Tweedle CD, Cohen MJ (1972) Electrical responses of insect central neurons: Augmentation by nerve section or colchicine. *Science* 178:507–509.

Robertson RM (1986) Neuronal circuits controlling flight in the locust: Central generation of the rhythm. *Trends Neurosci* 9:278–280.

Selverston AI (1985) Oscillatory neural networks. *Ann Rev Physiol* 47:29–48.

Siegler MVS, Burrows M (1984) The morphology of two groups of spiking local interneurones in the metathoracic ganglion of the locust. *J Comp Neurol* 224:463–482.

Siegler MVS, Pousman CA (1990) Motor neurons of grasshopper metathoracic ganglion occur in stereotypic anatomical groups. *J Comp Neurol* 297:298–312.

Thomas MV (1984) Voltage-clamp analysis of calcium-mediated potassium conductance in cockroach *Periplaneta americana* central neurones. *J Physiol (Lond)* 350:159–178.

Trimmer BA (1994) Characterization of a muscarinic current that regulates excitability of an identified insect motoneuron. *J Neurophysiol* 72:1862–1873.

Watson AHD (1984) The dorsal unpaired median neurons of the locust metathoracic ganglion: Neuronal structure and diversity, and synapse distribution. *J Neurocytol* 13:303–327.

Watson AHD (1992) Presynaptic modulation of sensory afferents in the invertebrate and vertebrate nervous system. *Comp Biochem Physiol* 103A:227–239.

Watson AHD, Burrows M (1982) The ultrastructure of identified locust motor neurones and their synaptic relationships. *J Comp Neurol* 205:383–397.

Watson AHD, Burrows M (1985) The distribution of synapses on the two fields of neurites of spiking local interneurones in the locust. *J Comp Neurol* 240:219–232.

Watson AHD, Burrows M (1987) Immunocytochemical and pharmacological evidence for GABAergic spiking local interneurons in the locust. *J Neurosci* 7:1741–1751.

Watson AHD, Burrows M (1988) The distribution and morphology of synapses on nonspiking local interneurones in the thoracic nervous system of the locust. *J Comp Neurol* 272:605–616.

Wolf H, Burrows M (1995) Proprioceptive sensory neurons of a locust leg receive rhythmic presynaptic inhibition during walking. *J Neurosci* 15:5623–5636.

Part III

Generation and Formation of Motor Patterns: Computational Approaches

13

How Computation Aids in Understanding Biological Networks

Eve Marder, Nancy Kopell, and Karen Sigvardt

Abstract

Models are now integrated into all aspects of research on motor systems. One recurrent controversy, however, concerns the form models can or should take to be useful. We discuss the different roles that models can play and illustrate each of these roles with examples. *Speculative* models are designed to address a fundamental problem in neuroscience and to explore the consequences of an idea. These models often precede specific data and function to motivate new experimental approaches. *Confirmatory* models are intended to determine if an existing data set is sufficient to explain the phenomenon under investigation. *Interpretive* models consist of new ways of analyzing or interpreting data. Models also vary with regard to the degree of complexity and supposed biological realism. We discuss the risks, benefits, and strategies associated with implementing models of increasing complexity in two "test cases": (1) reciprocal inhibition and half-center oscillation, and (2) intersegmental coordination in the lamprey, leech, and swimmeret systems.

Theoretical methods now form an integral part of the compendium of techniques available to motor systems investigators. Theoretical and computational methods are employed in a variety of ways. Both theorists themselves and the experimental community have widely disparate expectations of what these methods can bring to their understanding of motor systems. It is often asserted that theory is useful to the extent that it makes specific predictions that can be directly tested by means of experimentation. However, the relationship between theory and experimental prediction will differ according to the use to which theory is put.

Marder and Abbott (1995) defined three general classes of models: *speculative, confirmatory*, and *interpretive*. The first part of this chapter describes and illustrates these classes with specific examples from recent work. The second part of this chapter discusses two problems relevant to motor control: (1) reciprocal inhibition and half-center oscillations, and (2) chains of coupled oscillators in the control of intersegmental coordination.

Speculative Models

Speculative models are intended to provide a formal exploration of the possible implications or potential consequences of an idea; they may also suggest a possible solution to a previously puzzling or inexplicable phenomenon. In creating a speculative model, the investigator often starts with a problem, then constructs a possible solution, which in turn may suggest a new avenue for experimental investigation. In some cases, the suggested experiments will be obvious. If the model addresses a large and broadly defined problem, however, the connection to new experimental work may be on a relatively long time scale and may not be readily apparent. In the long run, all good speculative models will stimulate new and more focused experimental work.

The model of activity-dependent regulation of the intrinsic properties of neurons (LeMasson et al., 1993; Abbott and LeMasson, 1993; Siegel et al., 1994) is an example of a speculative model that led to experimental work (Turrigiano et al., 1994, 1995). One motivation for this model was the difficulty in developing detailed "biophysically realistic" models of single neurons based on biophysical data (e.g., Buchholtz et al., 1992; Golowasch et al., 1992). The frustration in building such models is that regardless of how carefully one characterizes the biophysical properties of the cell, inevitable measurement errors occur, and numerous properties of the neurons remain unmeasured. Conductance-based models are often sensitive to small changes in the balance of their conductances, which raises the question of how neurons maintain essentially constant intrinsic electrical properties, even though channel proteins turn over many times during the neuron's lifetime.

LeMasson and colleagues (1993) proposed a speculative model in which a neuron's activity regulates the balance of its conductances. In this model, the mean level of intracellular Ca^{++} is used to monitor activity. When the intracellular Ca^{++} rises, the levels of the inward conductances are down-regulated and those of the outward conductances are up-regulated. This constitutes a negative feedback, intended to keep the neuron's level of activity relatively constant (over a long time) despite external or internal perturbations.

Does this model, however, describe the behavior of biological neurons? Turrigiano and colleagues (1994, 1995) used cultured stomatogastric ganglion (STG) neurons to address this question. Most STG neurons in the animal fire in bursts of action potentials because they receive modulatory inputs and rhythmic synaptic drive from other STG neurons, but they are not rhythmically active when isolated from their presynaptic inputs (Hooper and Marder, 1987; Miller and Selverston, 1982). Nevertheless, when placed in dissociated cell culture (Turrigiano and Marder, 1993; Panchin et al., 1993;

Turrigiano et al., 1995), the vast majority of STG neurons fire rhythmic bursts of action potentials, suggesting that, in the absence of the rhythmic inhibition that causes most STG neurons to fire in rebound bursts, these neurons may become intrinsic bursters to maintain their rhythmic activity patterns. Moreover, the STG neurons might lose their bursting behavior if they were to receive rhythmic inhibition, as they do in the intact ganglion. To test this theory, Turrigiano and colleagues (1994) gave strong inhibitory pulses to isolated cultured neurons that were intrinsically bursting. After one hour of inhibitory pulses that elicited rebound bursting, the neurons were no longer intrinsically bursting, but were instead firing tonically.

Speculative models also serve to focus attention on data that might otherwise seem difficult to explain. For example, Linsdell and Moody (1994, 1995) have shown altered levels of K^+ channel expression in *Xenopus* myocytes subsequent to Na^+ channel mRNA injection or TTX application. The data are consistent with the predictions of the activity-dependent models described in the previous paragraphs, because the models suggest that the balance of conductances is regulated, rather than the actual value of each individual conductance.

Confirmatory Models

Confirmatory models are used to ask whether a given data set is adequate to account for the behavior of a system. They are most commonly used to establish whether a given set of membrane currents measured with voltage clamp is sufficient to account for a neuron's current-clamp behavior (e.g., Buchholtz et al., 1992; Golowasch et al., 1992; Turrigiano et al., 1995). By their nature, confirmatory models are tightly connected to data; their most immediate function is to pinpoint missing data and to suggest avenues for finding them.

Although confirmatory models may initially be used to check the adequacy of data, they can also be used to speculate. Parameter searches that determine which properties of a model are crucial for its behavior often yield new insights into the interactions of nonlinear processes that are totally inaccessible to the experimentalist without confirmatory models (Guckenheimer and Rowat, chapter 14, this volume).

Interpretive Models

Theoretical methods are often used to provide new tools for analyzing data. In some cases, these methods may depend on assumptions about which features of data are likely to be significant. At their best, interpretive models provide ways of integrating, interpreting, or categorizing data. One interpretive model appears in the recent work of Sen and colleagues (1995, 1996), who used decoding methods to predict the response of a facilitating synapse to any temporal pattern of presynaptic activity.

The immediate impetus for Sen and colleagues' work is that the motor patterns of the stomatogastric ganglion are richly modulated (Marder and Weimann, 1992). Therefore, it is crucial to determine when modulation of a motor pattern translates into changes in movement. The crustacean foregut consists of more than 40 sets of striated muscles (Maynard and Dando, 1974). Each of these muscles is innervated by one or more motor neurons at junctions that show facilitation and depression to widely different degrees (Govind et al., 1975). One way to determine whether a change in motor pattern will produce a change in movement is to stimulate the motor neuron in each of the patterns. It is not possible, however, to do this for all possible changes in motor pattern. Sen and colleagues (1995, 1996) extended methods pioneered by Krausz and Friesen (1977) and used the excitatory junctional potentials (EJPS) evoked by random motor nerve stimuli to predict the amplitude of the EJPS that result from any temporal pattern of presynaptic activity.

Comparative Modeling: Reciprocal Inhibition

Reciprocal inhibition is a common feature in many motor systems (Calabrese and Feldman; Roberts et al.; Stein and Smith; Wallén; chapters 5–7, 11, this volume). Moreover, in most half-center oscillator theory derived from work with a long history in the motor control field (Grillner et al., 1983; Guckenheimer and Rowat, chapter 14, this volume; Friesen, 1994; Rowat and Selverston, 1993, 1997; Stein and Smith, chapter 5, this volume) reciprocal inhibition is regarded as *the* mechanism producing stable alternating bursts of activity. Nevertheless, recent theoretical work on the dynamics of networks of reciprocally connected inhibitory neurons has expanded our understanding of how such networks operate.

Early modeling of reciprocal inhibition established that such networks *can* produce alternating bursts of activity (Perkel and Mulloney, 1974; Friesen, 1994). The early work, however, neither dissected the mechanisms by which such behavior can happen nor elucidated the circumstances under which behaviors other than alternating bursts might occur with reciprocal inhibition.

Wang and Rinzel (1992) first used the terms *release* and *escape* to define two classes of mechanisms by which the transitions between the active and inhibited states might occur. Release occurs when the active neuron stops inhibiting its partner, and escape occurs when the inhibited neuron depolarizes past its synaptic threshold or burst threshold despite ongoing inhibition. Skinner and colleagues (1994) used Morris-Lecar (1981) model neurons to study the relationship between synaptic threshold and period in networks that produce alternating bursts. They found that period was insensitive to synaptic threshold when the transition depended on the intrinsic properties of the neurons. In contrast, the period was highly sensitive to synaptic threshold when the network was either in a synaptic release or a synaptic escape mode (figure 13.1A). The relationship between period and synaptic threshold is opposite in the two modes of operation (Skinner et al., 1994; figure 13.1A).

Skinner and colleagues' (1994) used two-dimensional oscillators with much simplified currents, raising the question of whether the phenomena uncovered in the model would occur in a pair of real cells. Motivated by this question, Sharp and colleagues (1996) used the dynamic clamp (Sharp et al., 1993a, 1993b) to construct half-center oscillators from two biological neurons. In a dynamic-clamp experiment, the membrane potential is monitored and then sent to a computer. The computer calculates the current that would flow at that membrane potential as a consequence of a modeled conductance and sends that current back into the neuron, where it acts in parallel with the other membrane currents. In effect, the dynamic clamp places the modeled conductance into the neuron at the tip of the electrode (Sharp et al., 1993a, 1993b). The dynamic clamp can also be used to create artificial synaptic connections between neurons. Here, the membrane potential of one neuron is used to control a modeled synaptic conductance in a second neuron. The investigator sets the threshold for the synaptic potential (the membrane potential at which the presynaptic neuron starts to influence the conductance of the postsynaptic neuron), the synaptic conductance, time course, and reversal potential.

Figure 13.1B shows the results of moving the synaptic threshold from −52 mV to −40 mV in a dynamic clamp–constructed two-cell circuit formed from two stomatogastric ganglion neurons that are not synaptically coupled in the ganglion. The figure shows an inverted U-shaped curve similar to that seen in the simpler model shown in figure 13.1A. The sweep from synaptic escape (the left-hand portion of the plots seen in figure 13.1A and B) to synaptic release (the right-hand portion of the

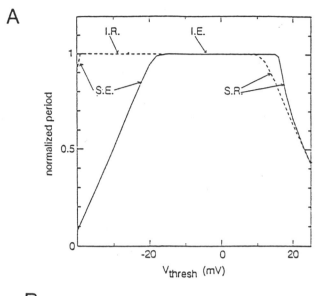

A

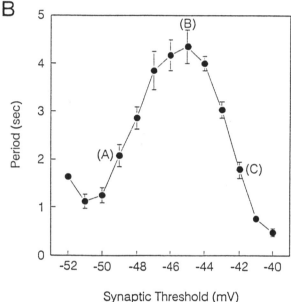

B

Figure 13.1

(A) Plots of the period as a function of synaptic threshold of a network consisting of two reciprocally inhibitory Morris-Lecar model neurons (Skinner et al., 1994). S.E. (Synaptic Escape regime), I.R. (Intrinsic Release regime), I.E. (Intrinsic Escape regime), and S.R. (Synaptic Release regime). The dashed and solid lines come from two different sets of simulations using different parameters. (Modified from Skinner et al., 1994; see it for details). (B) Plots of the period as a function of the synaptic threshold in two-cell reciprocally inhibitory networks formed using the dynamic clamp from two stomatogastric ganglion neurons. Region labeled A shows networks operating in the synaptic escape regime, B a narrow region of intrinsic escape, and C a region of synaptic release. Note that the inverted U spans the membrane potentials over which graded synaptic transmission in the stomatogastric nervous system is modulated. (Modified from Sharp et al., 1996.)

plots seen in figure 13.1A and B) takes place within a 5–10 mV range of synaptic thresholds, a range well within the documented effects of modulators on graded synaptic transmission in the stomatogastric nervous system (Johnson et al., 1995). Therefore, the same modulatory substance might actually increase or decrease the period of a network, depending on its mode of operation (i.e., escape or release).

Another potential implication for motor systems is seen in the simulations shown in figure 13.2. Here, a reciprocal inhibitory network of Morris-Lecar oscillators was constructed (simulations courtesy of M. Casey). One of the pair of neurons for networks operating at the same frequency in either the escape or the release mode is displayed in the figure. An excitatory synaptic input is applied at the same phase of the cycle in both cases. However, the response of the network is different in the two cases, as is illustrated in the phase response curves.

For most physiologists (especially those of us specializing in motor control), intuition tells us that reciprocal inhibition favors alternation between the inhibitory pair of neurons. Yet, simple models show that synchronization, not alternation, can be the outcome of reciprocal inhibition (Wang and Rinzel, 1992; Van Vreeswijk et al., 1994), an outcome which requires that there be a delay in the onset of inhibition and that the decay of the inhibition not be too fast compared with the recovery time of the cell and/or the time the cell is active. In this case, the distinction between escape and release is not as useful, and the models behave differently from those with instantaneous synapses. A recent study (Terman et al., submitted) on Morris-Lecar oscillators extended the geometric analysis used to describe the release/escape mechanisms and examined inhibition with a delay in onset and a decay time comparable to the time-to-threshold of an oscillating neuron. The analysis showed that, in different parameter regimes, different combinations of intrinsic and synaptic time constants govern whether synchrony is a stable outcome. It also showed that there can be a variety of other solutions.

The above models are intermediate level, in that they incorporate some aspects of biological realism, but they were not detailed, conductance-based models of all the currents of a given neuron. Different insights were obtained from biophysically realistic models of the half-center oscillator in the leech heartbeat system (Calabrese and Feldman, chapter 11, this volume; Nadim et al., 1995; Olsen et al., 1995). The realistic models showed that although graded synaptic transmission is easy to demonstrate experimentally, spike-mediated transmission is more important in determining the transitions

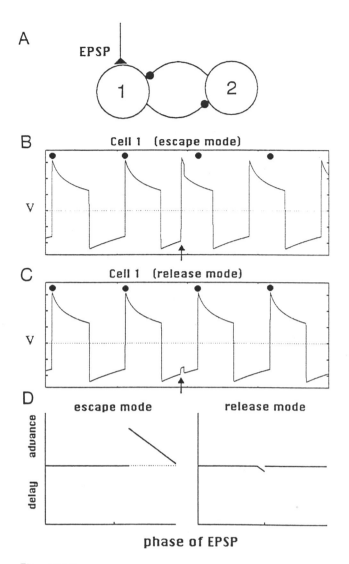

A

EPSP

1   2

B

Cell 1 (escape mode)

V

C

Cell 1 (release mode)

V

D

escape mode   release mode

advance

delay

phase of EPSP

Figure 13.2
(A) The circuit. Two identical Morris-Lecar (1981) model neurons (1 and 2) are connected by reciprocal inhibition (filled circles). An EPSP (filled triangle) is added to only neuron 1. (B) A neuron from a network in the escape mode. An EPSP is added to neuron 1 (upward arrow) in its inactive phase. Because the transition time in the escape mode depends on the neuron in the inactive state depolarizing past its synaptic release threshold, the EPSP depolarizes the cell and triggers an early transition, resulting in a stable phase advance. The dots denote the time of the onset of the burst in the unperturbed state. (C) A neuron from a network in the release mode. In the release mode, the transition occurs when the active cell falls below its synaptic threshold. Therefore, the EPSP in the inactive phase fails to change the transition time of the network, and no reset is obtained. (D) Full phase response curves for networks in both the escape and release modes. (Unpublished simulations done by Dr. Michael Casey.)

from inactive to active states (Olsen et al., 1995; Nadim et al., 1995). Olsen, Nadim, and colleagues found that the formal distinction between escape and release modes of operation was not particularly useful in the leech heartbeat system. Instead, the transitions between active and inactive states occur via multiple mechanisms that cannot be easily dissociated. It is likely that, in biological networks, multiple mechanisms always cooperate in stable network function, and the formal distinctions that are so instructive in the analysis of simple models are blurred in real situations.

Thus, as the level of analysis changes, we find that different models help us to find answers to different questions. More detailed models can give insight into the actual biological mechanisms by which groups of neurons interact. More simplified models allow us to see general principles, such as the relationship between the synaptic time constant and synchrony. Ideally, we wish to be able to move smoothly between levels of models and to understand how to reduce systematically more complex models into simpler forms that retain their essential properties.

Intersegmental Coordination: An Overview Strategy

The neural basis of intersegmental coordination has been studied in many animals, from the leech to higher vertebrates, and many kinds of theoretical models have been applied to its study, from detailed biophysical models to more abstract theories. The abstract theory developed by Kopell and Ermentrout (1986, 1988, 1990) for understanding intersegmental coordination shows how a general abstract theory can be developed for systems that share common properties and then adapted to fit their differences. This strategy has been used on networks that can be viewed as chains of coupled oscillators—networks related to undulatory locomotion and the crayfish swimmeret system. The object of the strategy is to determine how the models behave and to try to find which properties at this level of organization (i.e., oscillators and coupling) make a significant difference in determining the emergent behavior of the network. For a different approach to intersegmental coordination, see Lansner and colleagues (chapter 15, this volume).

Networks of neurons that produce and regulate undulatory locomotion have been studied in the lamprey (Cohen et al., 1992), leech (Friesen and Pearce, 1993), and *Xenopus* tadpoles (Tunstall and Sillar, 1993). The leech cord consists of a chain of twenty-one ganglia, each capable of producing an oscillation. In the crayfish swimmeret system, each swimmeret is controlled by its own local oscillatory network (Murchison et al., 1993). Although the lamprey vertebrate cord is not discrete, as few as two segments of the cord can also produce oscillations (Grillner et al., 1983). As yet, no evidence exists as to whether the functional organization of the lamprey spinal cord is continuous or discrete. Even without strict anatomical segmentation, if intersegmental coupling is provided by the same neurons that generate rhythmicity, but with smaller synaptic strengths (Williams, 1992), then the system can behave as if it were discrete. Thus, the lamprey, leech, and swimmeret networks can each be described as a chain of oscillators. The overview approach to these networks asks to what extent the behavior of such a chain is determined by variations in this structure (i.e., oscillators and coupling) alone, independent of the biophysical basis of the oscillation.

Complicated Equations Behave Like Simple Ones

If one describes each oscillator in the chain only by its phase, the interaction between oscillators, under very general conditions, depends only on the differences in the phases of the oscillators (Kopell and Ermentrout, 1986, 1988). When all the oscillators are locked at a common frequency, Ω, and each oscillator is connected only to its nearest neighbors, the complicated set of equations describing the behavior of the chain is reduced to the following set of simpler equations:

$$\Omega = \omega_1 + H_A(\phi_1) \qquad k = 1 \qquad (1)$$

$$\Omega = \omega_k + H_A(\phi_k) + H_D(-\phi_{k-1}) \quad 1 < k < n \qquad (2)$$

$$\Omega = \omega_n + H_D(-\phi_{n-1}) \qquad k = n \qquad (3)$$

Here ω_k is the intrinsic frequency of oscillator k and ϕ_k is the difference in phase between oscillator $k + 1$ and oscillator k. $H_A(\phi_k)$ and $H_D(-\phi_{k-1})$ give the frequency change in oscillator k by the coupling from oscillator $k + 1$ and oscillator $k - 1$ (see figure 13.3A). These equations were first applied to the lamprey spinal central pattern generator (CPG) by Cohen and colleagues (Cohen et al., 1982).

These "averaged phase difference" equations and the theory behind them are not as familiar as phase response curve (PRC) theory, which describes the effect—either a phase delay or a phase advance—on an oscillator due to a very brief incoming pulse as a function of when the pulse arrives in the cycle (see figure 13.3B for an example of a phase response curve). Thus, we digress to explain the relationship between the H-functions in the equations and phase response curves. PRC theory was

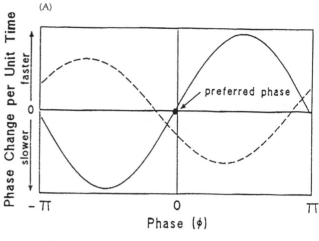

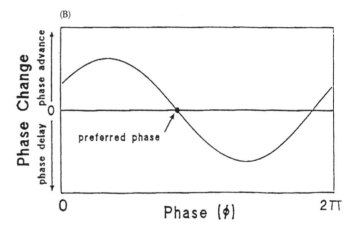

Figure 13.3
(A) Schematic H-functions. Change in frequency (phase per unit time) caused by the coupling as a function of the phase lag between the sending and receiving oscillators. (B) Schematic phase response curve (PRC). Delay (phase advance or phase delay) caused by the sending oscillator as a function of the time in the cycle at which the pulse arrives (time expressed as phase within the cycle, 0 to 2π).

developed to understand phase locking for an oscillator forced by a periodic sequence of identical short pulses, coming once per cycle (Pavlides, 1973). The theory predicts the phase in the cycle of the forced oscillator that the forcing pulse will arrive after transients have disappeared. For the special case in which the period of the forcing pulses equals the intrinsic period of the forced oscillator, PRC theory predicts that this "preferred" phase is the phase at which the incoming pulse has no effect on the forced oscillator (see figure 13.3B).

PRC theory is valid only when applied to a single short pulse per cycle and is analytically useful only if the coupling is unidirectional. In the lamprey and many other systems, however, the signals occupy a significant fraction of the cycle, more than one such signal per cycle occurs, and the coupling is bidirectional. Such complexities can be handled numerically, using PRC functions, by dividing signals up into little bits and then describing the full set of signals by the sum of such PRCs (e.g., Pearce and Friesen, 1985). Unhappily, when PRC theory has been used in this way, it can no longer be used to predict the behavior of the chain; one loses its original analytical advantage and must calculate the phase lags numerically. The numerical computation can be done only for some finite set of parameter values. Furthermore, it becomes difficult to understand why the results come out the way they do or to predict what would happen if the parameter values are changed.

If, however, the signals to the oscillators are spaced around the cycle, one can use "averaging theory" (Ermentrout and Kopell, 1991) to put all the PRCs together into a single function (for each coupling direction). The H-function captures what is in the sum of the PRCs. The advantage of working with the averaged functions is that one recovers the ability to do analysis and to gain insight into what the entire class of equations will do. The description of interactions in terms of averaged phase differences (H-functions) is a useful way to look at the undulatory locomotion in lamprey and leech, as well as swimmeret behavior. Nevertheless, these systems have major differences that require the framework to be used in different ways for each CPG.

Modeling the Lamprey CPG

In the lamprey, the intersegmental phase delay is constant along the length of the cord and independent of swimming speed. To describe more fully the framework used to understand the lamprey CPG, we need to specialize from the general formulation. The chain needs to be long and the coupling relatively local. Finally, it is assumed that, for the lamprey, the intrinsic frequencies of all the oscillators are the same; Cohen (1987) has shown that in the lamprey there is no systematic dependence of intrinsic frequency on the rostrocaudal position within the spinal cord.

A mathematical analysis of equations 1–3 for the lamprey system (with its equal intrinsic frequency and local coupling) showed that traveling waves of activity, with non-zero phase lags, occur for almost all equations of this form. The lags are constant along the chain, except for a small region (a "boundary layer") at one end. The mathematics predicts that, with bidirectional coupling, one direction of coupling usually "dominates" in determining the intersegmental phase lag, whereas the other direction plays essentially no role in determining the lag.

Dominance should not be taken to mean that one direction of coupling is stronger than the other; instead, the dominant coupling is defined as the coupling that determines the phase lag. The mathematical analysis also predicts that the phase lag of the network will be the phase lag at which the dominant coupling signal (either H_A or H_D) has no effect on the receiving oscillator (see figure 13.3A). Note the analogy between this prediction and PRC theory, which concludes that when the oscillators have equal intrinsic frequencies, the phase that the entrained oscillator assumes (the "preferred" phase) is the phase at which the coupling has no effect on the receiving oscillator (see figures 13.3A and 13.3B). For the preferred phase to be independent of frequency, it must be unaffected by a change in the activation of the oscillator (although the shape of the function could change). This conclusion requires that the coupling in the two directions be asymmetric; symmetry leads to a pair of waves traveling toward or away from the center of the chain. Several experimental results (described in the next section) support such a conclusion.

Modeling the Swimmeret CPG

The swimmeret CPG consists of four coordinated ganglia. In both the intact crayfish and the pharmacologically activated and isolated abdominal nerve cord, the activity in the motor roots to the swimmerets is characterized by a phase lag between segments that is constant at about 25% per segment and remains the same even with changes in the frequency of beating (Braun and Mulloney, 1993). Studies of the isolated abdominal nerve cord activated by pilocarpine or carbachol show no statistically significant differences in the intrinsic frequencies of the oscillators that control each segment (Mulloney and Hall, 1995). Because the chain has only a small number of oscillators, a boundary layer in phase lags would be dysfunctional; with only three phase lags determining the metachronal wave in the swimmeret system, a change in even one of them would greatly affect the system, whereas changing one in the lamprey would have little impact. To prevent a boundary layer, the ascending and descending coupling must individually produce the same preferred phase (Kopell and Ermentrout, 1986; see also Stein, 1970). However, the coupling must be asymmetric because the preferred phases would have opposite signs if coupling were symmetric.

Using their knowledge of both the asymmetry and the approximately equal (though not identical) strengths of coupling for the ascending and descending directions, Skinner and colleagues (1997) were able to account for both the phase lag and frequency data in differential activation experiments in the crayfish (Braun and Mulloney, 1995). For the swimmeret system, the notion of "dominance" does not appear to be a useful one; instead, the phase lag seems to be determined by the coupling in both directions.

Modeling the Leech CPG

Leech swimming movements, like those of the lamprey, are characterized by a rostrocaudal traveling wave, with the intersegmental phase lag independent of the swimming speed. However, unlike the lamprey system, the phase lags are not uniform along the length of the nerve cord; they increase from anterior to posterior segments (Pearce and Friesen, 1985). The connections from one ganglion extend both down and up a substantial portion of the chain of ganglia. Furthermore, there is evidence for a gradient in intrinsic frequencies. Finally, transmission delays are not negligible, as they are for the local coupling in the lamprey. Thus, the conclusions of the lamprey theory do not hold here.

In recent simulations, Hampson and Kopell (personal communication) have used the form of equations 1–3 and extended them to include transmission delays and multiple coupling that reach significant distances. Extremely important in determining the lags in this setting is the timing difference in the ascending and descending coupling—that is, the difference in the preferred phase that the ascending or descending coupling would create by themselves if there were only nearest neighbor coupling. The timing difference arises from the fact that the cells participating in the CPG can be grouped into three classes according to the relative phases at which they fire (Friesen and Pearce, 1993). Also, the origins and targets of the ascending fibers largely belong to different classes than those of the descending fibers.

In long chains with relatively short coupling (as in the lamprey), the timing difference is not relevant because only one direction of the coupling produces the phases. In the leech, as in the swimmeret system, the notion of dominance is not central. For chains in which the extent of the coupling is comparable to the lengths of the chain, the frequency gradient plays a very small role in the size of the lag, but the exact extent of the coupling *is* important.

Phase Difference Equations and Testable Predictions

The framework of equations 1–3 describes intrinsic frequencies and the ways in which the coupling affects natural frequencies. The solutions to the equations describe the patterns of phase lags in the coupled system. Thus, such a theory makes it possible to obtain testable predictions about observable quantities of the system, such as phase lags and frequencies.

When applied to the lamprey CPG, Kopell and Ermentrout's mathematical analysis led to three different kinds of experiments, all aimed at testing to see *if* there is dominance, and if so, which direction is dominant. It should be emphasized that the design of the experiments was heavily influenced by the modeling, which provided critical information about which data were useful to collect. In one of the three types of experiment (Sigvardt and Williams, 1996) the rostral and caudal pieces of the cord are bathed in different concentrations of D-glutamate. Because cycle frequency is a function of D-glutamate concentration, this changes the intrinsic frequency of the individual segmental oscillators in one half of the chain relative to the other. Mathematical analysis done by Kopell and Ermentrout (1990) indicated that this should lead to a pattern of phase lags in which the intersegmental phase lag within one of the two compartments would stay the same, whereas the lag in the other compartment would increase or decrease, depending on whether the intrinsic frequency of the chain in the latter compartment was higher or lower than that of the former compartment. The coupling direction originating in the compartment in which the lags stay fixed is then the dominant one. The experiments displayed the constant phase lags in one compartment and gave results that would be expected for ascending coupling dominant (Sigvardt and Williams, 1996).

The results of two other, quite different sets of experiments also match the predictions of the mathematical analysis, again suggesting that the phase lag is set by coupling in one direction and that ascending coupling is dominant (Kopell et al., 1990; Williams et al., 1990; Williams and Sigvardt, 1995).

Adding More Detail to the Current Lamprey Model

The current abstract model developed for the lamprey fits well for all the available data on phase lags. However, it does not hold well for the frequency data in the differential activation experiments (Sigvardt and Williams, 1996). The models of equations 1–3 predict (Kopell and Ermentrout, 1990) that the frequency of the differentially activated cord is determined by the frequency in the caudal compartment (if the ascending coupling is dominant in determining the phase lags). The data, however, imply that the network frequency is determined by the frequency of the rostral compartment.

No one has yet succeeded in producing a model that can simultaneously account for both the phase lag and the frequency data, which suggests that other degrees of freedom in the description of the unit oscillators—such as amplitude, duty cycle, and phases among cells within an oscillator—are relevant to the behavior.

Interaction between Modeling at Different Levels

The abstract theory gives a framework for addressing and answering questions about phase lags and frequencies. The answers to these questions are the same in all models that satisfy the hypotheses of the framework and are independent of the cellular and synaptic bases of the oscillations and the coupling. The theory, however, raises questions that must be addressed at the cellular level. For example, when activation is changed for the entire cord in the lamprey, the phase lags do not change (Sigvardt and Williams, 1996). The theory suggests that the phase lags are determined by the dominant coupling and raises the question of what kinds of circuits and connections among them allow the coupling to be unaffected by the changes in activation. If the neurons that provide intersegmental coordination are different from the local circuits that produce the oscillations, it is possible to change the frequency of the oscillators without changing the coupling, so that the preferred phase is unaffected by the different level of activation. However, if, as suggested (Williams, 1992), the intersegmental coupling is an extension of the intrasegmental coupling, then how the circuits are designed *can* make a difference. Williams (1992) has used the Buchanan-Grillner model (1987) of the segmental oscillator to explore this question, using different balances of excitatory and inhibitory, and ascending and descending coupling. This question can also be addressed in the biophysical models of the lamprey CPG developed by Grillner and his colleagues (e.g., Wallén et al., 1992; Lansner et al., chapter 15, this volume). Finally, general models are valuable in that the insights gained from them can be used to provide constraints on parameters in detailed biophysical models of the same system, especially when that model has large numbers of unknown parameters.

Conclusions

We face an apparent paradox. One the one hand, numerous mechanisms provide for plasticity and modulation of motor systems. Those mechanisms allow sensory and central signals to shape movements to the ongoing behavioral needs of the animal. On the other hand, the essential features of the circuits underlying rhythmic movement must be maintained so that we continue breathing and don't fall down when accelerating from a walk to a run. A great challenge for the future is to understand how the flexible modulation of motor circuits occurs without the loss of their essential stability. This problem is ideally suited for theoretical investigations because they can define precisely how and why qualitative transitions in behavior can occur.

Acknowledgments

The authors' research is supported by MH46742 (Marder), MH47150 (Kopell and Sigvardt), NS22360 (Sigvardt). Eve Marder would also like to acknowledge the support of the W. M. Keck Foundation.

References

Abbott LF, LeMasson G (1993) Analysis of neuron models with dynamically regulated conductances. *Neural Comp* 5:823–842.

Braun G, Mulloney B (1993) Cholinergic modulation of the swimmeret system in crayfish. *J Neurophysiol* 70:2391–2398.

Braun G, Mulloney B (1995) Coordination in the crayfish swimmeret system: Differential excitation causes changes in intersegmental phase. *J Neurophysiol* 73:880–885.

Buchanan JT, Grillner S (1987) Newly identified "glutamate interneurons" and their role in locomotion in the lamprey spinal cord. *Science* 236:312–314.

Buchholtz F, Golowasch J, Epstein IR, Marder E (1992) A mathematical model of an identified stomatogastric ganglion neuron. *J Neurophysiol* 67:332–340.

Cohen AH (1987) Effects of oscillator frequency on phase-locking in the lamprey central pattern generator. *J Neurosci Methods* 21:113–125.

Cohen AH, Ermentrout GB, Kiemel T, Kopell N, Mellen N, Sigvardt KA, Williams TL (1992) Modeling of intersegmental coordination in the lamprey central pattern generator for locomotion. *Trends Neurosci* 15:434–438.

Cohen AH, Holmes PJ, Rand RH (1982) The nature of the coupling between segmental oscillators of the lamprey spinal generator for locomotion: A mathematical model. *J Math Biol* 13:345–369.

Ermentrout GB, Kopell N (1991) Multiple pulse interaction and averaging in coupled neural oscillators. *J Math Biol* 29:195–217.

Friesen WO (1994) Reciprocal inhibition: A mechanism underlying oscillatory animal movements. *Neurosci Biobehav* 18:547–553.

Friesen WO, Pearce RA (1993) Mechanisms of intersegmental coordination in leech locomotion. *Semin Neurosci* 5:41–47.

Golowasch J, Buchholtz F, Epstein IR, Marder E (1992) The contribution of individual ionic currents to the activity of a model stomatogastric ganglion neuron. *J Neurophysiol* 67:341–349.

Govind CK, Atwood HL, Maynard DM (1975) Innervation and neuromuscular physiology of intrinsic foregut muscles in the blue crab and spiny lobster. *J Comp Physiol* 96:185–204.

Grillner S, Wallén P, McClellan A, Sigvardt K, Williams T, Feldman J (1983) The neural generation of locomotion in the lamprey: An incomplete account. In: *Neural Origin of Rhythmic Movements* (Roberts A, Roberts B, eds., 285–303. New York: Cambridge University Press.

Hooper SL, Marder E (1987) Modulation of the lobster pyloric rhythm by the peptide proctolin. *J Neurosci* 7:2097–2112.

Johnson BR, Peck JH, Harris-Warrick RM (1995) Distributed amine modulation of graded chemical transmission in the pyloric network of the lobster stomatogastric ganglion. *J Neurophysiol* 74:437–452.

Kopell N, Ermentrout GB (1986) Symmetry and phase coupling in chains of weakly coupled oscillators. *Comm Pure Appl Math* 39:623–660.

Kopell N, Ermentrout GB (1988) Coupled oscillators and the design of central pattern generators. *Math Biosci* 90:87–109.

Kopell N, Ermentrout GB (1990) Phase transitions and other phenomena in chains of coupled oscillators. *SIAM J Appl Math* 50:1014–1052.

Kopell N, Ermentrout GB, Williams TL (1990) On chains of oscillators forced at one end. *SIAM J Appl Math* 51:1397–1417.

Krausz HI, Friesen WO (1977) The analysis of nonlinear synaptic transmission. *J Gen Physiol* 70:243–265.

LeMasson G, Marder E, Abbott LF (1993) Activity-dependent regulation of conductances in model neurons. *Science* 259:1915–1917.

Linsdell P, Moody WJ (1994) Na$^+$ channel mis-expression accelerates K$^+$ channel development in embryonic *Xenopus laevis* skeletal muscle. *J Physiol* (Lond) 480:405–410.

Linsdell P, Moody WJ (1995) Electrical activity and calcium influx regulate ion channel development in embryonic *Xenopus* skeletal muscle. *J Neurosci* 15:4507–4514.

Marder E, Abbott LF (1995) Theory in motion. *Curr Opin Neur* 5:832–840.

Marder E, Weimann JM (1992) Modulatory control of multiple task processing in the stomatogastric nervous system. In: *Neurobiology of Motor Programme Selection: New Approaches to Mechanisms of Behavioral Choice* (Kien J, McCrohan C, Winlow W, eds.), 3–19. Oxford: Pergamon.

Maynard DM, Dando MR (1994) The structure of the stomatogastric neuromuscular system in *Callinectes sapidus, Homarus americanus,* and *Panulirus argus* (Decapoda Crustacea). *Phil Trans Roy Soc B* 268:161–220.

Miller JP, Selverston AI (1982) Mechanisms underlying pattern generation in lobster stomatogastric ganglion as determined by selective inactivation of identified neurons. II. Oscillatory properties of pyloric neurons. *J Neurophysiol* 48:1378–1391.

Morris C, Lecar H (1981) Voltage oscillations in the barnacle giant muscle fiber. *Biophys J* 35:193–213.

Mulloney B, Hall WM (1995) How are limbs on different segments of the body coordinated? A test of the "excitability gradient" hypothesis in the swimmeret system. *Soc Neurosci Abst* 21:1276.

Murchison D, Chrachri A, Mulloney B (1993) A separate local pattern-generating circuit controls the movements of each swimmeret in crayfish. *J Neurophysiol* 70:2620–2631.

Nadim F, Olsen OH, DeSchutter E, Calabrese RL (1995) Modeling the leech heartbeat elemental oscillator. I. Interactions of intrinsic and synaptic currents. *J Comput Neurosci* 2:215–235.

Olsen OH, Nadim F, Calabrese RL (1995) Modeling the leech heartbeat elemental oscillator. II. Exploring the parameter space. *J Comput Neurosci* 2:237–257.

Panchin YV, Arshavsky YI, Selverston AI, Cleland TA (1993) Lobster stomatogastric neurons in primary culture. I. Basic characteristics. *J Neurophysiol* 69:1976–1992.

Pavlides T (1973) *Biological Oscillators: Their Mathematical Analysis.* New York: Academic.

Pearce RA, Friesen WO (1985) Intersegmental coordination of the leech swimming rhythm. I. Role of cycle period gradient and coupling strength. *J Neurophysiol* 54:1444–1459.

Perkel DH, Mulloney B (1974) Motor pattern production in reciprocally inhibitory neurons exhibiting postinhibitory rebound. *Science* 185:181–183.

Rowat PF, Selverston AI (1993) Modeling the gastric mill central pattern generator of the lobster with a relaxation-oscillator network. *J Neurophysiol* 70:1030–1053.

Rowat PF, Selverston AI (1997) Oscillatory mechanisms in reciprocal inhibitory pairs of neurons, explored by means of phase portraits. *J Comput Neurosci* 4:103–127.

Sen K, Jorge-Rivera JC, Marder E, Abbott LF (1995) Synaptic response prediction using neural decoding. *Soc Neurosci Abst* 21:146.

Sen K, Jorge-Rivera JC, Marder E, Abbott LF (1996) Decoding synapses. *J Neurosci* 16:6307–6318.

Sharp AA, O'Neil MB, Abbott LF, Marder E (1993a) The dynamic clamp: Computer-generated conductances in real neurons. *J Neurophysiol* 69:992–995.

Sharp AA, O'Neil MB, Abbott LF, Marder E (1993b) The dynamic clamp: Artificial conductances in biological neurons. *Trends Neurosci* 16:389–394.

Sharp AA, Skinner FK, Marder E (1996) Mechanisms of oscillation in dynamic clamp constructed two cell half-center circuits. *J Neurophysiol* 76:867–883.

Siegel M, Marder E, Abbott LF (1994) Activity-dependent conductances produce nonuniform current distributions in spatially extended model neurons. *Proc Natl Acad Sci USA* 91:11308–11312.

Sigvardt KA, Williams TL (1996) Effects of local oscillator frequency on intersegmental coordination in the lamprey locomotor CPG: Theory and experiment. *J Neurophysiol* 76:4094–4103.

Skinner FK, Kopell N, Marder E (1994) Mechanisms for oscillation and frequency control in reciprocal inhibitory model neural networks. *J Comput Neurosci* 1:69–87.

Skinner FK, Kopell N, Mulloney B (1997) How does the crayfish swimmeret system work? Insights from nearest neighbor coupled oscillator models. *J Comput Neurosci* 4:151–160.

Stein PSG (1970) A neurophysiological study of two systems of coupled oscillators in the crayfish. Ph.D. thesis. Stanford University, Stanford, Calif.

Terman D, Bose A, Kopell N (submitted) Dynamics of two mutually coupled slow inhibitory neurons.

Tunstall MJ, Sillar KT (1993) Physiological and developmental aspects of intersegmental coordination in *Xenopus* embryos and tadpoles. *Semin Neurosci* 5:29–40.

Turrigiano GG, Abbott LF, Marder E (1994) Activity-dependent changes in the intrinsic properties of cultured neurons. *Science* 264: 974–977.

Turrigiano GG, LeMasson G, Marder E (1995) Selective regulation of current densities underlies spontaneous changes in the activity of cultured neurons. *J Neurosci* 15:3640–3652.

Turrigiano GG, Marder E (1993) Modulation of identified stomatogastric ganglion neurons in primary cell culture. *J Neurophysiol* 69:1993–2002.

Van Vreeswijk C, Abbott LF, Ermentrout GB (1994) When inhibition not excitation synchronizes neural firing. *J Comput Neurosci* 1:313–321.

Wallén P, Ekeberg Ö, Lansner A, Brodin L, Trávén H, Grillner S (1992) A computer based model for realistic simulations of neural networks. II. The segmental network generating locomotor rhythmicity in the lamprey. *J Neurophysiol* 68:1939–1950.

Wang X-J, Rinzel J (1992) Alternating and synchronous rhythms in reciprocally inhibitory model neurons. *Neural Comp* 4:844–897.

Williams TL (1992) Phase coupling by synaptic spread in chains of coupled neuronal oscillators. *Science* 258:662–665.

Williams TL, Sigvardt KA (1995) Intersegmental phase lags in the lamprey spinal cord: Experimental confirmation of the existence of a boundary region. *J Comput Neurosci* 1:61–67.

Williams TL, Sigvardt KA, Kopell N, Ermentrout GB, Remler MP (1990) Forcing of coupled nonlinear oscillators: Studies of intersegmental coordination in the lamprey locomotor central pattern generator. *J Neurophysiol* 64:862–871.

14

Dynamical Systems Analyses of Real Neuronal Networks

John Guckenheimer and
Peter Rowat

Abstract

Dynamical systems theory provides tools for the description and analysis of rhythmic behaviors of neuronal systems. We review several aspects of the theory and illustrate their use on simple models of reciprocally inhibiting neurons. We demonstrate that multiple time scales within a system can lead to bifurcations representing abrupt switches between different rhythms. Finally, we suggest that real neuronal networks have evolved to exploit mechanisms for pattern generation revealed by the theory.

Determining the function of biological structures is one of the primary goals of neuroscience. The structures underlying central pattern generators are neuronal networks, idealized as collections of compartments that interact through electrical and synaptic coupling. The function of these networks is to output patterned sequences of action potentials that stimulate muscular contraction. Network models that include single-compartment neuron models formulated in terms of intrinsic membrane conductances and ion concentrations can be used to study the contributions of the network architecture and the properties of intrinsic membrane conductances to the rhythmic behavior of pattern generators. One of the functional properties of a central pattern generator is to produce substantial changes in its rhythmic behavior in response to small inputs. The theory of bifurcations of nonlinear dynamical systems gives insight into how these changes occur and provides a geometric language for identifying the significant features of oscillatory mechanisms. As the state of a deterministic system evolves, it follows a trajectory in the multidimensional *phase space* formed from the time-dependent variables. The *phase portrait* is formed by partitioning the set of all trajectories into subsets that have the same asymptotic behavior; the different asymptotic behaviors are the *attractors* of the system. Models of a system are formulated as systems of (autonomous) ordinary differential equations that specify the rates of change of each variable for each point in the phase space. Integration of the differential equations yields the trajectories of the model. Dynamical systems theory elucidates general patterns observed in the partitioning of the trajectories in phase space. The theory gives substance to the geometric language revealing common features found in an astonishing array of different natural phenomena. The logic that stands behind dynamical systems analysis is subtle, so we describe a few assumptions of the theory. Furthermore, we assess the validity of the assumptions for neuronal systems.

Most applications of dynamical systems theory rely upon computer simulation and analysis. Differential equations seldom have solutions in terms of explicit analytic formulas, so numerical integration is the means of producing approximate solutions from the equations. The researcher amalgamates all of the solutions of a system into a phase portrait, so computational analysis of dynamical systems often involves integration of large number of trajectories. Moreover, we are interested in the effects of parameter variations and therefore want to compute many phase portraits. Figure 14.1, discussed in the third section ("An Example: Reciprocal Inhibition"), shows several phase portraits of a two-dimensional model neuron mapped to points of a plane representing values of two parameters. Figure 14.2 shows voltage traces of the model—solutions of the system—that map to trajectories in the phase portraits in figure 14.1. The primary goal of the mathematical analysis we describe is to extend such pictures to models with higher-dimensional phase spaces and more parameters. Simple estimates show that bruteforce computations to produce a coherent picture of system behavior are severely limited in their ability to solve this problem. To extend the usefulness of the models, we therefore seek additional tools for computing important properties of dynamical systems. Some of these tools exist, but many that we can imagine have not yet been built. The usefulness of dynamical systems methods for analyzing neuronal network models will be significantly enhanced by further development of algorithms that are more robust and more efficient than existing ones.

Dynamical models of neuronal systems span a wide range of sizes and degrees of biological realism. The Hodgkin-Huxley model for the action potential of squid giant axon is the foundation upon which most conductance-based models for neurons are constructed. These single compartmental models represent the electrical activity of a neuron through a summation of currents carried by individual conductances. Voltage-clamp techniques and pharmacological isolation of currents are used to measure those conductances. Evolutionary conservation of channel mechanism and function has ensured that the basic mechanisms utilized by most neuronal systems have common features. Thus, models built upon the Hodgkin-Huxley formalism to represent the dynamics of individual neurons have been successful in quantitatively reproducing the dynamics of neurons when the neurons are electrically compact. The development of such models is technically demanding and relies upon time-consuming experiments to characterize the conductances of individual neurons. Nonetheless, such models are invaluable in understanding important aspects of neuromodulation.

Buchholtz and colleagues (1992) constructed a Hodgkin-Huxley-type model for the LP cell in the stomatogastric ganglion of *Cancer borealis* that is based on the voltage-clamp measurements made by Golowasch (1991). Harris-Warrick and colleagues (1995a) offer a modification of this model that incorporates measurements on the LP cell in *Panulirus interruptus*. This thirteen-dimensional model incorporates all the main conductances that have been identified in the LP cell—namely, a sodium current, three potassium currents, a calcium current, a hyperpolarization-activated inward current (I_h), and a leak current. As a representation of the LP cell, the model appears to reproduce well the phenomenon of postinhibitory rebound in response to release from hyperpolarizing current injections. A smaller six-dimensional model of the AB cell in the stomatogastric ganglion of *Panulirus interruptus* was formulated by Guckenheimer and colleagues (1993) using more fragmentary voltage-clamp data. This model has a sodium current, three potassium currents, a calcium current, and a leak current, but no I_h current. Guckenheimer and colleagues conducted an extensive investigation of the dependence of the rhythmic behavior of the model neuron on the maximal conductance parameters for the potassium currents. They then compared their analysis with data from an isolated AB cell subjected to bath application of a potassium A current blocker.

Models with simplified representations of neurons that are not based directly upon conductance measurements are also useful. Rowat and Selverston (1993) developed a model for the gastric mill circuit of the lobster. Their model employs simplified representations of the individual neurons, but the network architecture includes all measured interactions among cells. This model has been used to test how modification of synaptic weights affects the phase relationships of the network rhythms. We reduce the model to a network of two cells interacting through reciprocal inhibition to illustrate the principles of dynamical systems theory discussed in this chapter.

Comparisons between model simulations and experimental data are a means of testing whether the components included within the models are sufficient to reproduce observations. In addition to "realistic" models of neuronal networks, there are models whose primary purpose is to provide test beds for the exploration of principles and mechanisms thought to be important in the construction of neuronal networks: "reduced" conductance-based models (e.g., the variation of the Morris-Lecar model studied by Rinzel and Ermentrout, 1989) and models directed at understanding specific dynamical mechanisms (e.g., the control of reciprocal inhibition studied by Skinner et al., 1994). Here, we explore how dynamical systems theory facilitates our understanding of the different types of models and their relationship to real neuronal systems. In the next section, we recall basic theoretical concepts.

Dynamical Systems Concepts

Dynamical systems theory gives a classification scheme for the solutions of systems of ordinary differential equations. The categories in the scheme are based upon an analysis of "generic" or typical systems. Qualitative features of such systems can be grouped in a manner that leads to a language that can describe system behavior. The syntax of this language rests upon a mathematical theory and provides a powerful guide to the development of numerical algorithms and the interpretation of simulations. The mathematical theory can be used as the foundation for modeling the dynamics of neural systems and for formulating principles that govern neural system function. This section provides an overview of dynamical systems concepts that are useful in the analysis of neuronal network models.

Principle 1: Genericity

The precise definition of *genericity* is technical, so we use an example to illustrate its meaning. The Lotka-Volterra equations are a simple model of interacting predator and prey populations. The equations that give the rates of change in host population h and prey population p are

$$\dot{h} = h(A - Bp)$$

$$\dot{p} = p(Ch - D)$$

The parameters A and D represent per capita rates of birth and death of the populations in the absence of interactions with the other species, whereas B and C represent the magnitude of the interactions. There is an equilibrium (steady-state) solution to the equations at $(h, p) = (D/C, A/B)$, but all other solutions to the system with positive h and p are periodic (Hirsch and Smale,

1974). Both predator and prey populations oscillate, with an amplitude that depends upon their initial values.

The property of having a whole family of periodic solutions is not generic. Small changes in the system produce large changes in the qualitative properties of the solutions. If the Lotka-Volterra system of equations is perturbed by adding a new term—for example, if we were to incorporate a term $-Eh^2$ representing density dependence of the population h into $\dot{h} = h(A - Bp - Eh)$—then the character of the solutions changes completely when $E > 0$. Instead of periodic solutions, all initial conditions with positive h and p tend to the equilibrium $(h, p) = (D/C, A/B - DE/BC)$. The Lotka-Volterra model is thus designated *structurally unstable* because its phase portrait changes qualitatively when the equations are perturbed. The list of properties known to be generic is very short. The second principle focuses upon the most important and immediate of these properties.

Principle 2: Hyperbolicity

Trajectories of dynamical systems come in three topological flavors: equilibrium points, periodic orbits, and regular trajectories (described further in the section called "Discussion"). The location of equilibrium points and periodic orbits is a prominent feature of the phase portrait of a dynamical system. In addition to locations, these special orbits have stable and unstable manifolds associated with them. The stable manifold for an equilibrium point or periodic orbit p is the set of trajectories that tend toward it as $t \to \infty$. Its unstable manifold is the set of trajectories that tend toward it as $t \to -\infty$. These invariant manifolds play a substantial role in the organization of the phase space of the system into regions of trajectories with similar long-time behavior.

In generic systems, the geometry of the stable and unstable manifolds near a periodic orbit is quite simple. Periodic orbits are hyperbolic, and the systems behave as if they were linear. For equilibrium points, hyperbolicity means that the locally linearized system separates the phase portrait into complementary subspaces of directions in which trajectories converge exponentially toward or diverge exponentially from the equilibrium. The stable and unstable manifolds of the equilibrium are tangent to the subspaces. Hyperbolicity for periodic orbits has a similar meaning, the primary difference being that the separation associated with the linearization has a one-dimensional subspace in the direction of the flow along the periodic orbit in addition to stable and unstable directions.

Dynamical Systems Analyses of Real Neuronal Networks

For two-dimensional vector fields, information about the invariant manifolds of special orbits characterizes the phase portrait of a generic system. In higher dimensions, there may be chaotic invariant sets, making more complex the geometric decomposition of the phase space into sets that reflect the long-time behavior of trajectories. Nonetheless, the spirit of the analysis is similar for both lower and higher dimensions. The complexity of the zoo of phase portraits of generic systems is bewildering, although some extensive theories apply to large classes of systems (Smale, 1967; Mañé, 1988). Fractals abound within the theory, and strange attractors were originally defined as attractors which were fractals.

We can view the phase portraits of dynamical systems as geometric descriptions in a language whose vocabulary and syntax are rooted in the theory. The language is powerful because the classification of objects depends on very general concepts of genericity. Therefore, even without specific models, one can analyze data for aspects that correspond to the general properties of dynamical systems. Relatively simple models, such as the iteration of one-dimensional mappings, produce geometric structures that have been widely observed in experimental data, including neural data (Hayashi and Ishizuka, 1992). Because the language arising from dynamical systems is constrained by the mathematics, it is not an easy language to master fluently. Nonetheless, we argue that the language is indeed relevant to the basic functioning of neuronal networks.

Principle 3: Normal Forms

In generic systems that depend upon parameters, periodic orbits that are not hyperbolic may occur at some parameter values. These particular values, as well as others in which the phase portrait of the system undergoes qualitative changes, are called *bifurcations*. For a neuronal model, a bifurcation might be associated with the emergence of a periodic state that has constant firing frequency from a quiescent state as some modulatory input is applied to the network. One goal of bifurcation theory is to produce maps of the parameter space for a system that show particular regions corresponding to different asymptotic states for the system. The maps develop a picture of the sensitivity of the system to individual differences as well as to modulation. Figure 14.1— discussed in more detail later in the chapter—shows such a map for a two-dimensional model neuron.

Linearization of a hyperbolic system near an equilibrium point transforms the system into one that has a simple analytic expression that can be solved in terms of elementary functions. Coordinate transformations can also be used to simplify the analytic expression of dynamical systems near points of bifurcation. The transformed systems are called *normal forms*. Analysis of normal forms leads to a catalog of dynamical behaviors that one expects to find in bifurcations of generic families of dynamical systems. The catalog is useful in a number of ways. First, it offers a way to make comparisons with experimental observations. For example, the "routes to chaos" (Eckmann, 1981) found in low-dimensional dynamical systems have been used to interpret phenomena displayed by fluids during transition from laminar to turbulent flow. The underlying principle behind this type of analysis is exemplified in the *Center Manifold Theorem* (Guckenheimer and Holmes, 1983), which gives a mathematical foundation for reducing the dynamics displayed by a high-dimensional vector field to one with only a few variables. This reduction capability is especially relevant to models of neural systems because often the function of such systems is to produce reliable rhythmic output that can be altered with small modulatory inputs.

The catalog of bifurcations for families of generic systems is also useful for the numerical analysis of example systems. Conductance-based models for neural networks produce relatively large dynamical systems, far larger than the two- and three-dimensional vector fields that have motivated much of the recent work on dynamical systems. Robust numerical algorithms that extend our ability to analyze these large systems are being developed with essential input from dynamical systems theory. The new computational methods have the potential to greatly expand our intuition and understanding of biological mechanisms that underlie "emergent behavior" in various networks.

Principle 4: Ergodicity

Some low-dimensional dynamical systems display chaos: their trajectories have aperiodic limit behavior and are sensitive to initial conditions. Chaos as a mechanism for generating unpredictability in a clockwork universe has received great attention, prompted by observations of unmistakable signs of chaos in many natural and laboratory phenomena, including neural output (Hayashi and Ishizuka, 1992). Investigation of the statistical properties of chaotic systems has led to the development of quantitative measures of the extent of chaotic behavior. Most of this analysis has been based upon the assumption that chaotic attractors have ergodic "natural measures"— intuitively equivalent to the assumption that most trajectories approaching the attractor have the same asymptotic density; in other words, they spend comparable amounts of time visiting the same regions near the attractor.

Three statistics of natural measures that quantify aspects of chaotic attractors are entropy, Lyapunov exponents, and fractal dimension. Algorithms for estimating these quantities from experimental data have been developed and widely used to examine time series ranging from global climate records to electrocardiograms. Substantial controversy has grown regarding the accuracy of such methods and the veracity of the conclusions drawn from them. Still, as an alternative to more traditional methods of time series analysis, which are based upon auto-regression models and power spectra, they are useful in detecting patterns that arise from nonlinear chaotic phenomena.

Principle 5: Multiple Time Scales

Neuronal systems have important time scales that range from the millisecond time scale of activation potentials to the month- or year-long developmental time scales. The theorist can adopt a working hypothesis that the separation of time scales is an important feature of neuronal system operation. Reliable responsiveness to stimuli is a process that must occur quickly, but adaptive mechanisms that regulate responses and reflect learning occur on much longer time scales. Understanding the impact of multiple time scales on the behavior of neuronal models is a major challenge to theorists. Here, we would like to extend the theory of generic families of dynamical systems to include a comprehensive description of singularly perturbed systems.

Singularly perturbed systems can be viewed from two perspectives. If the fast time scale of the system is taken as the basic time scale, then the limiting system is a parameterized family of vector fields. Moving away from the limit corresponds to a *slowly varying system* in which the variables that were parameters in the limiting equations now evolve on a slow time scale. If the slow time scale is taken as the basic time scale within the system, then the situation is more complicated. If the attractors of the fast subsystem are equilibrium points, then the motion of the limit system along the *slow manifolds* of equilibria are described by differential-algebraic equations. Such equations do not always have solutions: the dynamics of the fast equations are still important in describing the solutions of the limit equations. Furthermore, neuronal systems with bursting behavior have multiple time scale motions in which part of the fast motion occurs along limit cycles of the fast subsystem (Rinzel, 1987). We have little mathematics that can describe the dynamics of singularly perturbed systems near

the onset or termination of such bursts. Nor has there been much analysis that treats the properties of multiple time scale systems with regard to times that are long compared to the slow time scale within the system, despite the fact that the original constructions of chaotic systems by Cartwright and Littlewood (1947) were multiple time scale systems (Guckenheimer and Holmes, 1983).

An Example: Reciprocal Inhibition

To illustrate the principles presented in the previous section, we discuss models for reciprocal inhibition in small networks, adapted from the work of Rowat and Selverston (1993) on the gastric mill circuit of the stomatogastric ganglion. Their models are formulated abstractly, with no attempt to represent individual conductances within the model. Wang and Rinzel (1992) studied a similar model of a pair of reciprocally inhibiting cells—a model cast in terms of a single conductance that activates quickly and recovers slowly. Their analysis was extended by Skinner and colleagues (1994) to consider reciprocal inhibition in the context of a broader range of intrinsic properties for the individual cells. Oscillation based upon reciprocal inhibition between a pair of neurons is perhaps the oldest example of a dynamical behavior emerging from a neural network (Brown, 1911; Stein and Smith, chapter 5, this volume; Marder et al., chapter 13, this volume). Our purpose here is to emphasize that even the simplest differential equation models of such oscillators display a rich repertoire of different behaviors and that dynamical systems theory provides a sound substrate for exploring this behavior.

The equations we study here are

$$\dot{v}_1 = \rho_m(I_{1,\text{inj}} - (I_{1,\text{fast}} + I_{1,\text{slow}} + I_{1,\text{syn}}))$$

$$\dot{v}_2 = \rho_m(I_{2,\text{inj}} - (I_{2,\text{fast}} + I_{2,\text{slow}} + I_{2,\text{syn}})).$$

For each cell$_k$ ($k = 1, 2$), v_k is the membrane potential, $I_{k,\text{inj}}$ is the injected current, $I_{k,\text{fast}}$ is an idealized fast membrane current, $I_{k,\text{slow}}$ is an idealized slow membrane current, $I_{k,\text{syn}}$ is the postsynaptic current due to graded synaptic transmission from the presynaptic cell, and the time constant $1/\rho_m$ is proportional to the membrane capacitance. The fast current activates immediately with an N-shaped current-voltage (IV) curve defined by

$$I_{k,\text{fast}} = v_k - a_k \tanh(\sigma_k v_k / a_k).$$

This equation models the sum of an ohmic leak current, with unit slope ("v_k") and reversal potential 0 mV, and a saturating fast inward current whose activation curve has maximum slope σ_k and maximum amplitude proportional to a_k. The slope at the center of the 'N' is $1 - \sigma_k$, and the width of the N-shaped part is proportional to a_k. Only when $\sigma_k > 1$ is the IV-curve truly N-shaped because then the center segment has negative conductance. The slow current $q_k = I_{k,\text{slow}}$ approaches a steady-state value $s_k v_k$ with time constant $1/\rho_q$ if v_k is held fixed:

$$\dot{q}_k = \rho_q(-q_k + s_k v_k).$$

Thus, q_k combines the characteristics of two distinct types of slow currents, each with conductance s_k: a depolarization-activated $(v_k > 0)$ outward current and a hyperpolarization-activated $(v_k < 0)$, or I_h-like, inward current. For $(k, l) = (1, 2)$ or $(2,1)$, the postsynaptic current in cell_k has maximum conductance w_{kl} with reversal potential r_{kl}:

$$I_{k,\text{syn}} = f(\gamma_l, \theta_l, v_l)w_{kl}(v_k - r_{kl}),$$

where the proportion of w_{kl} active at any time is a sigmoidal function of the presynaptic potential v_l centered at θ with maximum slope γ:

$$f(\gamma, \theta, v) = 1.0/(1.0 + \exp(-4\gamma(v - \theta))).$$

The model is intended to portray slow oscillatory properties of a pair of cells, but not to represent action potentials. For reciprocal inhibition, the synaptic reversal potentials r_{kl} are taken below the usual lowest potential during oscillatory activity.

Understanding reciprocal inhibition requires a description of the response of a single cell to varying current for different values of the "steepness" parameter σ. The center of figure 14.1 displays a two-dimensional bifurcation diagram on the (σ, I) parameter plane. As σ and I vary, the model adopts ten distinct types of structurally stable phase portraits. In one of these, phase portrait 3, the horizontal axis is the membrane potential v, and the vertical axis is the slow current q. Some of the trajectories shown in the figure pass too close to one another for their separation to be resolved, but they never truly merge. The system in this region of the parameter space has three equilibrium points: the two denoted by triangles are stable (*sinks*), and the one denoted by a cross is a *saddle*. In addition, a stable periodic solution or *limit cycle* appears as the outermost curve in the phase portrait. Thus, there are three attractors: two sinks and a limit cycle. Each sink is surrounded by an unstable periodic solution (the dotted curve), which forms the boundary of its basin of attraction. The stable and unstable manifolds of the saddle point are also shown; the two steeply sloped branches of the stable manifold emerge

from unstable periodic orbits, and the nearly horizontal branches of the unstable manifold approach the limit cycle.

As is evident from figure 14.1, even this simple model displays a plethora of different phase portraits. The bifurcation diagram in the center of the figure organizes the information on how the different dynamical behaviors fit together. The numbers on the diagram correspond to the labels on the phase portraits. The curves in the bifurcation diagram locate where bifurcations occur with varying the parameters (σ, I), but three curves cannot be resolved at this scale. The large loop is a curve of Hopf bifurcations, at which an equilibrium gives birth to a periodic solution. In the outer region, all trajectories tend to a stable equilibrium. Region 1 has a single unstable equilibrium point, but all other trajectories in it tend to a stable limit cycle. The phase portraits for regions 0 and 1 are represented in figure 14.2. The cusp-shaped curve that divides regions 1 and 2 is a curve of saddle-node bifurcations at which a pair of new equilibrium points appear. The remaining, shorter bifurcation curves are curves of homoclinic bifurcations, along which branches of the stable and unstable manifolds of the saddle coalesce. Phase portrait 7 is located very close to such a bifurcation. Phase portraits 3 and 4 lie between phase portraits 2 and 5 on the horizontal line $I = 0$, which represents no current injection.

Figure 14.2 shows many traces from the model cell, each corresponding to a possible trajectory in a phase portrait of figure 14.1. Figure 14.2 includes a row for each phase portrait, and within each row there is a partition for each attractor in that phase portrait. In row 9, notice that both the fourth and fifth traces start on the unstable limit cycle; one, however, expands to the stable limit cycle; whereas the other contracts to the hyperpolarized equilibrium.

The bifurcation diagram and phase portraits can be used to interpret the progression of different states a cell will reach with increasing or decreasing current injection, for different values of σ. For example, in the range of σ in which the cell passes through regions 7 and 2 with increasing current injection, an initial hyperpolarizing current brings it to region 0 (h), where the only attracting state is a hyperpolarized equilibrium. When the saddle-node curve is crossed, a new pair of depolarized equilibria emerge, but they are unstable: hence, phase portrait 7. In one of the bifurcations between regions 7 and 8, a pair of periodic solutions (one stable and one unstable) is born, and there is bistability, shown in phase portrait 8. The unstable periodic solution contracts to-

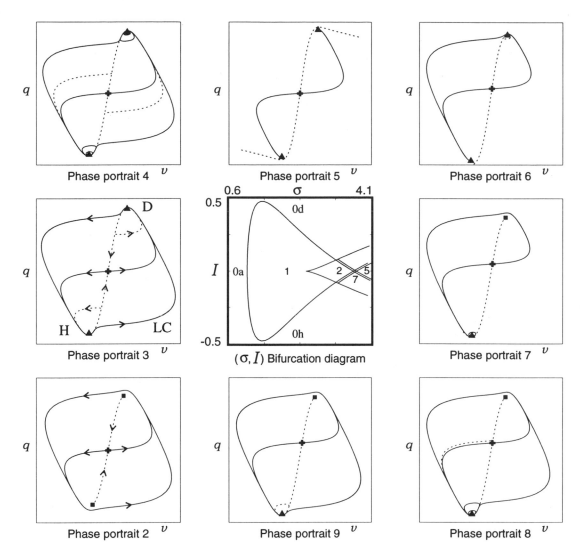

Figure 14.1

A two-parameter bifurcation diagram and its phase portraits for the dynamical system

$$\dot{v} = -8(v - \tanh(\sigma v) + q - I)$$

$$\dot{q} = 0.4(-q + 1.5v).$$

In the middle square, the (σ, I) plane is divided into regions by curves of Hopf, saddle-node, and homoclinic bifurcations. Each region has a topologically unique phase portrait. In each numbered region, a point has been selected and its phase portrait drawn in an outer square. Phase portraits for regions 0 and 1 appear in figure 14.2. Regions 3 and 4 are small diamonds between 2 and 5, region 6 is the strip between regions 5 and 7, and regions 8 and 9 are substrips between regions 7 and 2.

Some regions cannot be resolved in this diagram. In each phase portrait: triangles depict stable equilibrium points (*sinks*), crosses depict saddle points, and squares depict unstable equilibrium points (*sources*); solid curves depict the stable manifolds of periodic orbits and unstable manifolds of saddle points; dotted curves depict unstable periodic orbits and stable manifolds of saddle points. Arrows added in phase portraits 2 and 3 indicate the direction of motion associated with these manifolds. The parameter values for phase portraits 0–9 are (0.7, 0), (2.3, 0), (3.25, 0), (3.742, 0), (3.74252, 0), (4, 0), (3.95, −0.04), (3.52, −0.04), (3.51068, −0.04), (3.5, −0.04). In phase portrait 3, D, H, and LC label the attractors.

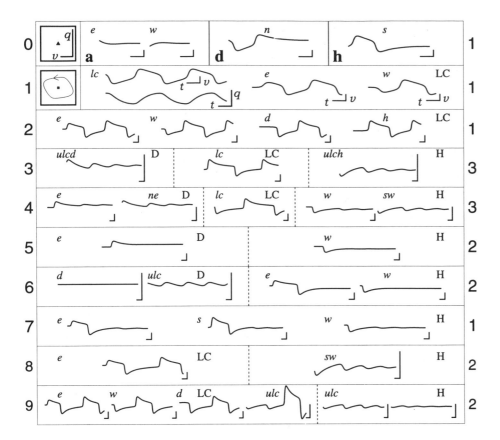

Figure 14.2

Voltage traces arising from trajectories in the figure 14.1 phase portraits. The row_j traces are obtained with parameters of the jth phase portrait. Rows 0 and 1 begin with their phase portraits. The righthand numerals give the number of attractors for each phase portrait. Row_0 is subdivided into subtypes corresponding to positions a, d, h within region_0. At a, large perturbations e and w from the single sink cause passive responses while at d or h, similar perturbations, n and s, cause excitable responses. The traces in row_i, $i > 0$, are partitioned and labeled according to the attractor they converge to: LC, limit cycle; D, depolarized sink; H, hyperpolarized sink. Traces are labelled by their initial point in the phase plane: points e and w are small perturbations from the central saddle; ne and sw are close to the saddle; s is below the sink; points d and h are the depolarized and hyperpolarized sources; lc is on the limit cycle; and ulc ($ulcd$, $ulch$) are on the unstable (depolarized, hyperpolarized) limit cycles. For the row_1 limit cycle, we show the v- and q-traces. Scalebars: 1 unit in each direction.

ward the stable equilibrium: phase portrait 9. Following the Hopf bifurcation while entering region 2, the hyperpolarized equilibrium loses its stability, and the only attractor is the periodic solution: phase portrait 2. When the upper Hopf bifurcation curve is crossed as the cell leaves region 2, the most depolarized equilibrium becomes stable: phase portraits 9 and 8, inverted. Shortly afterward, the stable limit cycle disappears by colliding with an unstable periodic solution, and the only remaining attractor is the depolarized equilibrium: phase portrait 7, inverted, followed by phase portrait 0 (d).

Brief transitory inputs that affect the values of q and v can cause a switch between attractors when the cell is in a multistable region of parameter space. This switch occurs in phase portrait 5, which depicts a cell with simple plateau potentials. If the cell is at the depolarized equilibrium, any perturbation that takes the state to the left

of the dotted curve will result in a switch to the hyperpolarized equilibrium, but not if the state remains on the right of this curve. A small hyperpolarizing current moves the cell to phase portrait 6. Here, the small unstable limit cycle around the depolarized equilibrium D ensures that most perturbations will cause the state to switch to the hyperpolarized equilibrium.

We now turn to the full four-dimensional model for reciprocal inhibition. Our intuition about reciprocal inhibition is cast largely in terms of fast switches between slowly varying states. Wang and Rinzel (1992), as well as Skinner and colleagues (1994) placed emphasis upon how the oscillation period is affected by where the transitions take place relative to the individual cell's intrinsic transitions. Here, we concentrate on adjusting the parameters of our model to vary both the timescales associated with the transitions and the sharpness of the

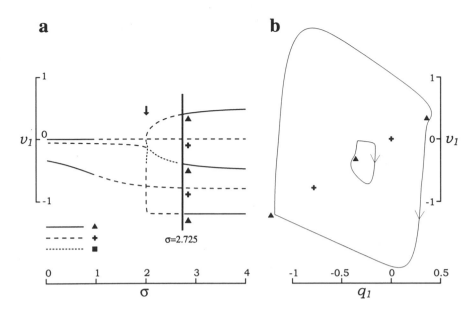

a

σ=2.725

b

Figure 14.3
Equilibrium point diagram and a phase portrait for the reciprocal inhibition model. (a) Equilibrium point curves plotted as a function of the parameter σ. Only v_1, of the four coordinates (v_1, q_1, v_2, q_2), is plotted. A change in the format of a curve between solid, dashed, or dotted indicates a change in the type of equilibrium. The parameters are symmetric between the two cells: $\rho_m = 8$, $\rho_q = 0.4$, $\gamma = 10$, $\theta = 0.013333$, $s = 1.0$, $w = 0.5$, $a = 1.0$, $I = 0$, $r = -4$. Symbols as in figure 14.1. (b) A partial phase portrait projected onto the (q_1, v_1) plane at σ = 2.725, with other parameters as in a. There are five attractors: three stable equilibrium points (triangles) and two limit cycles. The intersections of the grey line in A with the equilibrium point curves correspond to the equilibrium points in B. The v_1 scales are identical in a and b.

voltage range in which synaptic activation occurs. We have performed only a fragmentary analysis but have already found tantalizing questions lurking in this simple model of reciprocal inhibition, questions whose answers require the framework provided by dynamical systems theory.

We have investigated parameters in which the two cells have identical properties. The model has varied complex dynamical features. As the steepness parameter σ is varied, the model displays as many as seven equilibrium points (see arrow in figure 14.3a). In addition to the bistability associated with multiple equilibria, combinations of oscillatory and stable equilibrium behavior occur at the same parameter values. Figure 14.3b shows the projection of such a phase portrait onto the (q_1, v_1) coordinate plane. There are five equilibrium points, three of which are stable. In addition, there are two stable limit cycles. The large limit cycle is a half-center oscillation in which one cell is depolarized and the other is hyperpolarized. In the second limit cycle the two cells are synchronous; this limit cycle lies in the plane $v_1 = v_2$, $q_1 = q_2$, which is invariant under the flow because the model is symmetric with respect to interchanging the two cells. The half-center oscillations have a more complex symmetry that comes from both interchanging the two cells and advancing points a half period. Thus, the

system has at least three distinct types of attractors, and different regions of initial conditions can lead to any of the described behaviors.

We seek to follow the half-center oscillation to understand how it appears and vanishes with changing parameters. Its symmetry constrains the types of bifurcations that can occur. As we increase the parameters σ, the half-center oscillation disappears—not by colliding with an equilibrium point, but rather by colliding with an unstable limit cycle of the same symmetry type. When the latter event occurs, the trajectories that were attracted to the half-center oscillations now approach an equilibrium point in which the cells are at different potentials. Determining the character of the bifurcation that terminates the half-center oscillations can be done only by numerically integrating the equations for the model. Furthermore, simulations of the network appear rather mysterious without a theoretical understanding of what is happening. The limit cycle simply seems to vanish at a particular parameter value. The dynamical mechanism for the disappearance of the half-center oscillations is not immediately associated with a "switch" in which one cell becomes active while the other falls silent. The unstable cycle is difficult to find without algorithms that track the family of periodic oscillations through the bifurcation point (Doedel, 1986), so effort is required to understand how this bifurcation occurs. A similar bifurcation occurs as we reduce σ, at values for which there are only two stable equilibria. If we vary the injected current to the cells instead of changing the parameter σ, the half-center oscillations are terminated in the same manner.

The symmetry of the half-center oscillations precludes its bifurcation by period doubling. However, if we adjust the parameter values of the model so that the system is no longer symmetric, then period doubling becomes possible and indeed occurs. Cascades of period-doubling bifurcations may lead to chaotic behavior of the system. We have located a very narrow strip of parameter values in which this appears to occur, but iterations of a one-dimensional mapping do not approximate very well the return map of this chaotic behavior. Strong contraction takes place in one pair of directions in the four-dimensional phase space, but the motion along the unstable direction does not give a simple mapping with a few critical points, perhaps due to numerical artifacts. The period-doubling transition, however, is clear. The different time scales in the model contribute to the difficulty of the numerical analysis of the model. Whatever the causes of the numerical chaos in this model, we cannot discount the effects of both the deterministic dynamics of the system and stochastic fluctuations in contributing to aperiodicity in experimental observation.

Elson and Selverston (1992) studied the gastric mill circuit in the stomatogastric ganglion when modulated by muscarinic inputs. A subnetwork of three cell types—the LG, DG, and LPG neurons—provides the kernel of the rhythm-generating mechanism for this circuit. The three cell types are connected by five inhibitory synapses, the synapse from the LPG neuron onto the DG neuron being absent. Understanding the rhythms displayed by this network in response to modulatory inputs is considerably more difficult than understanding the behavior of a pair of cells. The model described above can be extended to a model for three cells that are interacting by pairwise reciprocal inhibition. In such a network, exploration of how synaptic weights affect the rhythmic output involves five synaptic weights rather than just two. Moreover, the different cell types in the stomatogastric ganglion have distinct intrinsic properties. Representing this detail in a model and relating it to the observed dynamics of the network is a substantial undertaking. It is difficult to predict how changes in the many model parameters will change the network properties. Nonetheless, the dynamical mechanisms that produce changes in qualitative behaviors are likely to be those identified by the study of generic systems.

We have investigated a three-cell network with this architecture. There are abrupt transitions between different rhythmic patterns. The observed changes of pattern, as well as the transition shown in figure 14.4, are apparently examples of *canards* that occur in systems with multiple time scales. Systems with multiple time scales have unstable "slow" manifolds in which the velocity of the motion is comparable to the slow time scale. Because the motion along the manifolds happens on the slow time scale, but the exponential separation of points in these regions occurs on the fast time scale, trajectories dramatically diverge from nearby initial points. The divergence can manifest itself in an apparent discontinuity in where trajectories go. In practical terms, the discontinuity appears as a switch in which tiny changes in a parameter seem to produce dramatically different trajectories. Trajectories that follow the unstable slow manifolds are called canards. Simple examples of this phenomenon can be seen in the single-cell model (figures 14.1 and 14.2). Near the equilibrium points D and H in phase portraits 3 and 4, the limit cycle follows the unstable manifold for a short distance, causing an increase in the limit cycle period. These phase portraits appear in the transition from a single attracting limit cycle (phase portrait 2) to widely separated equilibrium points (phase portrait 5). A similar canard appears in phase portraits 8 and 9 in the transition between the single-equilibrium behavior of phase portrait 7 and the single limit cycle of phase portrait 2. Note that the use of standard numerical integration methods for stiff systems to compute canards is problematic because the methods are adapted to deal primarily with strong exponential convergence of trajectories rather than divergence. The extreme sensitivity of canards to perturbations of parameters allows them to function as switches between well-defined behaviors.

Discussion

Dynamical systems theory has been used for data analysis without the intervention of specific models. Statistical properties of chaotic attractors and mechanisms of bifurcation in dynamical systems are sufficiently universal that a theorist can search for patterns in data that reflect aspects of the theory. The bifurcation diagrams that partition parameter spaces contain such universal patterns. Of course, mechanistic models are useful in obtaining a deeper understanding of a phenomenon, but the development of improved computational tools is required for dealing with more complex models than the model of reciprocal inhibition discussed in the previous section. For

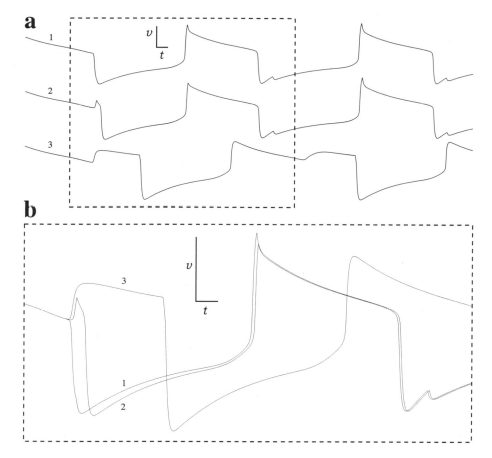

Figure 14.4

A "canard" phenomenon in a three cell model for the LG, DG, LPG subnetwork of the gastric mill circuit. (a) Three voltage traces showing a transition between behaviors corresponding to attractors in different phase portraits: σ was increased by 10^{-5} between the traces. (b) The traces in the dotted rectangle in (a) have been enlarged and overlaid to emphasize the canard in trace 2: first it follows trace 3, then switches back and synchronizes with trace 1.

example, Guckenheimer and colleagues (1993) gave a bifurcation analysis of a conductance-based model for the AB neuron of the stomatogastric ganglion. They used multidimensional bifurcation diagrams to compare the response of the model to conductance changes with data on the response of the AB cell to 4-AP, a blocker of the potassium A current in this neuron.

Initial parameter values for the model were chosen for regions close to degenerate bifurcations. Bifurcation curves can indicate regions of parameter space where small changes in parameter values result in qualitative changes in system behavior. Near degenerate bifurcations, sensitivity to small parameter changes is even greater, and there are often more regions of different types of qualitative behavior nearby. In view of the need for the nervous system to be maximally sensitive to its environment and to modify its motor behavior in response to small parameter changes, it is natural to speculate that many neuronal systems have evolved to operate in a parameter region close to a degenerate bifurcation.

We go further than suggesting that dynamical systems theory is a useful tool: we hypothesize that the language of dynamical systems may have deeper functional significance for neuronal systems. In particular, we assert that evolutionary changes in neuronal systems may have exploited the properties of multiple time scale dynamical systems that are close to points of degenerate bifurcation.

Our argument for the relevance of dynamical systems theory to the analysis of neuronal networks is based upon the following observations.

1. Much of the information in neuronal systems is carried by the timing of action potentials. The machinery that generates the action potentials is noisy, but the behavior resulting from the underlying neural activity is often very reliable.

2. Neural systems are adaptable. Their patterns of behavior can be modified in response to learning and conditioning, which indicates that the underlying mechanisms are quite flexible.

3. Neuronal systems are capable of switching behaviors in response to small inputs with low energetic cost.

4. Well-separated time scales seem to operate in neuronal systems. The duration of an action potential is a small fraction of the duration of a burst of repetitive firing, which in turn is of shorter duration than the periods associated with complex rhythmic bursting activity.

How can we assess whether neuronal systems make use of the principles of dynamical systems theory (defined more fully in the section "Dynamical Systems Concepts")? Our remarks do not constitute evidence for our hypothesis. Indeed, the hypothesis cannot be verified directly. Nonetheless, it provides a motivating strategy for studies of neuronal systems, one that leads to testable predictions. It is a truism that neuronal networks can support a varied functional repertoire. Central pattern generators must be able to output rhythmic patterns that coordinate all of the behaviors of the structures that they innervate. Such flexibility implies that the architecture of a network will often fail to determine the output. The modulation of inputs, synaptic strengths, and intrinsic properties of a network's neurons produces different outputs. Dynamical systems theory is well suited to contribute to our understanding of the relationship between modulation and behavioral changes.

The perspective offered by dynamical systems theory complements other approaches for examining neuronal systems. The amount of detail in our knowledge of neuronal systems is staggering. Neuroscience integrates the numerous data collected from the studies of the structure of individual neurons, connectivity properties of networks, molecular structure of channels and neurotransmitters, cascades of reactions involving second messengers, electrophysiological recordings from single channels, cells and extracellular potential fields, as well as from cognitive and behavioral studies. Overarching principles are needed to organize all of this information, but the systems do not decompose themselves into subunits as neatly as the machines that we build. We are left with a quandary as to whether top-down or bottom-up approaches will be more effective in discovering the principles of organization. As we build models, we need to remain vigilant to the possibility that there are many potential ways of carrying out the functional tasks performed by neuronal networks; therefore, the models that reproduce important features of neuronal function may

do so in ways that are different than the real system's methods. Thus, it is worthwhile to seek models that have the ability to integrate and explain disparate data. Dynamical systems theory highlights qualitative aspects of models directly related to neuromodulation, and this information can be used to constrain models for neuronal systems.

The analogy between multiple time scale dynamical systems and neuronal systems can be pursued in two different ways: (1) classify the generic behaviors of this class of dynamical systems and relate them to specific experimental observations, or (2) construct dynamical models for particular neuronal systems and relate them to experimental observations of these systems. Both tasks are useful. The first approach can lend insight into general mechanisms that appear to be critical in the functioning of pattern generators and other neuronal systems. Ideas can be explored more efficiently and more easily on simplified models, thus also allowing for more exploration of theoretical concepts. We have given a new example of such a mechanism, illustrating how a sensitive switch between two well-defined behaviors of a system might depend on the canard phenomenon in dynamical systems with two time scales. The second approach requires extensive effort to measure the properties of individual neurons within a network, even for a small network. Therefore, the second approach is feasible only in conjunction with supporting laboratory investigations. The coordination of laboratory and modeling studies of a system presents the practical problem of keeping the two in synchrony. Nonetheless, such studies can be very important in drawing attention to important biological detail easily overlooked in other approaches to the analysis of motor behavior.

Acknowledgments

John Guckenheimer was partially supported by the Department of Energy, the Office of Naval Research, and the National Science Foundation. Peter Rowat was supported by the National Science Foundation and the Okun Fund.

References

Brown T (1911) The intrinsic factors in the act of progression in the mammal. *Proc Roy Soc Lond B* 84:308–319.

Buchholtz F, Golowasch J, Epstein IR, Marder E (1992) Mathematical model of an identified stomatogastric ganglion neuron. *J Neurophysiol* 67:332–339.

Cartwright ML, Littlewood JE (1947) On non-linear differential equations of the second order. II. The equation $\ddot{y} + kf(y)\dot{y} + g(y, k) = p(t) = p_1(t) + kp_2(t); k > 0, f(y) \geq 1$. Ann Math 48:472–494.

Doedel E (1986) AUTO: Software for Continuation and Bifurcation Problems in Ordinary Differential Equations. Pasadena: CIT Press.

Eckmann JP (1981) Roads to turbulence in dissipative dynamical systems. Rev Mod Phys 53:643–654.

Elson RC, Selverston AI (1992) Mechanisms of gastric rhythm generation in the isolated stomatogastric ganglion of lobsters: Bursting, pacemaker potentials, synatic interactions and muscarinic modulation. J Neurophysiol 68:890–907.

Epstein IR, Marder E (1990) Multiple modes of a conditional neural oscillator. Biol Cybern 63:25–34.

Golowasch JP (1991) Characterization of a stomatogastric ganglion neuron. A biophysical and mathematical interpretation. Thesis, Brandeis University, Waltham, Mass.

Guckenheimer J, Gueron S, Harris-Warrick RM (1993) The dynamics of a conditionally bursting neuron. Philos Trans Roy Soc Lond B 341:345–359.

Guckenheimer J, Holmes P (1983) Nonlinear Oscillations, Dynamical Systems, and Bifurcation of Vector Fields. New York: Springer.

Harris-Warrick RM, Coniglio L, Barazangi N, Guckenheimer J, Gueron S (1995a) Dopamine modulation of transient potassium current evokes phase shifts in a central pattern generator network. J Neurosci 15:342–358.

Harris-Warrick RM, Coniglio L, Levini R, Gueron S, Guckenheimer J (1995b) Dopamine modulation of two subthreshold currents produces phase shifts in activity of an identified neuron. J Neurophysiol 74:1404–1420.

Hayashi H, Ishizuka S (1992) Chaotic nature of bursting discharges in the onchidium pacemaker neuron. J Theor Biol 156:269–291.

Hirsch M, Smale S (1974) Differential Equations, Dynamical Systems, and Linear Algebra. San Diego: Academic.

Mañé R (1988) A proof of the C^1 stability conjecture. Publ IHES 66:161–210.

Rinzel J (1987) A formal classification of bursting mechanisms in excitable systems. In: Proceedings of the 1986 International Congress of Mathematicians (Gleason AM, ed.), 1578–1594. Providence, R.I.: American Math Society.

Rinzel J, Ermentrout B (1989) Analysis of neural excitability and oscillations. In: Methods in Neuronal Modelling (Koch C, Segev I, eds.), 135–171. Cambridge, Mass.: MIT Press.

Rowat P, Selverston AI (1993) Modelling the gastric mill central pattern generator of the lobster with a relaxation-oscillator network. J Neurophysiol 70:1030–1053.

Skinner FC, Kopell N, Marder E (1994) Mechanisms for oscillation and frequency control in reciprocally inhibitory model neural networks. J Comput Neurosci 1:69–88.

Smale S (1967) Differentiable dynamical systems. Bull Am Math Soc 73:747–817.

Wang X-J, Rinzel J (1992) Alternating and synchronous rhythms in reciprocally inhibitory neurons. Neural Comput 4:84–97.

15

Realistic Modeling of Burst Generation and Swimming in Lamprey

Anders Lansner, Örjan Ekeberg, and Sten Grillner

Abstract

During the last ten years, the lamprey spinal swimming generator has been the subject of extensive experimental studies, mathematical modeling, and computer simulation. Models of the local central pattern generator have been investigated with respect to such issues as burst frequency range, the roles of different transmitters and receptors, brainstem control and sensory input, and the significance of population effects. Recent modeling results suggest that active 5-hydroxytryptamine modulation of the late afterhyperpolarization may be more important for burst generation than previously appreciated. The first models of intersegmental co-ordination in undulatory locomotion were formulated as a chain of discrete coupled oscillators. Such highly abstract models are useful because they allow analysis. In some respects, however, they are difficult to relate to biological reality. We have developed a set of continuous network models that include more biological detail at the single-cell as well as the network level. To describe the entire swimming behavior, we designed a neuro-mechanical model that incorporates characteristics of the central pattern generator, descriptions of the body with its musculo-skeletal apparatus, and the interaction with the surrounding water. A two-dimensional model was capable of producing forward, backward, and narrow swimming as well as turning. This model was recently extended to three dimensions. A hypothesized crossed-diagonal central pattern generator configuration added pitching and rolling to the movement repertoire. The modeling work presented illustrates the value of computer simulation as a research tool, the importance of interaction between modeling and experiments, and the need to work with models at different levels of abstraction.

The body of knowledge relating to cellular properties and interactions in different neuronal systems is rapidly growing. Purely conceptual models are not able to organize our available knowledge into a functionally meaningful whole. Computational neuroscience (i.e., mathematical modeling and computer simulation of neuronal systems) offers new possibilities to assist those aspects of experimental research that require synthesis (Sejnowski and Churchland, 1992; Koch and Davis, 1994). Modeling in close interaction with experiments have focused on motor systems of invertebrates and primitive vertebrates because those systems remain among the most well-known with respect to system properties.

A model of a particular system can be formulated in many different ways. We focus here on "realistic" models—that is, models with descriptions at the cellular level. We consider the structure and function of the neural circuitry that underlies lamprey undulatory swimming. We describe work that uses spiking neuron models of the local and distributed lamprey central pattern generator (CPG), as well as a neuro-mechanical model of the entire swimming behavior.

Outline of the Lamprey Swimming CPG

The lamprey is a primitive, eel-like aquatic vertebrate that swims with undulatory movements. It has served as an experimental model for the neural generation of locomotion (Grillner et al., 1995; Grillner et al., 1991). The "fictive swimming" preparation of this system offers a major advantage: when stimulated by excitatory amino acids, an isolated piece of spinal cord generates rhythmic bursts of activity that resemble natural swimming activity. This preparation makes the neural circuitry experimentally available in an extraordinary way. The lamprey locomotor CPG and the frog embryo CPG have been the subject of numerous modeling and simulation studies (see also Marder et al., chapter 13, this volume); they are currently among the best-understood vertebrate motor systems (Roberts and Tunstall, 1990; Arshavsky et al., 1993; Roberts et al., chapter 7, this volume; Dale, chapter 8, this volume).

The lamprey swimming movements are produced by a laterally directed wave of muscular activity that travels from head to tail. Its wavelength is about the same as the length of the body. The spinal swimming rhythm CPG is distributed along the spinal cord. It drives the muscles via the motor neurons, the axons of which form the ventral roots. Each ventral root pair is associated with a spinal cord segment. The entire cord has about one hundred ventral root pairs and thus the same number of segments. In order to maintain the one cycle per body length over the entire frequency range, the phase lag of activity must be constant with a value near 1% of a cycle per segment.

Local and Distributed Burst Generation

The Local CPG: Burst Generation

The neuronal circuitry responsible for rhythm generation in a small piece of spinal cord is here referred to as the *local CPG*. It consists of two halves that have reciprocal inhibition between them. Each half consists of a set of premotor interneurons: excitatory interneurons (EINs),

contralaterally and caudally projecting interneurons (CCINs), and lateral interneurons (LINs) (Buchanan and Grillner, 1987; Grillner et al., 1991; Grillner et al., 1995; Wallén, chapter 6, this volume). The entire network is activated by glutamate projections from brainstem neurons that produce bursts of activity that alternate between the two sides (Otha and Grillner, 1989). The fast excitatory EIN action is glutamatergic; CCIN and LIN inhibition is glycinergic. Slower G-protein-mediated modulators such as 5-HT (serotonin), GABA$_B$, and dopamine are also found in this system. Further, stretch receptor neurons (edge cells) in the cord itself provide sensory feedback to the local CPG (Viana di Prisco et al., 1990).

The first attempts to model the local swimming CPG showed that moderate- to high-frequency bursting could easily be produced by the proposed network (Grillner et al., 1988). The decrease in burst frequency seen during bath application of 5-HT could be replicated. Later simulations used a simulation program, SWIM, that incorporated a compartmentalized Hodgkin-Huxley-type cell model with the most relevant ion channels (Ekeberg et al., 1991; Wallén et al., 1992; Ekeberg et al., 1994). Using this simulator, we replicated the activity induced by bath application of excitatory amino acids as well as the intrinsic NMDA-induced oscillations of the cells (Brodin et al., 1991). In a later study, brainstem and sensory input to the local CPG was included (Tråvén et al., 1993). Results suggested that the relative importance of AMPA/kainate receptor activation over NMDA progressively increased with increasing brainstem drive to the CPG. In addition, simulations of rhythmic sensory input resulted in shifts of the local oscillator to either higher or lower frequencies as compared to its intrinsic frequency.

A parallel series of simulations examined the effect of having several cells of each type in the model network (Hellgren et al., 1992). This "population model" produced a stable bursting activity over a large frequency range even without LINs in the network. The result forced a reconsideration of the importance of LINs in burst generation. Later experiments also support the hypothesis that the LIN may not be of primary importance in burst termination (Grillner et al., 1995).

In a new simulation study, using simplified but nevertheless dynamic and adapting spiking model neurons, we have further examined the mechanisms responsible for burst termination in the lamprey network. We found that dynamic modulation of the late afterhyperpolarization (AHP) of EINs and CCINs gives a stable burst generator with an adequate frequency range (figure 15.1). We assume that the lamprey spinal cord midline neurons that

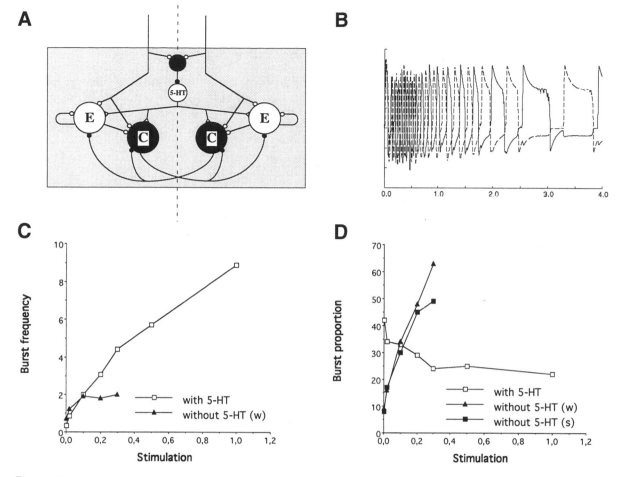

Figure 15.1
A. Local CPG network with excitatory interneuron (E), contralaterally inhibitory interneuron (C), 5-HT neurons, and brainstem drive. B. Sample of burst generation at high to low levels of stimulation. Population EIN activity on y-axis, arbitrary time on x-axis. Left and right sides are shown in solid and dashed lines respectively. Burst frequency (C) and burst proportion (D) as a function of tonic input. Curves in C and D are with and without 5-HT modulation and with weak (w) and strong (s) reciprocal inhibition.

release 5-HT are responsible for AHP modulation. In this model, 5-HT release is gradually reduced at higher frequencies so that the AHP becomes more pronounced and can build up more rapidly to terminate the burst. This burst-generating network differs from ones developed in previous models in that accumulated late AHP is the dominant burst termination factor throughout the entire frequency range. Neither LIN nor reciprocal CCIN inhibition need to be present. A simulated half-segment is itself capable of producing bursting throughout the entire frequency range.

Our results so far clearly demonstrate the importance of including relevant cell properties in the model to help us understand the burst generation mechanisms of this network. However, the mechanism suggested here remains a hypothesis until it has been critically examined and verified experimentally.

The Distributed CPG: Intersegmental Co-ordination

The spinal pattern generator can be seen as a number of local CPGs, connected in order to produce a traveling wave of motor activity along the body. The intersegmental co-ordination has been the subject of a number of mathematical and simulation studies. Even before the neuronal network was known in any detail, it was possible to utilize the mathematics of non-linear oscillators to make predictions about the nature of the coupling (Cohen et al., 1982; Cohen et al., 1992; Marder et al., chapter 13, this volume). More recently, discrete segmental oscillators made up of simplified neuron models have been used to study the consequences of different coupling schemes (Buchanan, 1992; Williams, 1992).

Anatomical data do not support the supposition that each local CPG is distinct at the level of the premotor neurons, however. The premotor interneurons seem to

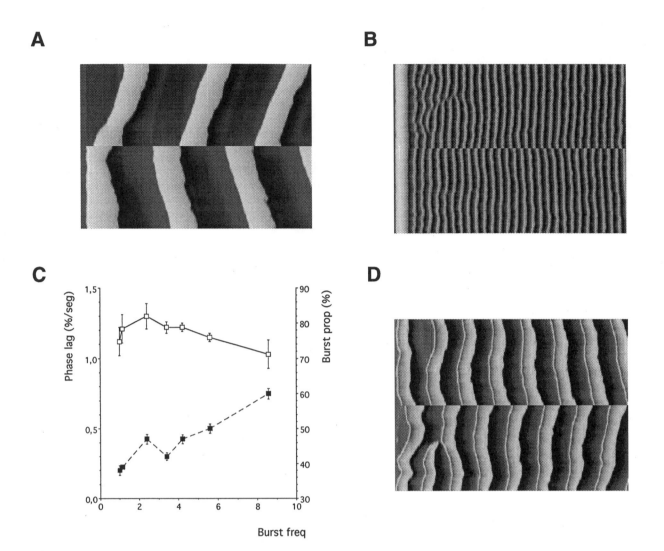

Figure 15.2

(A) Slow swimming. (B) Fast swimming. (C) Phase lag (upper curve) and burst proportion (lower curve) versus bursting frequency. (D) Backward swimming. In A, B, and D, activation at different levels of the spinal cord as a function of time is shown. White corresponds to maximum activity and black to maximum inhibition. Time is indicated along the horizontal dimension. Activity on the right and left side is shown in the upper and lower half, respectively. The rostral end is at the center, with progressively more caudal parts toward the top and bottom respectively.

comprise a continuous column-like structure that extends along the entire cord. Such a network was simulated by Ekeberg (1993) in the context of a neuro-mechanical model. This network structure has the basic connectivity patterns of the local CPG extended longitudinally: the EINs project in the local neighborhood of about two segments rostrally and caudally; the CCIN inhibition distributes about the same amount rostrally but extends caudally some twenty segments.

The local CPG model with dynamic AHP modulation was recently incorporated into a simulation of a continuous network of this type, generating stable bursting and a constant phase lag (about 1%) along the body throughout a wide frequency range (figure 15.2). If the

lack of connections from neighboring segments in the most rostral and caudal ends is compensated for by making the remaining connections stronger, phase lag becomes zero. Additional excitation to some part of the network produces a phase lag with the stimulated part leading. Non-end-compensated caudally extending CCIN connections give a bias for forward "swimming." They also tend to stabilize activity, especially at higher frequencies. Nevertheless, it is still possible to control the phase lag and even to reverse it by adding extra inhibition and excitation respectively to the head and tail part of the CPG.

In addition, a more detailed model of the entire distributed CPG has been simulated (Wadden et al., 1997).

A

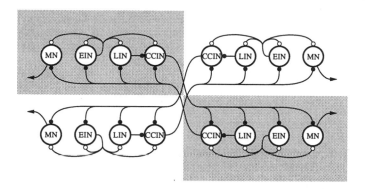

B

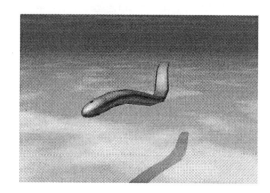

Figure 15.3

(A) Crossed-diagonal CPG configuration hypothesized for the 3-D neuro-mechanical model. The spinal CPG neurons are subdivided into separate dorsally and ventrally controlling populations. A preferred crossed-diagonal connectivity forms a dual-oscillator system. (B) One

frame from a video of the swimming 3-D lamprey model demonstrating a roll maneuver produced by the diagonal stimulation indicated (shaded) in A.

It includes about 2,400 neurons and 700,000 synapses, which approaches the upper limit of what is possible to simulate using currently available computers and software. This model replicates many of the properties of the real system, but it still includes a frequency dependency of the phase lag. Work is in progress to add features of the model that generated constant phase lag to the more detailed simulation.

A Neuro-Mechanical Model

In most simulation studies, the lamprey CPG has been described in isolation—that is, without any feedback from its surroundings: the "fictive swimming" experimental condition. By adding a model of the mechanical properties, however, further aspects of the swimming act can be analyzed, such as the role of sensory feedback. In a recent study, the continuous neuronal network model of the lamprey CPG was connected to a two-dimensional mechanical model that described the body, including its interaction with the surrounding water (Ekeberg, 1993). All components of the system (neurons, mechanosensors, muscles, body, and surrounding water) were simplified considerably. Nevertheless, the combined neuro-mechanical model displays surprisingly realistic swimming movements. Its repertoire includes the ability to make turns, a maneuver previously not known to be captured by the currently mapped circuitry alone. In the presence of external disturbances, sensory feedback had a stabilizing effect on locomotion (Ekeberg et al., 1995).

The combined neuro-mechanical model was recently extended to three dimensions to enable study of yaw,

pitch, and roll movement control. The spinal CPG neurons were subdivided into separate dorsally and ventrally controlling populations, an arrangement that has some biological support. The assumption of a preferred crossed-diagonal connectivity formed a dual-oscillator system (figure 15.3A). Simulations based on this crossed-oscillator hypothesis show that tonic brainstem input to selected parts of the CPG is able to elicit all three kinds of turning movements (figure 15.3B; see also Ekeberg et al., 1995).

Abstract and Detailed Models

The lamprey swimming CPG has been modeled at several different levels of abstraction: as a chain of coupled mathematical oscillators, as a network of simplified nonspiking as well as spiking neurons, and as a network of compartmental Hodgkin-Huxley model neurons.

The most abstract coupled oscillator models are valuable because they allow formal analysis of the system. They are formulated in such a way, however, that makes it difficult to relate them to biological reality at the cellular level. On the other hand, detailed models that relate directly to the cellular level comprise a large number of parameters, thus exerting a high demand on the availability of data. Even a detailed model represents a simplification, and many of its parameter values are based on estimates. Yet, the results presented here on the possible role of 5-HT-mediated AHP modulation in the lamprey CPG clearly illustrate what we can gain by taking relevant cellular properties into account. Ideally, models at different levels of abstraction should complement each other. Current models are still quite far apart, however, and the connections between them need to be developed further. Simulation results must always be interpreted cautiously. A model that fits currently available data and produces reasonable output should not be taken as the only possibility or the ultimate truth. It is always necessary to go back to experiments to verify and improve the model. In fact, one of the most important roles of modeling and simulation is to serve as a tool for identifying critical experiments.

Conclusions

Our understanding of the neural control of undulatory swimming in lamprey has increased dramatically in the past ten years. Mathematical modeling and computer simulation have been and will continue to be highly valuable in this research. We are now approaching models that connect overt behavior with the underlying cellular processes for the complete behavior of lamprey swimming.

We are likely to witness a fast improvement in methods, simulation software, and tools for analysis and presentation of large amounts of simulation data. We are still many years away, however, from the time when models of complex neuronal networks and systems will exhibit the same level of correspondence with the actual physical system as the models currently available in physics and chemistry.

Acknowledgments

This work was supported in part by the Swedish Natural Science Research Council (NFR) and the Swedish National Board for Technical Development (NUTEK).

References

Arshavsky YI, Orlovsky GN, Panchjin YV, Roberts A, Soffe SR (1993) Neuronal control of swimming locomotion. *Trends Neurosci* 16:227–232.

Brodin L, Tråvén H, Lansner A, Wallén P, Ekeberg Ö, Grillner S (1991) Computer simulation of N-Methyl-D-Aspartate (NMDA) receptor induced membrane properties in a neuron model. *J Neurophysiol* 66(2):473–484.

Buchanan JT (1992) Neural network simulations of coupled locomotor oscillators in the lamprey spinal cord. *Biol Cybern* 66:367–374.

Buchanan JT, Grillner S (1987) Newly identified "glutamate interneurons" and their role in locomotion in the lamprey spinal cord. *Science* 236:312–314.

Cohen AH, Ermentrout GB, Kiemel T, Kopell N, Sigvardt K, Williams TL (1992) Modelling of intersegmental coordination in the lamprey central pattern generator for locomotion. *Trends Neurosci* 15:434–438.

Cohen AH, Holmes PJ, Rand RH (1982) The nature of the coupling between segmental oscillators of the lamprey spinal generator for locomotion. *J Math Biol* 13:345–369.

Ekeberg Ö (1993) A neuro-mechanical model of undulatory swimming. *Biol Cybern* 69:363–374.

Ekeberg Ö, Hammarlund P, Levin B, Lansner A (1994) SWIM: A simulation environment for realistic neural network modeling. In: *Neural Network Simulation Environments* (Skrzypec J, ed.), 47–71. Hingham, Mass.: Kluwer.

Ekeberg Ö, Lansner A, Grillner S (1995) The neural control of fish swimming studies through numerical simulations. *Adaptive Behavior*, 3(4)363–384.

Ekeberg Ö, Wallén P, Lansner A, Tråvén H, Brodin L, Grillner S (1991) A computer based model for realistic simulations of neural networks. I. The single neuron and synaptic interaction. *Biol Cybern* 65:81–90.

Grillner S, Buchanan JT, Lansner A (1988) Simulation of the segmental burst generating network for locomotion in lamprey. *Neurosci Lett* 89:31–35.

Grillner S, Deliagina T, Ekeberg Ö, El Manira A, Hill RH, Lansner A, Orlovsky GN, Wallén P (1995) Neural networks that co-ordinate locomotion and body orientation in lamprey. *Trends Neurosci* 18(6):270–279.

Grillner S, Wallén P, Brodin L, Lansner A (1991) The neuronal network generating locomotor behavior in lamprey: Circuitry, transmitters, membrane properties, and simulation. *Annu Rev Neurosci* 14:169–199.

Hellgren J, Grillner S, Lansner A (1992) Computer simulation of the segmental neural network generating locomotion in lamprey by using populations of network interneurons. *Biol Cybern* 68:1–13.

Koch C, Davis JL (1994) *Large-Scale Neuronal Theories of the Brain*. Cambridge, Mass.: MIT Press.

Otha Y, Grillner S (1989) Monosynaptic excitatory amino acid transmission from the posterior rhombencephalic reticular nucleus to spinal neurons involved in the control of locomotion in lamprey. *J Neurophysiol* 62:1079–1089.

Roberts A, Tunstall MJ (1990) Mutual re-excitation with postinhibitory rebound: A simulation study on the mechanism for locomotor rhythm generation in the spinal cord of *Xenopus* embryos. *Eur J Neurosci* 2:11–23.

Sejnowski T, Churchland P (1992) *The Computational Brain*. Cambridge, Mass.: MIT Press.

Tråvén H, Brodin L, Lansner A, Ekeberg Ö, Wallén P, Grillner S (1993) Computer simulations of NMDA and non-NMDA receptor–mediated synaptic drive: Sensory and supraspinal modulation of neurons and small networks. *J Neurophysiol* 70:695–709.

Viana di Prisco G, Wallén P, Grillner S (1990) Synaptic effects of intraspinal stretch receptor neurons mediating movement-related feedback during locomotion. *Brain Research* 530:161–166.

Wadden T, Hellgren J, Lansner A, Grillner S (1997) Intersegmental coordination in the lamprey: Simulations using a network model without segmental boundaries. *Biol Cybern* 76:1–9.

Wallén P, Ekeberg Ö, Lansner A, Brodin L, Tråvén H, Grillner S (1992) A computer-based model for realistic simulations of neural networks. II. The segmental network generating locomotor rhythmicity in the lamprey. *J Neurophysiol* 68:1939–1950.

Williams TL (1992) Phase coupling in simulated chains of coupled oscillators representing the lamprey spinal cord. *Neural Comput* 4:546–558.

16

Integrate-and-Fire Simulations of Two Molluscan Neural Circuits

William N. Frost, James R. Lieb, Jr.,
Mark J. Tunstall, Brett D. Mensh,
and Paul S. Katz

Abstract

We constructed realistic simulations of neural circuits in two marine molluscs to explore basic network operation and to examine learning-related circuit plasticity. In both cases, we used a single-compartment, integrate-and-fire approach, which allows modeling of cellular and synaptic properties from a readily acquired data set.

In *Tritonia diomedea*, a brief noxious stimulus elicits a rhythmic central pattern generator–driven escape swim lasting tens of seconds. Previous modeling had concluded that the swim CPG consists of three cell types: C2, DSI, and VSI. Our recent studies of learning and intrinsic neuromodulation in the swim network prompted us to construct a new three-cell simulation, using data obtained from non-sensitized, non-modulated preparations. The new CPG simulation was unable to generate a rhythmic output, suggesting that the *Tritonia* swim CPG is more complex than previously envisioned; further simulations specifically implicate roles for intrinsic neuromodulation and for additional neurons in the normal operation of the swim network.

In *Aplysia californica*, a brief tactile stimulus to the animal's respiratory siphon elicits the siphon withdrawal reflex. We modeled the detailed reflex circuitry underlying this response, then used the simulation to evaluate the functional roles of three different sites of circuit plasticity that have been determined, by previous experimental work, to underlie behavioral sensitization. We found that the three sites have distinct roles in transforming sensory input into motor neuron firing patterns, indicating that the information acquired in learning is itself stored in fragmented fashion.

Because of their large, accessible neurons and relatively simple nervous systems, invertebrates have been widely used to investigate the neural basis of motor pattern generation (Getting, 1988). A comparatively new tool in this work is the use of realistic network modeling (Calabrese and De Schutter, 1992; Selverston, 1993; Mulloney and Perkel, 1988; Lansner et al., chapter 15, this volume), which uses experimental data to construct a computer simulation similar enough to the real network that it can be used to test directly the functional roles of the real neurons and their synaptic connections in the biological circuit.

A study by Getting (1983b) was very influential in demonstrating the value of realistic network modeling. He constructed an integrate-and-fire simulation of a three-cell circuit in the marine mollusc, *Tritonia diomedea*, in order to test whether the neurons and their known synaptic connections constituted the central pattern generator (CPG) for the animal's escape swim.

We have used Getting's realistic simulation approach as an integral tool in our further studies of the *Tritonia* swim CPG, as well as in studies of the circuit underlying the siphon withdrawal reflex in another marine mollusc, *Aplysia californica* (Lieb and Frost, 1997). In both cases, we collected the necessary data, constructed the simulation, and then asked whether the modeled cells and synapses would generate a network response similar to that observed in the animal. For *Tritonia*, the answer was no, and the network simulation is currently being used to guide our experimental efforts to identify missing elements in the biological circuit. For *Aplysia*, the network simulation did perform very similarly to the biological network, so we have proceeded to use it to explore both the basic functional organization of the circuit and the behavioral roles of different sites of learning-related circuit plasticity.

Integrate-and-Fire Modeling Scheme

Two commonly used, but very different, approaches to realistic network modeling can be described as the *Hodgkin-Huxley* and *integrate-and-fire* schemes (Segev, 1992). Each approach has different strengths, so specific issues of interest usually determine which to use. Hodgkin-Huxley modeling schemes have a high degree of *mechanistic realism* because they are constructed based on the properties of the actual voltage- and Ca^{2+}-dependent conductances in each cell. Hodgkin-Huxley models are thus well suited for studies of the biophysical mechanisms of neuronal behavior. This realism comes at a cost, however. Creating accurate simulations of each neuron in a given circuit requires extensive voltage-clamp characterization of their various conductances and careful adjustment of large numbers of free, interacting parameters for each neuron. Integrate-and-fire approaches, on the other hand, aim at *phenomenological realism* only: the simulated neurons are designed to closely mimic the firing responses of their biological counterparts, but via a much simpler computational means that does not usually require voltage-clamp characterization of the different neurons. Integrate-and-fire schemes, therefore, can be the preferred method for network-level issues, in which the functions of various synaptic connections and neuronal firing properties, but not the details of their biophysical underpinnings, are under direct investigation.

Integrate-and-fire methodologies vary widely in complexity, but their defining feature is that neither action potentials nor threshold are emergent properties of a set of voltage-dependent conductances. In our particular implementation, whenever membrane potential reaches threshold potential, the program notes that an action potential has occurred, abruptly resets threshold to a more positive potential (from where it exponentially decays to its resting level), and activates a pair of potassium conductances that generate a spike undershoot. By adjusting the free parameters that control threshold and the spike undershoot, it is relatively easy to construct model neurons that have the same excitability and spike-frequency accommodation properties as their biological counterparts (see figure 16.1A and B).

In the work reviewed here, we collected data for each cell and synapse in the circuit from several preparations and constructed the model counterpart to represent the mean or typical example (see figure 16.1C and D). This procedure prevented us from modeling our favorite or strongest examples, thus avoiding data selection that could have biased network performance. Also, after we constructed each model neuron and synapse, we did not permit any further changes of their free parameters. This procedure allowed us to use the model network to ask how well the known cells and synaptic connections account for the behavior of the real network and precluded our adjusting any parameter values to bias the network toward a desired outcome.

Simulation of the *Tritonia* Swim CPG

The motor program driving the escape swim response in *Tritonia* originates from a central pattern generator—a group of interneurons that, through their endogenous properties and synaptic interconnections, generate a prolonged rhythmic discharge without the need for sensory feedback (Getting, 1989a; Dorsett et al., 1969). The CPG was initially thought to be composed of just three cell types: the dorsal swim interneurons (DSIs), ventral swim interneuron A (VSIA), and cerebral cell 2 (C2) (Getting, 1989a; see also figure 16.2A and B). Based on these cells' membrane and synaptic properties, Getting (1981) suggested that the *Tritonia* swim CPG is an example of a network oscillator—a circuit whose rhythm arises from the synaptic connections among otherwise non-bursting neurons. His initial use of realistic modeling was to test this hypothesis (Getting, 1983b). He found that he was able to get the circuit to oscillate, but only by setting certain synaptic strengths at values different than their experimentally observed values. Getting resolved some of the discrepancies between the real and model networks when he subsequently discovered the

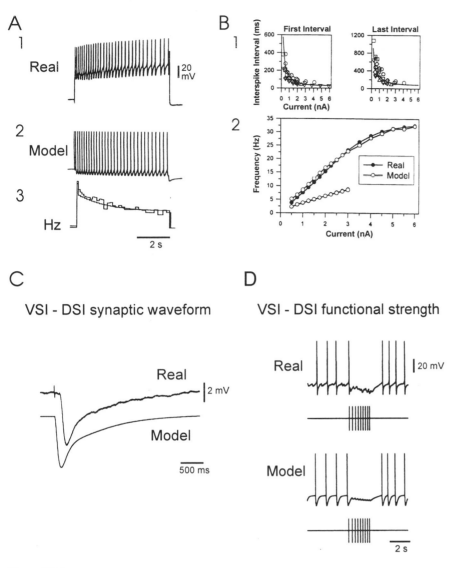

Modeling DSI excitability

A

1 Real

2 Model

3 Hz

2 s

B

1 First Interval   Last Interval

2

Frequency (Hz)

● Real
○ Model

Current (nA)

C

VSI - DSI synaptic waveform

Real

Model

2 mV

500 ms

D

VSI - DSI functional strength

Real

20 mV

Model

2 s

Figure 16.1

Construction of model cells and synapses. (A) Comparison of the real (1) and model (2) dorsal swim interneurons (DSIs) of the *Tritonia* swim CPG. 3 shows instantaneous firing frequency of the two responses. (B) Procedure for modeling the cell. Best-fit curves were drawn through firing response data for a number of different cells, for a range of current pulses (1). These curves were then converted to instantaneous frequency (2) and used as templates against which to construct the model cell. 2 shows a comparison of firing behavior of the real and model DSIs to different injected currents. The upper and lower curves depict the instantaneous frequency at the start and end, respectively, of the different firing responses. The lower two curves are exactly superimposed. (C) Comparison of real and model VSI-DSI synaptic potential waveforms in response to a single VSI action potential. (D) Comparison of real and model VSI-DSI synaptic strength. The lower traces of each pair represent the VSI firing train; the upper traces represent the DSI response.

VSIB neuron (Getting, 1983a), which replaced VSIA in a revised network model (Getting, 1989b).

Two recent findings led us to undertake the construction of a new model of the *Tritonia* CPG. First, we found that the DSIs play a previously unsuspected neuromodulatory role in the network. In addition to performing their conventional synaptic actions, the DSIs release serotonin to produce potent heterosynaptic enhancement of the chemical synaptic connections made by C2, both within and outside the CPG (Katz et al., 1994; Katz and Frost, 1995a; Katz and Frost, 1995b). DSI stimulation also enhances C2 excitability (Katz and Frost, 1994). Because the DSIs fire intensely at the onset of the swim motor program, this modulation may play an important role in the initial transformation of the resting network into a rhythmic CPG. Second, our studies of sensitization in *Tritonia* have shown that a single swim from a state of rest results in the sensitization of the

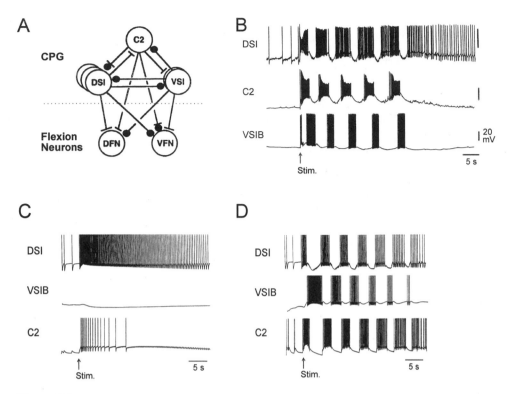

Figure 16.2

Simulation of the *Tritonia* CPG. (A) The escape swim neural circuit. Excitatory connections are represented as bars, inhibitory connections by circles. Mixed component synaptic connections are represented by combinations of the two (C2, DSI, VSI: defined in text; DFN: dorsal flexion neurons; VFN: ventral flexion neurons). (B) The swim motor program recorded in the isolated brain preparation in response to a brief (1 s, 10Hz) stimulus to a peripheral nerve. (C) Failure of the reconstructed three-cell model to oscillate, based upon values obtained in a well-rested preparation. (D) Behavior of the model after adding DRI (not shown), strengthening two synaptic connections, and adding the effects of intrinsic neuromodulation of C2 by DSI (see text).

swim circuit for subsequent swims (Brown et al., 1996) and is associated with persistent cellular changes in the swim circuit (Frost et al., 1988a). In order to evaluate the circuit in the absence of these features, we constructed a three-cell CPG simulation from a new set of data collected from preparations that had not produced a swim motor program for at least three hours. By modeling the rested circuit, we hoped to test whether intrinsic neuromodulation is necessary for normal circuit function and whether a non-sensitized model network would oscillate.

After carefully constructing the new network, we found that it failed to generate an oscillatory output, no matter how large the input stimulus (see figure 16.2C), indicating that the cellular properties and monosynaptic connections of the model's three neurons, as measured in well-rested preparations, are not sufficient to generate the swim motor program. Clearly, we were missing something. One answer to what the missing element might be came from our recent discovery of a long-sought element of the circuit: Getting's hypothesized "ramp" cell (Frost and Katz, 1996). In addition to providing the major excitatory drive to the CPG, the ramp cell is recruited by feedback connections from C2 and is responsible for C2's strong indirect excitatory connection onto the DSIs.

After adding this recruited pathway to the simulation, we found that the basic three-cell network could generate at least one swim cycle if we artificially strengthened two synapses, the DSI-C2 and the C2-VSIB connections. The result suggested that additional recruited elements may be present at these two points in the network when it is excited and generating a swim rhythm, or that these connections may have non-linear properties. We then added the effects of the intrinsic modulation of C2 by DSI to the modified network and found that this addition substantially increased the number of cycles in the oscillation (see figure 16.2D; see also Tunstall et al., 1995). Our finding here is consistent with the idea that the intrinsic modulation plays an important role in configuring or maintaining the resting network in its oscillatory state. We are currently using this simulation approach to guide our experimental efforts to identify the missing components of the escape swim central pattern generator.

Simulation of the *Aplysia* Siphon Withdrawal Reflex Circuit

The siphon withdrawal reflex circuit of the marine mollusc *Aplysia californica* has been widely used to study the cellular basis of sensitization, which is a simple form of learning. Our research has incorporated realistic network simulations to explore how this well-defined circuit functions and, especially, how different known sites of learning-related circuit modification contribute to sensitization. In our simulated circuit, unlike in the biological network, we were able to alter individual components of the circuit selectively to evaluate their relative contributions to the production of the behavior.

The circuit consists of two parallel pathways, a monosynaptic sensory-to-motor neuron connection and a polysynaptic pathway in which excitatory and inhibitory interneurons are interposed between the sensory and motor neurons (Frost and Kandel, 1995). Our simulation (Lieb and Frost, 1997) focused on the best understood subset of the circuit: the LFS motor neurons, three different groups of interneurons (L29, L30, L34), and the synaptic connections made by the known sensory neurons onto these cells (figure 16.3A). A comparison of the respective outputs of the real and simulated networks showed that they produce a very similar motor neuron firing response to siphon sensory input (see figure 16.3B). The LFS neurons in both networks fired with an initial high-frequency burst of action potentials (the *phasic component*), followed by a lower-frequency spike train lasting several seconds (the *tonic component*). The correspondence between real and biological networks suggests that, qualitatively at least, many of the key interneuronal elements of the siphon withdrawal reflex circuit have now been identified.

We next explored the roles of different circuit elements in producing the characteristic phasic and tonic components of the motor neuron firing response. By systematically removing individual cells or synapses from the model network, we demonstrated that the phasic component is mediated by both the sensory neurons and the interneurons, whereas the long-lasting tonic firing response is mediated entirely by the interneurons—primarily L29 (Frost et al., 1991; see also White et al., 1993). We also found that recurrent inhibition among the interneurons demonstrably attenuates the sensory excitation of the motor neurons (Lieb and Frost, 1995; see also Trudeau and Castellucci, 1993; Blazis et al., 1993), an effect that is greatest at low stimulus intensities.

Finally, we used our network simulation to investigate the nature of the information stored at the different circuit sites modified during sensitization. Our simulation showed (Lieb and Frost, 1992) that the enhancement of the monosynaptic sensory-to-motor neuron connection that occurs during sensitization (Kandel and Schwartz, 1982) increases only the phasic component of the motor neuron firing response, whereas the changes in interneuronal connections that occur (Frost et al., 1988b) primarily increase the tonic response component, with just a small effect on the phasic component (see figure 16.3C). Based on physiological experiments that use these simulation outputs to drive real LFS motor neurons—which allowed us to insert the effect of a single site of plasticity back into the preparation—we have shown that the enhancement of the sensory-to-motor neuron monosynaptic connection seen in sensitization specifically acts to enhance the amplitude of the siphon contraction (see figure 16.3D, panel 1). The interneuronal modifications, on the other hand, act to enhance both the amplitude and the duration of the contraction (see figure 16.3D, panel 2). Our findings indicate that the different circuit modifications that occur in sensitization contribute differently to the enhanced withdrawal response, suggesting that the information acquired in learning is itself stored in fragmented fashion.

Concluding Comments

Realistic network simulation is a powerful tool for evaluating the completeness of our knowledge of a given circuit, for exploring the functional roles of specific circuit elements, and for determining the functional significance of learning-related plasticity and other forms of modulation. In both of the molluscan circuits reviewed here, modeling served not to confirm but to challenge our previous understanding of the circuits. In each case, realistic simulations yielded results not anticipated in advance—results that are broadening our understanding of motor circuit function.

Acknowledgments

This work was supported by MH48536, MH49563 and NS36500. The authors wish to thank David Lawrence for programming work, and Lise Eliot, Javier Medina, Clint Morris, and Ling-Gang Wu for their contributions to this work.

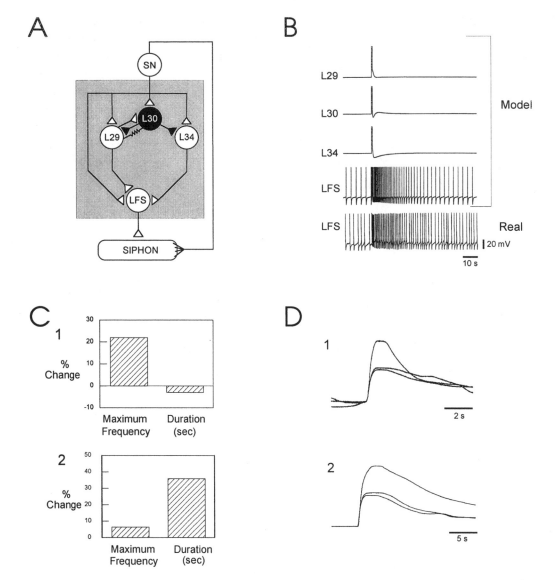

Figure 16.3

Simulation of the *Aplysia* siphon withdrawal reflex circuit. (A) The known circuitry by which siphon stimulation excites the LFS motor neurons. The gray box indicates the circuit components simulated in our model network. (B) Response of the network simulation and of a real LFS neuron to a sensory input (modified from Lieb and Frost, 1997). (C) Contributions of different sites of circuit plasticity to the enhanced motor neuron firing response. 1. Introducing the enhanced sensory neuron to motor neuron connection alone acts to enhance the peak motor neuron firing frequency, with no enhancement of the duration of motor neuron firing. 2. Introducing the enhanced L29 connections alone acts to increase the duration of motor neuron firing and slightly increase the peak motor neuron firing frequency. (D) Behavioral effects of driving real motor neurons with the output of the simulation. The traces represent displacement transducer recordings of siphon movements. 1. The enhanced sensory neuron to motor neuron connection acts to enhance only the amplitude of the siphon contraction. 2. The enhanced L29 connections act to enhance both the amplitude and the duration of the siphon contraction. In both 1 and 2, the upper trace is the siphon contraction produced by the indicated plasticity. The lower two traces are control responses obtained before and after the upper trace.

References

Blazis DEJ, Fischer TM, Carew TJ (1993) A neural network model of inhibitory information processing in *Aplysia*. *Neural Computation* 5:213–227.

Brown G, Frost WN, Getting PA (1996) Habituation and iterative enhancement of multiple components of the *Tritonia* swim response. *Behav Neurosci* 110:478–485.

Calabrese RL, De Schutter E (1992) Motor-pattern-generating networks in invertebrates: Modeling our way toward understanding. *Trends Neurosci* 15:439–445.

Dorsett DA, Willows AOD, Hoyle G (1969) Centrally generated nerve impulse sequences determining swimming behavior in *Tritonia*. *Nature* 224:711–712.

Frost WN, Brown G, Gettintg PA (1988a) Sensitization of the *Tritonia* escape swim: Behavioral and cellular modifications. *Soc Neurosci Abstr* 14:607.

Frost WN, Clark GA, Kandel ER (1988b) Parallel processing of short-term memory for sensitization in *Aplysia*. *J Neurobiol* 19:297–334.

Frost WN, Kandel ER (1995) Structure of the network mediating siphon-elicited siphon withdrawal in *Aplysia*. *J Neurophysiol* 73:2413–2427.

Frost WN, Katz PS (1996) Single neuron control over a complex motor program. *Proc Natl Acad Sci USA* 93:422–426.

Frost WN, Wu LG, Lieb J (1991) Simulation of the *Aplysia* siphon withdrawal reflex circuit: Slow components of interneuronal synapses contribute to the mediation of reflex duration. *Soc Neurosci Abstr* 17:1390.

Getting PA (1981) Mechanisms of pattern generation underlying swimming in *Tritonia*. I. Neuronal network formed by monosynaptic connections. *J Neurophysiol* 46:65–79.

Getting PA (1983a) Mechanisms of pattern generation underlying swimming in *Tritonia*. III. Intrinsic and synaptic mechanisms for delayed excitation. *J Neurophysiol* 49:1036–1050.

Getting PA (1983b) Mechanisms of pattern generation underlying swimming in *Tritonia*. II. Network reconstruction. *J Neurophysiol* 49:1017–1035.

Getting PA (1988) Comparative analysis of in vertebrate central pattern generators. In: *Neural Control of Rhythmic Movements in Vertebrates* (Cohen AH, Rossignol S, Grillner S, eds.), 101–127. New York: Wiley.

Getting PA (1989a) A network oscillator underlying swimming in *Tritonia*. In: *Neuronal and Cellular Oscillators* (Jacklet JW, ed.), 215–236. New York: Marcel Dekker.

Getting PA (1989b) Reconstruction of small neural networks. In: *Methods in Neuronal Modeling: From Synapses to Networks* (Koch C, Segev I, eds.), 171–194. Cambridge, Mass.: MIT Press.

Kandel ER, Schwartz JH (1982) Molecular biology of learning: Modulation of transmitter release. *Science* 218:433–443.

Katz PS, Frost WN (1994) Evidence that serotonergic neuromodulation intrinsic to the *Tritonia* swim CPG is due to presynaptic enhancement of release. *Soc Neurosci Abstr* 20:1201.

Katz PS, Frost WN (1995a) Intrinsic neuromodulation in the *Tritonia* swim CPG: The serotonergic dorsal swim interneurons act presynaptically to enhance transmitter release from interneuron C2. *J Neurosci* 15:6035–6045.

Katz PS, Frost WN (1995b) Intrinsic neuromodulation in the *Tritonia* swim CPG: Serotonin mediates both neuromodulation and neurotransmission by the dorsal swim interneurons. *J Neurophysiol* 74:2281–2294.

Katz PS, Getting PA, Frost WN (1994) Dynamic neuromodulation of synaptic strength intrinsic to a central pattern generator circuit. *Nature* 367:729–731.

Lieb JR, Frost WN (1992) Interneuronal plasticity contributes significantly to enhanced motor neuron firing during sensitization of the *Aplysia* siphon-withdrawal reflex. *Soc Neurosci Abstr* 18:1390.

Lieb JR, Frost WN (1995) Dynamic representation of learned information in a distributed memory in *Aplysia*. *Soc Neurosci Abstr* 21:1458.

Lieb JR, Frost WN (1997) Realistic simulation of the *Aplysia* siphon-withdrawal reflex circuit: Roles of circuit elements in producing motor output. *J Neurophysiol* 77:1249–1268.

Mulloney B, Perkel DH (1988) The roles of synthetic models in the study of central pattern generators. In: *Neural Control of Rhythmic Movements In Vertebrates* (Cohen AH, Rossignol S, Grillner S, eds.), 415–453. New York: Wiley.

Segev I (1992) Single neurone models: Oversimple, complex, and reduced. *Trends Neurosci* 15:414–421.

Selverston AI (1993) Modeling of neural circuits: What have we learned? *Annu Rev Neurosci* 16:531–546.

Trudeau L-E, Castellucci VF (1993) Functional uncoupling of inhibitory interneurons plays an important role in short-term sensitization of *Aplysia* gill and siphon withdrawal reflex. *J Neurosci* 13:2126–2135.

Tunstall MJ, Katz PS, Frost WN (1995) A revised model of the *Tritonia* swim CPG suggests a role for intrinsic neuromodulation and predicts missing neurons. *Soc Neurosci Abstr* 21:146.

White JA, Ziv I, Cleary LJ, Baxter DA, Byrne JH (1993) The role of interneurons in controlling the tail-withdrawal reflex in *Aplysia*: A network model. *J Neurophysiol* 70:1777–1786.

Part IV

Modulation and Reconfiguration

17

Chemical Modulation of Vertebrate Motor Circuits

Keith T. Sillar, Ole Kiehn, and
Norio Kudo

Abstract

Vertebrate locomotion is driven by neuronal networks intrinsic to the spinal cord, called central pattern generators (CPGs). The basic building blocks of the CPGs comprise synaptic connections between spinal neurons and the membrane properties of the constituent neurons themselves (Kiehn et al., chapter 4, this volume). Knowledge of those components may be sufficient to explain the stereotyped motor output that the neuronal networks often produce under experimental conditions, but they cannot fully account for the intrinsic flexibility in the performance of the same networks during real behavior. Much of this flexibility is likely to derive from the influences of modulatory neurons that act on the CPGs to control various aspects of the locomotor rhythm, including cycle period as well as the duration and intensity of bursts of motoneuron firing. Here, we review current appreciation of the neurons, modulators, and receptors that shape the final output of locomotor CPGs. Our focus is on two systems that are important in both the development and the intrinsic modulation of ongoing locomotion. GABAergic and serotonergic inputs adapt the rhythmic output of locomotor CPGs by targeting a range of cellular and synaptic mechanisms in the spinal cord. Both transmitter systems activate metabotropic, postsynaptic receptor subtypes to alter the firing properties of spinal motoneurons and premotor interneurons. By these means, the conversion of a presynaptic input to a postsynaptic response is modified in gain. In addition, however, the same modulators can use presynaptic mechanisms actively to regulate the strength of synaptic connections between CPG neurons. We try to address why it is necessary for a modulator to access so many different mechanisms in order to accomplish its global effects on the locomotor system. Finally, we review a range of other newly discovered modulators that have also been shown to influence locomotion, but these have yet to be studied in detail.

Vertebrate locomotor central pattern generators (CPGs) comprise spinal neurons, the ensemble of ionic conductances and transmitter receptors present in their membranes, and their synaptic interconnections (see Kiehn et al., chapter 4, this volume). Together, these building blocks form a neuronal network that is able to generate and sustain a well-coordinated, rhythmic motor output pattern that drives locomotor movements. Diagrams that represent CPGs with fixed characteristics, however, are not able to explain the variability in frequency and intensity that is characteristic of many locomotor behaviors. During locomotion, the speed and strength of movement, its direction, and even coordination are continuously changing. Many of these changes are most likely mediated by modulatory inputs that add flexibility to the motor output generated by CPGs. Thus, both the intrinsic response properties of the neurons and the synaptic connections between them are actively regulated by inputs from modulatory neurons. A detailed knowledge of such influences is needed to understand how the basic rhythmic output of CPGs is adapted to suit differing behavioral requirements. Here, we review the current knowledge of neuromodulatory inputs to locomotor CPGs: where do the inputs originate, what transmitters do they use, what properties of the networks do they change, and how do these changes translate into an alteration in the motor pattern?

Locomotor Parameters Targeted by Neuromodulators

Neuromodulators alter one or more of the parameters of the locomotor pattern. The frequency of locomotion may vary by an order of magnitude; changes in the duration and intensity of motor bursts in each cycle influence the force of muscle contractions; and finally, with changes in locomotor frequency, the phase relationships between motoneuron pools must be modified to accommodate the concomitant changes in coordination and gait. A large (and ever growing) number of modulators—including amino acids, amines, and peptides—have been shown to influence one or more of these locomotor rhythm parameters. The effects are almost always exerted via metabotropic receptors that alter the integrative electrical properties of neurons and also act on presynaptic terminals to control the release of neurotransmitters operating within the CPG. Metabotropic receptors are membrane-spanning molecules that usually exert their effects on other molecules via intracellular G-proteins. These receptors act in contrast to ionotropic receptors whose receptor sites and associated channels are formed by a shared set of membrane-spanning molecules. Our review focuses on the roles of metabotropic serotonin (5-HT) and gamma-aminobutyric acid type B (GABA$_B$) receptors, about which most is known. We also consider the possible contribution of other, less well-understood modulators.

Neuromodulation by 5-HT

Sources and Actions of 5-HT on Locomotor Rhythms

In a wide range of vertebrate preparations, 5-HT modulates the basic locomotor pattern by increasing the intensity and duration of each burst of motoneuron activity—for example, in amphibian tadpoles (Sillar et al., 1992b; Woolston et al., 1994), lampreys (Christenson et al., 1989), neonatal rats (Sqalli-Houssaini et al., 1993; Kiehn and Kjaerulff, 1996), rabbits (Viala and Buser, 1969), and cats (Barbeau and Rossignol, 1990). This equivalent action in such phylogenetically and ontogenetically diverse species suggests an ancestral role for 5-HT in the modulation of vertebrate locomotion, a notion supported by the presence of homologous 5-HT-containing neurons in a similar location in the central nervous system (CNS) of all vertebrates.

The principle source of 5-HT acting upon locomotor circuitry in the spinal cord is the raphe region of the brain stem. Located in the ventral medulla, the raphe region consists of several nuclei, each containing neurons that are predominantly, but not exclusively, serotonergic. In some raphe neurons 5-HT co-localizes with substance P (Ozaki et al., 1992), a peptide, and with thyrotropin-releasing hormone (TRH) (Johansson et al., 1981). A large proportion of raphe neurons (over 70% in the cat; Wiklund et al., 1981) possess axonal projections that extend into both the dorsal and ventral horns of the spinal cord. In some species, however, 5-HT-containing neurons are also present in the spinal cord itself—for example, in the lamprey (van Dongen et al., 1985) and the turtle (Kiehn et al., 1992). Both sources of 5-HT may be responsible for the modulatory actions of the amine on locomotor rhythm generation. Although much has yet to be learned about the role of serotonergic neurons in relation to locomotor control, unit recordings from raphe neurons indicate that they are normally tonically active and exhibit an increased firing rate during motor behavior, properties that may be modulated in relation to the locomotor cycle (reviewed in Jacobs, 1994).

Actions of 5-HT on Cellular Conductances

The principal effects of 5-HT are to alter the timing and intensity of motoneuronal discharge during locomotion. These effects are due, in part, to the actions of 5-HT on selected voltage-gated conductances in the motoneurons, which influence their firing properties. Overwhelming evidence supports the conclusion that, in the lamprey spinal cord, the blockade of an apamin-sensitive Ca^{2+}-dependent K$^+$ current (I$_{K(Ca)}$) by 5-HT is of paramount importance (Wallén et al., 1989; Hill et al., 1992; El Manira et al., 1994; see, however, Meer and Buchanan, 1992). I$_{K(Ca)}$ contributes to the slow spike afterhyperpolarization (sAHP) that regulates the firing frequency of neurons (see Kiehn et al., chapter 4, this volume). Reduction of the sAHP decreases spike accommodation and allows more action potentials to occur in response to a given depolarizing input. Because a progressive activation of $I_{K(Ca)}$ within a burst of action potentials is also thought to contribute to the self-termination of the burst, a reduction of $I_{K(Ca)}$ by 5-HT will impair burst termination; it will both lengthen the burst and increase the firing rate within the burst. This effect occurs in many members of the motoneuron pool and accounts for a large part of 5-HT's modulatory actions on the lamprey swimming rhythm. In addition, 5-HT also slows, in a dose-dependent manner, the frequency of the lamprey rhythm induced by excitatory amino acids (EAAs; Harris-Warrick and Cohen, 1985), which suggests a 5-HT modulation of the CPG itself and could be explained if the amine similarly reduced $I_{K(Ca)}$ in premotor interneurons (Wallén et al., 1989).

In other systems, 5-HT is known to exert a range of effects on other motoneuron membrane properties, (reviewed in Kiehn, 1991) including depolarization, presumably through closure of a resting K^+ conductance (Vandermaelen and Aghajanian, 1982); hyperpolarization, either through the opening of a K^+ conductance or activation of an electrogenic Na^+-K^+ pump (Zhang and Krnjevic, 1989); and enhancement of a low voltage-activated Ca^{2+} conductance (Berger and Takahashi, 1990). Neither the extent to which such mechanisms are activated during locomotor activity, nor the consequences of their incorporation into modulation at the network level have been elucidated, however.

One important property of spinal cord motor and interneurons, first described in lamprey spinal cord, that may contribute to the generation of the locomotor rhythm is the expression of intrinsic (TTX-resistant) oscillations in membrane potential in the presence of the glutamate receptor agonist, NMDA (Sigvardt et al., 1985; Wallén and Grillner, 1985, 1987). The oscillations are expressed as long as Mg^{2+} ions and NMDA are present in the bathing solution; they display voltage dependence due to a region of negative slope resistance in the current-voltage relationship imparted by Mg^{2+} ions. Similar oscillatory membrane behaviour has subsequently been noted in neurons of other vertebrate CPGs, including amphibian tadpoles (Sillar and Simmers, 1994a, 1994b; Wedderburn and Sillar, 1994) and mammals (Hochman et al., 1994). It has been proposed that the intrinsic oscillatory properties in the lamprey system are normally expressed during locomotor rhythm generation, at which point they contribute to the cycle-by-cycle fluctuations in membrane potential. However, the oscillations are slow (1 Hz or less) as compared to the cycle frequencies (up to 10 Hz) attained during fictive

locomotion, suggesting that they might contribute to locomotor activity only at the lower end of the behavioral frequency range (Grillner et al., 1991). Nevertheless, these conditional oscillatory properties provide an effective target for neuromodulatory inputs that can control the basic parameters of locomotion by triggering the onset and offset of consecutive oscillatory cycles. In the lamprey, 5-HT can indeed modulate the frequency of TTX-resistant oscillations by interacting with $I_{K(Ca)}$ channels that not only control spike frequency, but also contribute to the slow repolarizing plateau phase of the intrinsic oscillatory cycle (Wallén et al., 1989). The latter phase is prolonged in the presence of 5-HT, and it might provide the amine with an additional mechanism to lengthen the duration of rhythmic bursts. However, for this argument to be valid, TTX-resistant oscillations must indeed contribute to cyclical fluctuations during fictive swimming, a possibility that needs to be established with certainty (see, however, Wallén and Grillner, 1987).

Actions of 5-HT on Transmitter Receptors

NMDA receptor–mediated intrinsic oscillations in membrane potential are present in the spinal neurons of two closely related amphibian species, *Rana* and *Xenopus*; in these animals, the expression of oscillations is also conditional upon the presence of 5-HT (figure 17.1; Sillar and Simmers, 1994a, 1994b; Wedderburn and Sillar, 1994). In *Xenopus*, the ability of 5-HT to induce oscillations in the presence of NMDA depends upon the animal's developmental stage. It may occur only when larval neurons have developed a sufficient number of 5-HT receptors, but not before. The oscillations in *Rana* and *Xenopus* always appear in the hyperpolarizing direction from the depolarized plateau induced by NMDA (see figure 17.1B), thereby suggesting that 5-HT enables the repolarizing phase of each oscillation, in a manner as yet to be determined. This repolarizing effect contrasts with the effects of 5-HT in the lamprey, where the amine prolongs the depolarizing plateau phase. Presumably, the interaction between 5-HT and the NMDA receptors, which triggers the oscillations, is accomplished via a 5-HT enhancement of the region of negative slope resistance of these spinal neurons. We do not know if oscillations in other species also rely upon 5-HT and NMDA receptor co-activation. It is conceivable, however, that intraspinal serotonergic neurons in the lamprey are strongly depolarized by NMDA and that a sufficient amount of 5-HT is released from these neurons to influence the expression of NMDA oscillations during

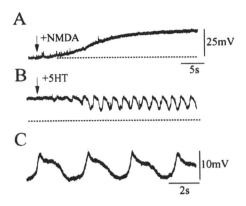

Figure 17.1
Induction of TTX-resistant, NMDA receptor–mediated membrane potential oscillations by 5-HT in embryonic *Rana temporaria* spinal neurons. (A) In the presence of 0.5 μM TTX in the saline bath, the presumed motoneuron located ventrally in the spinal cord (rhythmically active during fictive swimming prior to TTX) was depolarized by 25 mV from its resting level (−68 mV; dotted line) following application of NMDA (100 μM), but it did not produce membrane potential oscillations (cf. lamprey motoneurons; Sigvardt et al., 1985; Wallén and Grillner, 1987). (B) Addition of 5 μM 5-HT to the saline caused induction of sustained oscillations in membrane potential at frequency of 0.5 Hz. The oscillations were sustained as long as 5-HT (or the 5-HT$_1$ receptor agonist, 5-CT) was present, but were blocked by APV, zero Mg^{2+}, or the 5-HT$_{1A}$ receptor antagonist, NAN190 (see Sillar and Simmers, 1994a, 1994b). Note that the oscillations emerged in the hyperpolarizing direction from the depolarized plateau attained by NMDA (see text for further details). (C) Similar oscillations in a different neuron in *Rana* shown with a different voltage scale. Compare the waveform here with similar waveforms recorded in adult lampreys in the presence of NMDA and TTX (e.g., figure 2A in Wallén and Grillner, 1987). (Adapted from Sillar and Simmers, 1994a, 1994b).

NMDA-induced locomotion. The reliance of the oscillatory mechanism upon activation of a specific subtype of 5-HT receptor in immature locomotor systems (e.g., *Xenopus* swimming; Wedderburn and Sillar, 1994) should allow the contributory role of the oscillations in locomotion to be explored directly through the use of appropriate 5-HT receptor antagonists.

Modulation of Synaptic Connections by 5-HT

In addition to acting upon a range of conductances that alter the intrinsic electrical properties of neurons in locomotor networks, certain neuromodulators—including 5-HT—are able to alter the strength of the synaptic connections between spinal neurons. Exploration of the diversity of such influences, their underlying molecular mechanisms, and their functional roles in the development and control of locomotor behavior is still in its infancy, but it offers an important focus for future studies on neuromodulation. Many of the known modulatory effects are mediated presynaptically and involve a de-

crease in voltage-activated Ca^{2+} conductances, a direct action upon the release machinery, or both.

5-HT impairs glycinergic reciprocal inhibition during swimming in *Xenopus* tadpoles (Sillar and Wedderburn, 1994, and unpublished). The inhibition is not mediated postsynaptically because 5-HT does not significantly affect the amplitudes of spontaneous, TTX-resistant glycinergic inhibitory postsynaptic potentials (IPSPs). 5-HT does, however, dramatically reduce the frequency of the occurrence of the spontaneous IPSPs, thus providing direct evidence for a presynaptic site of action. The role of this 5-HT-dependent modulation of glycine release is unclear. Possibly, reciprocal inhibition is decreased by the amine during swimming in order to delay the termination of each burst, which would allow burst durations to increase not only in absolute terms, but also in relation to the cycle period. It is not known, however, if a similar mechanism contributes to the observed effects of 5-HT on the ongoing rhythm in other vertebrate locomotor systems.

In the lamprey locomotor system, 5-HT has been shown to modulate the strength of connections between glutamatergic reticulospinal interneurons and motoneurons (Buchanan and Grillner, 1990). The unique morphology and large size of the reticulospinal axons, as well as of their connections onto motoneurons, have enabled very direct examination of the effects of 5-HT on the release process (Shupliakov et al., 1995). 5-HT reduces the extent of spike-mediated, synaptic vesicle depletion not by effecting calcium influx, but rather by directly effecting the release machinery. Thus, in the presence of the amine, the number of vesicles available for release is dramatically increased. Reticulospinal neurons are not a part of the swimming CPG. They are mostly silent during swimming but are activated to convey transient commands for steering and escape.

Pharmacological Profile of 5-HT Effects

The effects of 5-HT are mediated via numerous pharmacologically distinct receptor subtypes (Peroutka, 1988). Of the subtypes described so far, all but one—the 5-HT$_3$ receptor—operates through a G-protein. 5-HT$_3$ receptors do not appear to be present on rhythmically active, spinal cord locomotor neurons. Rather, they are expressed at quite high density in the dorsal horn, where they may be involved in the modulation of sensory synaptic transmission (Alhaider et al., 1991). In lower vertebrates, receptors with a pharmacological profile resembling the mammalian 5-HT$_{1A}$ receptor may be exclusively involved in modulating the locomotor pattern (*Xenopus* tadpole:

Scrymgeour-Wedderburn and Sillar, 1994; lamprey: Wikström et al., 1995). 5-HT$_{1A}$ receptors, with some 5-HT$_2$ involvement (reviewed in Wallis, 1994), also affect the modulation of mammalian locomotor rhythm generation.

Neuromodulatory Effects of GABA

Sources and Effects of GABA on the Motor Pattern

Although glycine appears to be the transmitter mainly responsible for reciprocal coupling between antagonistic motor centers in the spinal cord (see Kiehn et al., chapter 4, this volume; Roberts et al., chapter 7, this volume; Wallén, chapter 6, this volume), another inhibitory amino acid transmitter, GABA, plays a range of subsidiary modulatory roles. Like 5-HT, the source of GABA is neurons that are either intrinsic or extrinsic to the spinal cord. Among the intrinsic spinal GABAergic neurons, some are involved in sensory processing in the dorsal horn, whereas others are located more ventrally and have processes that intermingle with motor pattern–generating neurons (e.g., Christenson et al., 1990). GABAergic neurons extrinsic to the spinal cord are present throughout the brain, and several populations innervate the spinal cord. With the exception of a population in the hindbrain of *Xenopus* embryos that is involved in the termination of swimming (see Roberts et al., chapter 7, this volume), however, their precise roles in locomotor behavior have yet to be determined.

Pre- and Postsynaptic Effects of GABA

GABA's effects are mediated by two main types of pharmacologically distinct receptors: ionotropic GABA$_A$ receptors that gate a Cl$^-$ ion channel and metabotropic GABA$_B$ receptors that are G-protein coupled. In general, the activation of GABA$_A$ receptors causes membrane hyperpolarization, which either reduces the excitability of the spinal locomotor networks or completely blocks the ongoing rhythm (see Kiehn et al., chapter 4, this volume). It has been suggested that, in the lumbar spinal cord of the neonatal rat, tonic activation of GABA$_A$ receptors suppresses rhythm generation because such rhythms can be elicited by the application of bicuculline (Cazalets et al., 1994). In the lamprey, activation of presynaptic GABA$_B$ receptors causes modulation of synaptic transmission from excitatory and inhibitory spinal neurons (Alford and Grillner, 1991), whereas postsynaptic GABA$_B$ receptors reduce Ca^{2+} currents to decrease indirectly the activation of I$_{K(Ca)}$ channels. The

reduction of both synaptic transmission and Ca^{2+} currents changes the input-output properties of the spinal neurons in a fashion analogous to the effects of 5-HT and ultimately reduces the swimming frequency (Tegnér et al., 1993).

In *Xenopus* embryos, GABA$_B$ receptor activation modulates motoneuron spike threshold and reciprocal glycinergic inhibition during fictive swimming (Wall and Dale, 1993; Dale, chapter 8, this volume). Bath application of the GABA$_B$ receptor agonist baclophen reduces the amplitude of midcycle, glycinergic IPSPs in motoneurons during fictive swimming. Baclophen also reduces the frequency of spontaneous, TTX- and cadmium-resistant glycinergic IPSPs in motoneurons, suggesting that GABA$_B$ receptors on the terminals of glycinergic commissural interneurons can decrease the probability of transmitter release. Moreover, baclophen blocks ω-conotoxin-sensitive Ca^{2+} channels, which presumably contributes to the presynaptic inhibition of evoked release (Wall and Dale, 1994). A function for spinal GABAergic neurons during *Xenopus* embryo swimming remains unknown. As a result, the role of the GABAergic, presynaptic regulation of reciprocal inihibition during swimming is unclear. Nonetheless, *Xenopus* embryo spinal neurons do possess both GABA$_A$ and GABA$_B$ receptors, and spinal interneurons with GABA-like immunoreactivity are present in the spinal cord (Roberts et al., 1987).

Modulatory Effects of Other Transmitters

Recent research on the lamprey spinal cord has revealed the modulatory actions of several other transmitters, including EAAs that activate metabotropic glutamate receptors, whose activation leads to an increase in the frequency of the swimming rhythm (Krieger et al., 1994). The peptide neurotensin has the opposite effect: it slows down the rhythm and increases motor bursts durations (Barthe and Grillner, 1995). Neurotensin's effects on the locomotor rhythm thus resemble those of both 5-HT and GABA$_B$ receptor activation. The underlying mechanisms of action, though not yet studied in detail, appear to be quite different, however, because neurotensin depolarizes spinal neurons and does not block the sAHP.

The monoamine dopamine, which co-localizes with 5-HT in ventral plexus neurons of the lamprey spinal cord, slows the swimming rhythm. Like 5-HT, dopamine impairs I$_{K(Ca)}$ to reduce the sAHP (Schotland et al., 1995). Interestingly, however, the mechanism by which it accomplishes the impairment is distinct from that used by 5-HT because dopamine reduces Ca^{2+} entry during the action potential in a fashion analogous to the way in which GABA$_B$ receptor activation works.

Modulation of Spinal Networks during Development

The networks that drive rhythmic motoneuron activity are formed in the spinal cord at very early stages of development, often before birth (or hatching) and prior to the expression of locomotion—for example (reviewed in Sillar, 1994), in agnathans (Cohen et al., 1990), fish (Batty, 1984; Kuwada, 1986), amphibians (Kahn and Roberts, 1982), birds (Bekoff, 1992; Bekoff and Lau, 1980; O'Donovan, 1989), mammals (Kudo and Yamada, 1987; Kudo et al., 1991; Hernandez et al., 1991). Rat fetuses can generate rhythmic, swimming-like movements when 20 days old (Bekoff and Lau, 1980), whereas rat neonates can swim at postnatal day 1 (Bekoff and Trainer, 1979) and can step overground at postnatal day 11 (Westerga and Gramsbergen, 1990). Furthermore, in newborn rats, sensory inputs can reset the ongoing locomotor activity (Kiehn et al., 1992; Sqalli-Houssaini et al., 1993); also, both electrical and chemical stimulation of the brain stem can induce locomotion of hindlimbs (Atsuta et al., 1988; Atsuta et al., 1990; Atsuta et al., 1991). Those findings in rats suggest that sensory feedback and descending signals are capable of modulating the activity of spinal locomotor circuits at a developmental stage when swimming behavior is expressed, and prior to the onset of stepping. It is likely that, in many different vertebrates, the building blocks of spinal locomotor circuits are put in place early in development, and as development proceeds, they are progressively modulated by intrinsic spinal and descending control systems that themselves continue to develop after birth or hatching.

Early rhythmic movements in young locomotor systems, like those in adult systems, are produced by intrinsic spinal networks that require neither sensory feedback nor descending inputs for basic rhythm generation. At the level of the underlying neural circuitry, similar transmitter receptors (e.g., EAA receptor–mediated excitation and glycinergic inhibition) are involved in the generation and coordination of both young and mature locomotor rhythms. In some cases, some evidence also exists for the participation of homologous types of neurons in young and adult preparations. For example, in both *Xenopus* embryos (Dale, 1985) and adult lampreys (Buchanan, 1982), reciprocal inhibition of antagonistic motoneurons during swimming is mediated by glycine release from inhibitory interneurons with commissural projections. Apparently, the primitive networks are retained and adapted to perform more complex locomotor functions at later stages in development. In the chick, for example, hatching and walking behaviors are distinctly different, but the basic muscle synergies remain similar, suggesting that the output of a common rhythm-generating circuit is modulated during development to accommodate the switch from one behavior to the other (Bekoff, 1992). In other cases—in the rat, for example—the rhythmic motor activity induced by activating NMDA receptors with the racemic mixture N-methyl-D,L-aspartate (NMA) changes from a synchronous pattern to an alternating one during prenatal development (Kudo et al., 1991; Ozaki et al., 1996). The switch may be due to the development of commissural, glycinergic inhibitory pathways because a pattern of rhythmic activity with left/right synchrony is expressed early in development (at day E16.5; figure 17.2Aa) but is subsequently (at day E20.5) replaced by an alternating one (see figure 17.2Ba). In the presence of NMA, pharmacological block of glycine receptors with strychnine has no effect on the early synchronous pattern (figure 17.2Ab), but it does abolish alternation and cause the synchronous pattern to resume when bath applied at E20.5 (figure 17.2Bb). The latter experiments suggest that, although the basic rhythm-generating units are in place early in mammalian development, major changes may occur in specific aspects of the fetal networks. After birth, however, the output of the network seems to remain relatively stable (Kiehn and Kjaerulff, 1996).

The output of the *Xenopus* embryo CPG also undergoes dramatic developmental changes. Myotomal motoneurons usually discharge a single impulse on each and every cycle of embryonic swimming activity (Kahn and Roberts, 1982; Sillar and Roberts, 1993), so that the duration and intensity of muscle contractions during swimming cannot normally be varied on a cycle-by-cycle basis. However, the motor output develops rapidly. Within twenty-four hours after hatching has occurred, the larval swimming pattern involves a burst of discharge in each cycle, during which motoneurons can fire more than once (Sillar et al., 1991, 1992a). This modulation in neuronal firing properties is responsible for a significant increase in rhythm flexibility because the output to the muscles can now be varied in different cycles. The firing capability of embryonic neurons is thought to be restricted by a voltage-dependent K$^+$ conductance that renders the neurons refractory after impulse generation (Soffe, 1990). Presumably, the relative contribution of this conductance to the firing behavior of

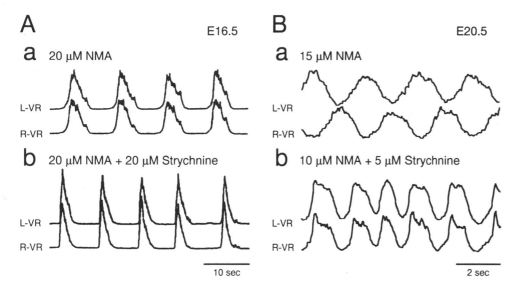

Figure 17.2

Effects of strychnine on NMA-induced rhythmic motor activity in the neonatal rat from two stages of embryonic development, at days E16.5 (A) and E20.5 (B). Integrated ventral root discharges are recorded from the fourth lumbar segment on the left (L-VR) and right (R-VR) sides, respectively. Aa. At day E16.5, 20 μM NMA induced a rhythmic motor pattern that was synchronous across the body. Ab. The basic coordination of the synchronous rhythm was unaffected by relatively high concentrations of strychnine (20 μM). Ba. At stage E20.5, 15 μM NMA elicited a motor pattern that now alternated between the two sides of the body. Bb. Lower concentrations of strychnine (5 μM) disrupted the coordination across the body and led to a synchronous motor pattern, similar to that recorded at the earlier stage (cf. Aa). (See text for further details.)

larval neurons gradually decreases during development to allow multiple firing to occur. Interestingly, the postembryonic development of the swimming circuit is coincident with the growth of serotonergic, raphespinal projections into the ventral aspect of the cord (van Mier et al., 1986). Like the growth of these fibers, the development of the rhythm follows a rostrocaudal path throughout the first day after hatching. Furthermore, a bath application of 5-HT, or its metabolic precursor 5-HTP, mimics the normal timetable of axial rhythm development (Sillar et al., 1992b), suggesting that the transition from a simple embryonic motor pattern to a more flexible adult-like form is causally linked to the incorporation of a descending monoaminergic system in the spinal cord, the same system that modulates ongoing locomotion later in life (Sillar et al., 1995).

Neuroanatomical studies in the chick have also suggested an important role for 5-HT in the development of spinal circuitry (Okado et al., 1992). Pharmacological deletion of serotonergic fibers near the time of hatching causes a significant reduction in non-serotonergic axosomatic synapses on spinal motoneurons, both in the course of development and in adulthood. Thus, in addition to controlling the development of spinal synaptic connections, 5-HT may sustain synaptic connectivity in mature animals. In isolated spinal cord preparations from fetal as well as newborn rats, bath application of 5-HT can also activate, sustain, and stabilize the rhythmic output of the spinal networks for locomotion (Sqalli-Houssaini et al., 1993; Iizuka et al., 1995). Bath application of NMA and 5-HT together induces more stable and long-lasting episodes of rhythmic activity than does NMA or 5-HT alone (Sqalli-Houssaini et al., 1993). The 5-HT-induced rhythm is completely suppressed by APV, a selective antagonist of NMDA receptors, whereas the NMDA-induced rhythm is not blocked by ketanserin, a selective antagonist of 5-HT₂ receptors. Those results suggest that 5-HT modulates CPG function at early stages of mammalian development (Iizuka et al., 1992). In the immature rat, the raphespinal tract descends to the lumbar segment and 5-HT-positive fibers grow into the motor nucleus prenatally (Ozaki et al., 1992; Kudo et al., 1993). It remains to be elucidated, however, whether 5-HT plays an important role in the formation and differentiation of CPGs during prenatal mammalian development. We do know that the 5-HT system affects postnatal locomotor development in the rat because the deletion of 5-HT by intraperitoneal administration of p-chlorophenylalanine (PCPA) in newborn rats retards general locomotor capability (Myoga et al., 1995).

GABA is also involved in the maturation of locomotor circuitry. In the chick, for example, GABAergic neurons appear in the ventral horn early in embryogenesis, only to disappear later in development (Antal et al., 1994a, 1994b). The rhythmic depolarizing synaptic drive to sartorius motoneurons in the chick is dominated by depolarizing inhibition early in development, but excitatory drive predominates later on (O'Donovan, 1989; O'Donovan et al., 1992), as is consistent with the eventual disappearance of GABA neurons. This is interesting in view of the apparent suppression by GABA of lumbar rhythm generation in newborn rats (Cazalets et al., 1994). Perhaps the transient occurrence of GABA neurons in the ventral horn of the chick and rat is linked to a trophic role in the development of the locomotor networks, in addition to the role they play in rhythm generation.

Conclusions

Two types of neuron, one GABAergic and one serotonergic, have emerged as particularly important in both the development and intrinsic modulation of vertebrate locomotor circuitry. Through the actions of metabotropic, pre- and postsynaptic receptors on spinal motoneurons and interneurons, these two types of modulatory neurons target a very wide range of cellular and synaptic mechanisms that comprise the basic building blocks of the spinal CPGs for locomotion. The details about such GABAergic and serotonergic modulation are beginning to unfold from research on a relatively wide range of motor systems. Far less is known, however, about how parallel mechanisms merge to accomplish the global effects of a given neuromodulator on the circuitry and how different neuromodulatory systems interact. In the case of 5-HT, much of our knowledge derives from work on the lamprey and the *Xenopus* tadpole. In both systems, global effects on the swimming circuitry appear to be accomplished by a single, pharmacologically distinct 5-HT receptor, which has a profile resembling the mammalian 5-HT_{1A} receptor. Activation of this 5-HT receptor appears to be responsible for the modulation of conductances that control repetitive firing in the lamprey and *Xenopus*. Furthermore, in *Xenopus*, the same receptor also appears to be responsible for the induction of bistable membrane properties, membrane hyperpolarization, and the modulation of glycinergic reciprocal inhibition.

The unexpected diversity of 5-HT's effects raises two important issues that should become useful focuses for future studies on the modulation of locomotor networks. The first issue concerns the molecular mechanisms that are activated by a single class of receptor. Perhaps the diversity of functional effects is accomplished by a differential distribution of 5-HT_{1A} receptors throughout the neuronal membrane and by changing the nature of second messenger–receptor linkages in different cellular compartments. The second issue concerns the functional significance of the incorporation of so many different modulatory mechanisms. Presumably, separate mechanisms differentially modulate various aspects of the motor rhythm, but the simultaneous activation of all mechanisms in concert is necessary for 5-HT to accomplish its global influence on locomotion. Conceivably, such specific questions can be addressed in further experiments on simple vertebrate preparations, such as the *Xenopus* tadpole. Whether the findings of the experiments will be generally applicable can only be addressed by subsequent searches for similar features in more complex locomotor circuitry. Nonetheless, the challenge to be faced in research on adult and higher vertebrate systems is to assess how a given neuromodulator, such as 5-HT, activates multiple postsynaptic receptor subtypes and how it operates in concert with other modulatory inputs. 5-HT and GABA are clearly important modulators that act on spinal CPGs, but we know far less about many other influences, including the metabotropic glutamate receptors and the numerous peptide and amine receptors.

Acknowledgments

We thank the following for their support of research carried out in our laboratories: the Royal Society (London), the BBSRC, and the Wellcome Trust (Sillar); the Human Frontier Science Program (Kiehn and Kudo); the Novo Nordic Foundation and the Danish MRC (Kiehn). Ole Kiehn is a Hallas Møller Senior Research Fellow. Keith T. Sillar is a Royal Society 1983 University Research Fellow.

References

Alford S, Grillner S (1991) The involvement of GABAb receptors and coupled G-proteins in spinal GABAergic presynaptic inhibition. *J Neurosci* 11:3718–3726.

Alhaider AA, Lei SZ, Wilcox GL (1991) Spinal 5-HT₃ receptor-mediated antinociception: Possible release of GABA. *J Neurosci* 11:1881–1888.

Antal M, Berki ACS, Horvarth L, O'Donovan MJ (1994a) Developmental changes in the distribution of GABA-immunoreactive neurons in the embryonic chick lumbosacral spinal cord. *J Comp Neurol* 343:228–236.

Antal M, Polgar E, Berki ACS, Biryani A, Poskar Z (1994b) Development of specific populations of interneurons in the ventral horn of the embryonic chick lumbosacral spinal cord. *Eur J Morphol* 32:201–206.

Atsuta Y, Abraham P, Iwahara T, Garcia-Rill E, Skinner RD (1991) Control of locomotion in vitro. II. Chemical stimulation. *Somatosens Mot Res* 8:55–63.

Atsuta Y, Garcia-Rill E, Skinner RD (1988) Electrically induced locomotion in the in vitro brain stem–spinal cord preparation. *Dev Brain Res* 42:309–312.

Atsuta Y, Garcia-Rill E, Skinner RD (1990) Characteristics of electrically induced locomotion in rat in vitro brain stem–spinal cord preparation. *J Neurophysiol* 64:727–735.

Barbeau H, Rossignol S (1990) The effects of serotonergic drugs on the locomotor pattern and on cutaneous reflexes of the adult chronic spinal cat. *Brain Res* 514:55–67.

Barbeau H, Rossignol S (1991) Initiation and modulation of the locomotor pattern in the adult chronic spinal cat by noradrenergic, serotonergic, and dopaminergic drugs. *Brain Res* 546:250–260.

Barthe J-Y, Grillner S (1995) Neurotensin-induced modulation of spinal neurons and fictive swimming in the lamprey. *J Neurophysiol* 73:1308–1312.

Batty RS (1984) Development of swimming movements and musculature of larval herring (*Clupea harengus*). *J Exp Biol* 110:217–229.

Bekoff A (1992). Neuroethological approaches to the study of motor development in chicks: Achievements and challenges. *J Neurobiol* 23:1586–1505.

Bekoff A, Lau B (1980) Interlimb coordination in 20-day-old rat fetuses. *J Exp Zool* 214:173–175.

Bekoff A, Trainer W (1979) The development of interlimb co-ordination during swimming in postnatal rats. *J Exp Biol* 83:1–11.

Berger AJ, Takahashi T (1990) Serotonin enhances a low-voltage-activated calcium current in rat spinal motoneurons. *J Neurosci* 10:1922–1928.

Buchanan JT (1982) Identification of interneurons with contralateral caudal axons in the lamprey spinal cord: synaptic interactions and morphology. *J Neurophysiol* 47:961–975.

Buchanan J, Grillner S (1990) 5-hydroxytryptamine depresses reticulospinal excitatory postsynaptic potentials in motoneurons of the lamprey. *Neurosci Lett* 112:71–74.

Cazalets JR, Grillner P, Menard I, Cremieux J, Clarac F (1990) Two types of motor rhythm induced by NMDA and amines in an in vitro spinal cord preparation of neonatal rat. *Neurosci Letts* 111:116–121.

Cazalets JR, Sqali-Houssaini Y, Clarac F (1994) GABAergic inactivation of the central pattern generator for locomotion in isolated neonatal rat spinal cord. *J Physiol* 474:173–181.

Christenson J, Bongianni F, Grillner S, Hokfelt T (1990) Putative GABAergic input to axons of spinal interneurons in the lamprey spinal cord as shown by Lucifer Yellow and GABA immunohistochemistry. *Brain Res* 538:313–318.

Christenson J, Franck J, Grillner S (1989) Increase in endogenous 5-hydroxytryptamine levels modulates the central network underlying locomotion in the lamprey spinal cord. *Neurosci Lett* 100:188–192.

Cohen AH, Tamara A, Dobrov GL, Kiemel T, Baker MT (1990) The development of the lamprey pattern generator for locomotion. *J Neurobiol* 21:958–969.

Dale N (1985) Reciprocal inhibitory interneurons in the spinal cord of *Xenopus laevis*. *J Physiol* 363:527–543.

El Manira A, Tegnér J, Grillner S (1994) Calcium-dependent potassium channels play a critical role for burst termination in the locomotor network in lamprey. *J Neurophysiol* 72:1852–1861.

Grillner S, Wallén P, Brodin L, Lansner A (1991) Neuronal network generating locomotor behavior in lamprey. *Ann Rev Neurosci* 14:169–199.

Harris-Warrick RM, Cohen AH (1985) Serotonin modulates the central pattern generator for locomotion in the isolated lamprey spinal cord. *J Exp Biol* 116:27–46.

Hernandez P, Elbert K, Droge MH (1991) Spontaneous and NMDA evoked motor rhythms in the neonatal mouse spinal cord: An in vitro study in comparison with in situ activity. *Exp Brain Res* 85:66–74.

Hill RH, Matsushima T, Schotland J, Grillner S (1992) Apamin blocks the slow AHP in lamprey and delays the termination of locomotor bursts. *Neuroreport* 3:943–945.

Hochman S, Jordan LM, MacDonald JF (1994) N-methyl-D-aspartate receptor–mediated voltage oscillations in neurons surrounding the central canal in slices of rat spinal cord. *J Neurophysiol* 72:565–577.

Iizuka M, Nishimaru H, Kudo N (1995) Developmental changes in the pattern of the 5-HT-induced locomotor rhythm in the spinal cord of fetal rats. *Jap J Physiol* 45:S179.

Iizuka M, Watanabe Y, Kudo N (1992) Differential role of NMDA and non-NMDA receptors in the neuronal networks for locomotion. *Neurosci Res Suppl* 17:S209.

Jacobs B (1994) Serotonin, motor activity, and depression-related disorders. *Am Sci* 82:456–463.

Johansson O, Hökfelt T, Pernow B, Jeffcoat SL, White N, Steinbusch HWM, Verhofstad AAJ, Emson PC, Spindel E (1981) Immunohistochemical support for three putative transmitters in one neuron: Coexistence of 5-hydroxytyptamine, substance P, and thyrotropin releasing hormone like immunoreactivity in medullary neurons projecting to the spinal cord. *Neuroscience* 6:1857–1881.

Kahn JA, Roberts A (1982). The central nervous origin of the swimming motor pattern in embryos of *Xenopus laevis*. *J Exp Biol* 99:185–196.

Kiehn O (1991) Plateau potentials and active integration in the "final common pathway" for motor behavior. *Trends Neurosci* 14:68–73.

Kiehn O, Iizuka M, Kudo N (1992) Resetting from low threshold afferents of N-methyl-D-aspartate-induced locomotor rhythm in the isolated spinal cord–hindlimb preparation from newborn rats. *Neurosci Letters* 148:43–46.

Kiehn O, Kjaerulff O (1996) Spatiotemporal characteristics of 5-HT and dopamine-induced hindlimb locomotor activity in the in vitro neonatal rat. *J Neurophysiol* 75:1472–1482.

Krieger P, Tegnér J, El Manira A, Grillner S (1994) Effects of metabotropic glutamate receptor activation on the cellular and network level in the lamprey spinal cord. *Neuroreport* 5:1760–1762.

Kudo N, Furukawa F, Okado N (1993) Development of descending fibers to the rat embryonic spinal cord. *Neurosci Res* 16:131–141.

Kudo N, Ozaki S, Yamada T (1991) Ontogeny of rhythmic activity in the spinal cord of the rat. In: *Neurobiological Basis of Human Locomotion* (Shimamura M, Grillner S, Edgerton VR, eds.), 127–136. Tokyo: Japanese Scientific Society Press.

Kudo N, Yamada T (1987) N-methyl-D,L-aspartate-induced locomotor activity in a spinal cord–hindlimb muscles preparation of the newborn rat studied in vitro. *Neurosci Lett* 75:43–48.

Kuwada JY (1986) Cell recognition by neuronal growth cones in a simple vertebrate embryo. *Science* 233:740–746.

Meer DP, Buchanan JT (1992) Apamin reduces the late afterhyperpolarization of lamprey spinal neurons, with little effect on fictive swimming. *Neurosci Lett* 143:1–4.

Myoga H, Nonaka S, Matsuyama K, Mori S (1995) Postnatal development of locomotor movements in normal and para-chlorophenylalanine-treated newborn rats. *Neurosci Res* 21:211–221.

O'Donovan MJ (1989) Motor activity in the isolated spinal cord of the chick embryo: Synaptic drive and firing pattern of single motoneurons. *J Neurosci* 9:943–958.

O'Donovan MJ, Sernagor E, Sholomenko G, Ho S, Antal M, Yee W (1992) Development of spinal motor networks in the chick embryo. *J Exp Zool* 261:261–273.

Okado M, Cheng L, Tanatsugu Y, Hamada S, Hamaguchi K (1992) Synaptic loss following removal of serotoninergic fibers in newly hatched and adult chickens. *J Neurobiol* 24:687–698.

Ozaki S, Kudo N, Okado N (1992) Immunohistochemical study on development of serotonin-, substance P-, and enkephalin-positive fibers in the rat spinal motor nucleus. *J Comp Neurol* 325:462–470.

Ozaki S, Yamada T, Iizuka M, Nishimaru H, Kudo N (1996) Development of locomotor activity induced by NMDA receptor activation in the lumbar spinal cord of the rat fetus studied in vitro. *Dev Brain Res* 97:118–125.

Peroutka SJ (1988) 5-hydroxytryptamine receptor subtypes: Molecular, biochemical, and physiological characterization. *Trends Neurosci* 11:496–501.

Roberts A, Dale N, Ottersen OP, Storm-Mathisen J (1987) The early development of neurons with GABA immunoreactivity in the CNS of *Xenopus laevis* embryos. *J Comp Neurol* 261:345–449.

Schotland J, Shupliakov O, Wikström M, Brodin L, Srinivasan M, You Z, Herrera-Marschitz M, Zhang W, Hökfelt T, Grillner S (1995) Control of lamprey locomotor neurons by co-localized monoamine transmitters. *Nature* 374:266–268.

Scrymgeour-Wedderburn JF, Sillar KT (1994) Modulation of rhythmic swimming activity in post-embryonic *Xenopus laevis* tadpoles by 5-hydroxytryptamine acting at 5-HT$_{1a}$ receptors. *Proc Roy Soc Lond B* 255:139–145.

Shupliakov O, Pieribone VA, Gad H, Brodin L (1995) Synaptic vesicle depletion in reticulospinal axons is reduced by 5-HT: Direct evidence for presynaptic modulation of glutamatergic transmission. *Eur J Neurosci* 7:1111–1116.

Sigvardt KA, Grillner S, Wallén P, van Dongen PAM (1985) Activation of NMDA receptors elicits fictive locomotion and bistable membrane properties in the lamprey spinal cord. *Brain Res* 336:390–395.

Sillar KT (1994) Synaptic specificity: Development of locomotor rhythmicity. *Curr Opin Neurobiol* 4:101–107.

Sillar KT, Roberts A (1993) Control of frequency during swimming in *Xenopus* embryos: A study on interneuronal recruitment in a spinal rhythm generator. *J Physiol* 472:557–572.

Sillar KT, Simmers AJ (1994a) 5-HT induces NMDA receptor–mediated intrinsic oscillations in embryonic amphibian spinal neurons. *Proc Roy Soc Lond B* 255:139–145.

Sillar KT, Simmers AJ (1994b) Oscillatory membrane properties of spinal cord neurons that are rhythmically active during fictive swimming in *Rana temporaria* embryos. *Eur J Morphol* 32:185–192.

Sillar KT, Simmers AJ, Wedderburn JFS (1992a) The post-embryonic development of cell properties and synaptic drive underlying locomotor rhythm generation in *Xenopus laevis*. *Proc Roy Soc Lond B* 249:65–70.

Sillar KT, Wedderburn JFS (1994) Presynaptic modulation of glycine neurotransmission by 5-HT in the spinal cord of *Xenopus laevis* embryos. *Eur J Neurosci Supp* 7:167.

Sillar KT, Wedderburn JFS, Simmers AJ (1991) The development of swimming rhythmicity in post-mebryonic *Xenopus laevis*. *Proc Roy Soc Lond B* 246:147–153.

Sillar KT, Wedderburn JFS, Simmers AJ (1992b) Modulation of swimming rhythmicity by 5-hydroxytryptamine during post-embryonic development in *Xenopus laevis*. *Proc Roy Soc Lond B* 250:107–114.

Sillar KT, Woolston A-M, Wedderburn JFS (1995) Involvement of brainstem serotonergic interneurons in the control of a vertebrate spinal locomotor circuit. *Proc Roy Soc Lond B* 259:65–70.

Soffe SR (1990) Active and passive membrane properties of spinal cord neurons that are active during swimming in *Xenopus* embryos. *Eur J Neurosci* 2:1–10.

Sqalli-Houssaini Y, Cazalets JR, Clarac F (1993) Oscillatory properties of the central pattern generator for locomotion in neonatal rats. *J Neurophysiol* 70:803–813.

Tegnér J, Matsushima T, El Manira A, Grillner S (1993) The spinal GABA system modulates burst frequency and intersegmental coordination in the lamprey: Differential effects of GABA$_A$ and GABA$_B$ receptors. *J Neurophysiol* 69:647–657.

Vandermaelen CP, Aghajanian GK (1982) Serotonin-induced depolarization of rat facial motoneurons in vivo: Comparison with amino acid transmitters. *Brain Res* 239:139–152.

Van Dongen PA, Hökfelt T, Grillner S, Verhofstad AA, Steinbusch HW, Cuello AC, Terenius L (1985) Immunohistochemical demonstration of some putative neurotransmitters in the lamprey spinal cord and spinal ganglia: 5-hydroxytryptamine-, tachykinin-, and neuropeptide-Y-immunoreactive neurons and fibres. *J Comp Neurol* 234:501–522.

Van Mier P, Joosten HWJ, van Rheden R, ten Donkelaar HJ (1986) The development of serotonergic raphe spinal projections in *Xenopus laevis*. *Int J Dev Neurosci* 4:465–476.

Viala D, Buser P (1969) The effects of DOPA and 5-HTP on rhythmic efferent discharges in hindlimb nerves in the rabbit. *Brain Res* 12:437–443.

Wall MJ, Dale N (1993) GABA$_B$ receptors modulate glycinergic inhibition and spike threshold in *Xenopus* embryo spinal neurons. *J Physiol* 469:275–290.

Sillar, Kiehn, and Kudo

Wall MJ, Dale N (1994) GABA$_B$ receptors modulate an ω-conotoxin-sensitive calcium current that is required for synaptic transmission in the *Xenopus* embryo spinal cord. *J Neurosci* 14:6248–6255.

Wallén P, Buchanan S, Grillner S, Hill RH, Christenson J, Hökfelt T (1989) Effects of 5-hydroxytryptamine on the afterhyperpolarization, spike frequency regulation, and oscillatory membrane properties in the lamprey spinal cord. *J Neurophysiol* 61:759–768.

Wallén P, Grillner S (1985) The effect of current passage on N-methyl-D-aspartate-induced, tetrodotoxin-resistant membrane potential oscillations in lamprey neurons active during locomotion. *Neurosci Letts* 56: 85–93.

Wallén P, Grillner S (1987) N-methyl-D-aspartate receptor–induced, inherent oscillatory activity in neurons active during locomotion in the lamprey. *J Neurosci* 7:2745–2755.

Wallis DI (1994) 5-HT receptors involved in the initiation or modulation of motor patterns: Opportunities for drug development. *Trends Pharmacol Sci* 15:288–292.

Wedderburn JFS, Sillar KT (1994) TTX-resistant, NMDA receptor–mediated membrane potential oscillations in spinal locomotor neurons of *Xenopus laevis* larvae are 5-HT-dependent. *Neurosci Abst* 20:763.

Westerga J, Gramsbergen A (1990) The development of locomotion in the rat. *Dev Brain Res* 57:163–174.

Wiklund L, Leger L, Persson M (1981) Monoamine cell distribution in the cat brainstem: A fluorescence histochemical study with quantification of indoleaminergic and locus coeruleus cell groups. *J Comp Neurol* 203:613–647.

Wikström M, Hill R, Hellgren J, Grillner S (1995) The action of 5-HT on calcium-dependent potassium channels and on the spinal locomotor network in lamprey is mediated by 5-HT$_{1A}$-like receptors. *Brain Res* 678:191–199.

Woolston A-M, Wedderburn JFS, Sillar KT (1994) Descending serotonergic spinal projections and modulation of locomotor rhythmicity in *Rana temporaria* embryos. *Proc Roy Soc Lond B* 255:73–79.

Zhang CL, Krnjevic K (1989) Apamin depresses selectively the afterhyperpolarization of cat spinal motoneurons. *Neurosci Lett* 74:58–62.

18

Modulation of Neural Circuits by Steroid Hormones in Rodent and Insect Model Systems

Janis C. Weeks and
Bruce S. McEwen

Abstract

Steroid hormones affect neural function and behavior throughout the animal kingdom. This review discusses recent progress in understanding steroid action in the popular model systems of rodents and insects. In rodents, gonadal and adrenal (stress) hormones affect a variety of central nervous system regions during development and in adulthood, producing changes that range from reversible modulation of neuronal activity to permanent structural alterations. In insects, steroid hormones regulate the reorganization of the central nervous system during metamorphosis, thus affecting neuronal structure and survival as well as electrophysiological function. Many steroid effects on neuronal phenotype occur in both rodents and insects, including dendritic remodeling, neurogenesis, neuronal death, and changes in excitability and neuropeptide expression. Although the genomic effects of steroids are mediated by members of the same receptor superfamily in both vertebrates and invertebrates, the extent to which specific cellular and molecular mechanisms are shared remains to be determined.

It is now widely accepted that neural circuits are not fixed, hard-wired entities; rather, they can be modulated and reconfigured throughout an animal's life (Getting, 1989; Meyrand et al., 1994; Harris-Warrick et al., chapter 19, this volume). Among the classes of molecules that profoundly affect neurons and behavior are the steroid hormones. In vertebrates, gonadal steroids such as testosterone and estradiol play key roles in sexual differentiation of the central nervous system (CNS) during development and regulate the expression of behaviors associated with mating and territoriality in adulthood. Other steroid hormones such as glucocorticoids (stress hormones) can also alter learning capacity and emotionality by affecting specific brain regions such as the hypothalamus and hippocampus. In insects, ecdysteroids regulate the dramatic changes in the CNS and behavior that accompany metamorphosis.

Similarities in steroid hormone action span the animal kingdom. Intracellular steroid receptors, which bind hormone and alter gene expression via specific DNA binding sites ("genomic actions"), belong to the same superfamily in vertebrates and insects (Koelle et al., 1991). More rapid steroid actions have also been described in vertebrates that alter membrane properties, ion movements, and second messenger systems via receptors

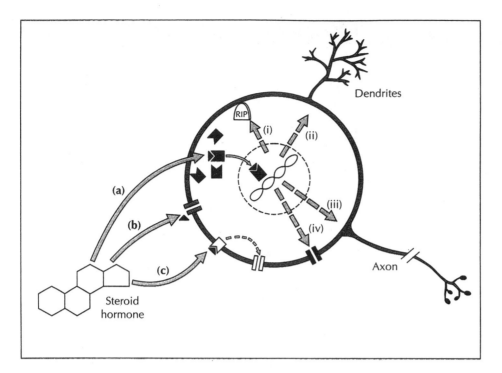

Figure 18.1

Summary of some physiological effects and mechanisms of action of steroid hormones on excitable cells. (a) Steroid hormones bind to intracellular receptors that alter gene expression. These genomic effects include (i) programmed cell death, (ii) growth or regression of dendrites, (iii) changes in synaptic function, and (iv) synthesis or modulation of ion channels. Two classes of non-genomic effects are also shown: (b) direct binding of steroids to a ligand-gated ion channel, (e.g., the GABA$_A$ receptor, which is modulated by steroids that differ from those that bind to the intracellular steroid receptors), and (c) binding of steroids to membrane receptors, which act via second messengers (e.g., glucocorticoid binding to a membrane receptor that inhibits reproductive behavior via G-proteins). The cell surface and intracellular receptors are structurally dissimilar. (Reprinted with permission from *Current Opinion in Neurobiology*; Weeks and Levine, 1995.)

located on or near the cell surface ("non-genomic actions"; figure 18.1; see also the review in McEwen, 1991a). Steroids exert similar effects on neuronal phenotype in vertebrates and invertebrates, including dendritic remodeling, neurogenesis, neuronal death, and alterations in excitability and neuropeptide expression. The neuronal changes are often accompanied by behavioral changes; one of the key challenges in the field is to determine how steroid-induced changes in neuronal properties alter the function of the neural circuits that subserve behavior. The nature and diversity of steroid-induced plasticity in CNS function, as well as its underlying mechanisms, are the subjects of this review.

Roles of Steroid Hormones in the Life Cycles of Insects and Vertebrates

A description of where hormones fit in the life cycles of vertebrate and invertebrate organisms sets the stage for our discussion of steroid-induced neuronal plasticity. The organization of the CNS of a vertebrate such as the rat reflects its ability to engage in complex social behaviors that require a definition of gender as well as social order. Those abilities depend on a brain organization in which higher cortical centers communicate with lower vegetative centers such as the hypothalamus and brain stem via a limbic system. The endocrine system and autonomic nervous system have evolved to play important roles in the communication processes. The hypothalamus serves a dual role by directing the activity of the autonomic nervous system and by regulating the hormonal output from the pituitary gland. The hypothalamus receives and integrates information from higher brain centers and passes this information on in the form of chemical signals that are released into the blood via the endocrine and autonomic nervous systems.

Hormones provide important signals to the brain; many hormone-sensitive brain structures are both developmentally programmed by the actions of hormones early in life and acted upon by circulating hormones in adulthood (Becker et al., 1992). It is therefore not surprising that hormones—especially sex hormones and adrenal hormones secreted in response to stress—play a major role in shaping the structure and function of the nervous system, a process which starts in utero when the brain begins to undergo sexual differentiation. Although sexual differentiation in mammals is confined to a restricted period of early development, it has life-long consequences that affect the structure of organs and tissues, including the brain, as well as the responses of many of these same cells and tissues to the reversible, activational effects of circulating hormones. The white rat, *Rattus norvegicus*, provides a useful model system in which to study the interactions between the developmental and activational effects of gonadal hormones. Sexual differentiation is controlled primarily by testosterone, which is secreted perinatally in males. Testosterone produces its effects via androgen receptors, and after being converted to estradiol by aromatizing enzymes in the brain, it also acts via estradiol receptors. The conversion of testosterone to either estradiol or dihydrotestosterone (the active androgen for androgen receptors) is a key, developmentally regulated event in the hypothalamus and limbic brain, including parts of cortical structures such as the hippocampus and cerebral cortex itself (see McEwen et al., 1995a). In the rat, sexual differentiation affects a number of brain regions that participate in the control of sexual and social behaviors.

Steroid hormones likewise exert profound effects on the insect nervous system. The most detailed information has come from studying metamorphosis in insects such as the hawk moth, *Manduca sexta*, and the fruitfly, *Drosophila melanogaster*. Metamorphosis is controlled by a small ensemble of hormones that includes the ecdysteroids—ecdysone and its biologically active hydroxylation product, 20-hydroxyecdysone (20-HE)—and juvenile hormone (JH), a sesqueterpenoid. Several peptide hormones also play key roles. Metamorphosis entails profound behavioral changes—with attendant changes in body form, musculature, appendages, sensory systems, and locomotory patterns—as insects progress through the larval, pupal and adult stages. *Drosophila* and *Manduca* offer complementary advantages for studying hormonally regulated neural plasticity: *Manduca* is ideal for endocrinological and electrophysiological studies, whereas *Drosophila* offers the best molecular-genetic system for investigating steroid-regulated gene expression. There is increasing convergence of research on these two species (reviewed by Riddiford and Truman, 1994; Levine et al., 1995). Our review focuses on *Manduca*, in which the relationship between hormonal effects on neurons and behavior is best understood.

Manduca is known as the "white rat of insect endocrinology" because of the wealth of information avail-able about its endocrinology (figure 18.2). Its life cycle lasts approximately 6 weeks and encompasses five larval stages (instars), the pupal stage, and adulthood. Each molt is triggered by an elevation of ecdysteroids in the hemolymph (blood), with the type of molt determined by the JH level and by the previous history of hormonal exposure. Molts from one larval instar to the next are triggered by a surge of ecdysteroids in the presence of JH. In the final larval instar, metamorphosis is initiated by a small pulse of ecdysteroids in the absence of JH; this *commitment pulse* commits cells to subsequent pupal development and triggers wandering behavior when the caterpillar burrows underground. The larval-pupal molt is then triggered by a *prepupal peak* of ecdysteroids in the presence of a low level of JH. Following pupation, the development of the adult moth is driven by a prolonged rise and fall of ecdysteroids in the absence of JH. Male and female *Manduca* have similar hormone titers during metamorphosis (Baker et al., 1987), and steroid hormones are not known to contribute to sexual differentiation.

Cellular Actions of Steroid Hormones

Steroid hormones alter a variety of neuronal properties in both invertebrate and vertebrate animals. In insects, ecdysteroids regulate the growth and regression of dendritic and axonal arbors, postembryonic neurogenesis, programmed neuronal death, neuronal excitability and neuropeptide expression (reviewed in Weeks and Levine, 1992). In most cases, JH is notable only by its absence. The effects of ecdysteroids on neuronal phenotype are the building blocks for the reconfiguration of neural circuits that accompanies metamorphosis. Like the vertebrate steroid hormones, ecdysteroids exert genomic effects via intracellular receptor molecules (see figure 18.1). The mapping of ecdysteroid receptor expression patterns in the insect CNS has been useful in identifying putative target neurons (Fahrbach, 1992; Truman et al., 1994). All of the ecdysteroid effects discussed in this chapter are believed to be genomic; non-genomic effects of ecdysteroids have not been reported, perhaps because few attempts have been made to investigate them.

Steroid hormones exert a similar range of phenotypic effects on vertebrate neurons. A prime example occurs during sexual differentiation, when androgenic effects on the male CNS produce sex differences in neural circuitry and behavior. One of the surprises of recent research on hormone action in the brain is the plasticity of adult neurons. In addition to affecting neuronal structure, steroid

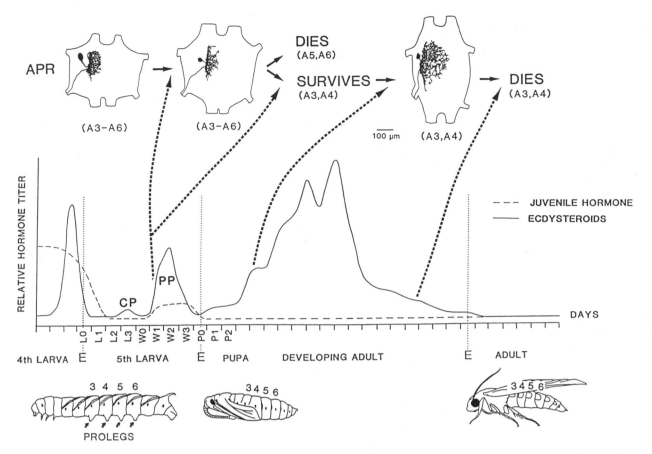

Figure 18.2

Metamorphic changes in *Manduca* hormones and neurons. Changes in hemolymph levels of ecdysteroids and juvenile hormone (JH; bottom) regulate phenotypic changes in neurons (top, linked by dashed arrows). The prepupal peak of ecdysteroids triggers regression of accessory planta retractor motoneurons (APRs) in all segments and death of APRs in a subset of segments. Regrowth of respecified APRs is triggered by the pupal rise in ecdysteroids, and, based on studies of other motoneurons (Truman and Schwartz, 1984), death of adult APRs results from the fall in ecdysteroids at emergence. Drawings show insects with segments A3–A6 labeled. E, ecdysis; CP, commitment pulse; PP, prepupal peak; W0, wandering. (Hormone titers modified from Riddiford and Truman, 1994.)

hormones regulate neuronal excitability and neurotransmission (see Orchinik and McEwen, 1995). Some of the mechanisms that underlie steroid hormone action are obscure, others are known to involve changes in specific gene products, and still others may be non-genomic (McEwen, 1991a). Non-genomic hormonal effects (see figure 18.1) include the modulation of the GABA$_A$ receptor by steroid metabolites of progesterone or deoxycorticosterone (which bind to a receptor site different from the GABA or benzodiazepine site) and a G-protein-coupled glucocorticoid receptor that has a steroid specificity different from that of the intracellular glucocorticoid receptor.

Among the most frequently studied genomic actions of steroid hormones is the regulation of expression of neuropeptide neuromodulators. For example, ovarian hormones regulate the expression of oxytocin, which plays a key role in the female rat's mating behavior (Flanagan and McEwen, 1995). Vasopressin, an impor-

tant modulator of social interactions, is influenced by androgens and glucocorticoids (DeVries, 1995; Miller et al., 1992; Insel et al., 1994; Winslow et al., 1993). Corticotropin Releasing Hormone (CRH), a powerful central activator of autonomic and behavioral responses related to fear and anxiety, is at least in part regulated by glucocorticoids (Koob et al., 1994). Other actions of steroids in vertebrates that are likely to have genomic mechanisms involve structural plasticity of the CNS during development and adulthood.

Actions of Sex and Stress Hormones in the Rat

The rat is the most commonly used vertebrate species for studying steroid effects on the CNS, although important information is also obtained from fish, amphibians and birds (see Weeks and Levine, 1995). Much of the information obtained from these various systems is transferable in some aspects among species; yet each species offers unique opportunities. The rat has provided a great deal of information about sexual differentiation, sexual behavior, and the effects of stress and stress hormones on the brain. Sex and stress hormones act on the adult brain to modify neuronal structure and neurochemical characteristics; these modulations are superimposed on the developmental actions of hormones, especially as they determine the structure and activity of the sexually differentiated brain. Here, we consider several neural systems in which such effects have been studied. We also discuss the mechanisms and functional significance of hormonal actions for behavior.

Spinal Nucleus of the Bulbocavernosus

Motoneurons of the spinal nucleus of the bulbocavernosus (SNB) innervate the bulbocavernosus muscle of the penis. During development and maturity androgen actions regulate the structure and function of this sexually dimorphic system (Forger and Breedlove, 1991). Female rats lack the bulbocavernosus muscle and have a smaller number of SNB motoneurons; in males, androgens prevent the developmental death of SNB motoneurons by preventing the degeneration of the target muscle (Nordeen et al., 1985). In the adult SNB, androgens regulate the dendritic extent of SNB motoneurons (Kurz et al., 1986) by acting, at least in part, via the target muscle itself (Rand and Breedlove, 1995), even though the SNB motoneurons are themselves targets for androgen action (Breedlove and Arnold, 1980). The shrinkage of SNB motoneuron arbors after castration may contribute to the concomitant loss of sexual behavior, but this possibility needs to be tested electrophysiologically.

Ventromedial Nucleus of the Hypothalamus

The ventromedial nucleus of the hypothalamus (VMN) is the principal hormone-sensitive brain region that mediates the lordosis (mating) response of the female rat (Pfaff, 1980). Ovarian hormones—estradiol and progesterone—regulate a number of key VMN features that are sexually dimorphic (McEwen, 1991b). Neurons of the ventrolateral VMN contain estrogen receptors; estradiol induces progestin receptors, oxytocin receptors, and new synapses in ovariectomized females. All three parameters fluctuate during the estrous cycle. Estradiol also induces preproenkephalin mRNA (Freidin and Pfaff, 1995) and modulates protein kinase C activity (Kow et al., 1994). In addition ovarian steroids modulate $GABA_A$ receptor binding in the VMN (Schumacher et al., 1989).

Estrogenic effects on the VMN are relatively rapid. Within 1–2 hours of estrogen exposure in an ovariectomized female rat, cell nuclear volume increases and ribosomal RNA increases in the nucleus and cytoplasm (McEwen et al., 1987). Progestin receptor and oxytocin receptor induction is evident within 6–8 hours, and new synapses on dendritic spines are evident within 24–48 hours (McEwen, 1991b). An increase in preproenkephalin mRNA also rapidly follows estrogen treatment and is closely correlated with the induction of lordosis (Freidin and Pfaff, 1995).

The functional significance of the estrogenic effects is considerable. Progestin receptor induction in the VMN is closely correlated with the ability of the rat to show lordosis behavior (Parsons et al., 1980). Oxytocin receptor induction also shows a close correlation with lordosis. Moreover, oxytocin and progesterone are linked in three ways to the lordosis response: (1) oxytocin can induce the lordosis reflex, but only in female rats primed with estrogen and progesterone; (2) oxytocin receptor antagonist treatment blocks the display of lordosis in female rats primed with estradiol and progesterone; and (3) deficient in progestin receptor induction, yet showing oxytocin receptor induction by estradiol, male rats do not display lordosis (Schumacher et al., 1992). Increased GABA activity in the VMN facilitates lordosis behavior (McCarthy et al., 1994). Likewise, increased synthesis of preproenkephalin may contribute to the enhancement of lordosis behavior; researchers speculate that this increase might occur via sigma opioid receptors (Freidin and Pfaff, 1995). It remains to be seen at what level the various neurotransmitter influences listed in this paragraph converge with the synaptic changes in the regulation of lordosis behavior.

The density of VMN synapses is higher in males than females; in female rats, synaptic density rises and falls during the estrous cycle (Frankfurt et al., 1990; Lewis et al., 1995). Male VMN synapse density increases after gonadectomy (compared to the decrease seen in females), and estrogen treatment reverses the increase of synapse density (McEwen, 1991b). Moreover, the male VMN has a larger number of synapses on VMN neurons than the female VMN (Matsumoto and Arai, 1986), but it is not known whether the afferent innervation for the male and female VMN are qualitatively different.

Hippocampus

The hippocampus is the cognitive arm of the limbic system and participates in contextual memory, spatial memory, and declarative memory. Both sex and stress hormones affect hippocampal structure and function;

moreover, the hippocampus shows developmentally programmed sex differences (see McEwen et al., 1995a,b). In addition, the dentate gyrus continues to undergo neurogenesis, which is regulated by adrenocotical secretions, during adult life (Cameron and Gould, 1996; Cameron et al., 1995).

Adrenocorticoids and Long-Term Potentiation

Adrenal steroids have short-term effects on hippocampal long-term potentiation (LTP) that indicate a biphasic dose-response curve. The two arms of this curve appear to be mediated by the two types of adrenal steroid receptors co-expressed within hippocampal neurons (see McEwen et al., 1995a). Within sixty minutes of application to awake or anaesthetized rats, steroid agonists for the Type I (mineralocorticoid) receptor enhance the magnitude and duration of LTP, whereas agonists for the Type II (glucocorticoid) receptor suppress LTP. Specific antagonists of the Type I and Type II receptors block these actions, indicating that they are likely to be mediated by the intracellular receptors.

These effects mimic a biphasic dose-response curve for corticosterone seen for hippocampal primed burst potentiation (PBP), a close relative of LTP (Diamond et al., 1992). The levels of corticosterone that facilitate PBP or LTP fall within the range of the levels measured during the rising phase of the diurnal rhythm that precedes the active or waking period of the day, whereas the levels of corticosterone that inhibit PBP or LTP are the same as those measured during acute stress. Rapid actions of glucocorticoids during the sleep-waking period may therefore modulate excitability in the hippocampus and contribute to fluctuations in cognitive performance and learning.

Dentate Granule Cell Neurogenesis and Apoptosis

The dentate gyrus is a unique structure, consisting of granule neurons that arise postnatally in the rat and that continue to be produced during adult life (Gould and McEwen, 1993; Cameron and Gould, 1996). Adrenal steroids inhibit or "contain" neurogenesis and neuronal death, and adrenalectomy increases both processes: neurons die in the outer or older zone of the granule cell layer, while new neurons are born in the inner and hilar regions of the dentate gyrus. The functional significance of granule neuron birth and death may be related to the long-term, seasonal fluctuations in the size of the hippocampus found in voles and deer mice (Sherry et al., 1992). It is not yet clear what signals control hippocampal volume—that is, whether seasonal differences

occur in adrenal steroid levels or in the expression of adrenal steroid receptors in the hippocampus. The Type I receptor seems to be primarily responsible for the adrenocorticoid actions that limit granule cell birth and death (Gould and McEwen, 1993; Cameron and Gould, 1996).

Glucocorticoids and Stress-Induced Atrophy of Dendrites

Repeated stress causes dendrites on the apical tree of pyramidal neurons in the CA3 region to atrophy (see McEwen et al., 1995a). The atrophic process takes approximately 3 weeks of daily treatment and results in mild cognitive impairment in learning a radial arm maze. Daily corticosterone administration mimics this effect, and in the tree shrew, social stress causes a similar phenomenon to occur over a period of 28 days. Although the dendritic atrophy is reversible, evidence indicates that prolonged and severe stress in primates and the wear and tear of aging in rats lead to a permanent loss of pyramidal neurons. Indeed, individual differences in aging of the hippocampus may be related to elevated activity of the stress axis and levels of glucocorticoids (Meaney et al., 1994; McEwen and Sapolsky, 1995). Evidence in humans also supports a relationship between cortisol elevations and hippocampal atrophy, which is associated with the impairment of short-term verbal memory (see McEwen and Sapolsky, 1995, for review). Moreover, hippocampal atrophy in elderly human subjects predicts later development of Alzheimer's disease, raising the possibility that reversible atrophy may be an initial event in the process of permanent pyramidal neurons loss (DeLeon et al., 1993).

Estradiol, Progesterone, and Cyclic Synaptogenesis

Excitatory synapses on dendritic spines of CA1 pyramidal neurons are induced by estradiol during the estrous cycle of the female rat (see McEwen et al., 1995b, for review). Progesterone secretion at the time of ovulation causes the newly induced synapses to disappear. Although we have almost no data on spatial learning ability of female rats in relation to estrogen levels, one report does show that LTP is enhanced on the afternoon of proestrus, when the peak density of excitatory synapses is reached in CA1. Moreover, the seizure threshold for the dorsal hippocampus is lowest on the day of proestrus (Teresawa and Timiras, 1968).

The male hippocampus shows a decrease of dendritic spine density after gonadectomy, but the decrease is not reversed by estrogen treatment unless the male rat has been treated with an inhibitor of testosterone aromatization at birth (Lewis et al., 1995). Indeed, the developing hippocampus transiently expresses both aromatizing enzymes and estrogen receptors at birth. Estrogen treatment of females at this time masculinizes spatial learning ability, whereas gonadectomy of males at birth produces a feminine spatial capability (Handa et al., 1994; see McEwen et al., 1995b, for further discussion and references).

Actions of Ecdysteroids in *Manduca*

One limitation of research on vertebrate systems is that steroid effects are typically studied in populations of neurons with distributed or undefined roles in behavior. In contrast, many individually identifiable insect neurons play demonstrable behavioral roles and are electrophysiologically accessible. In this section, we discuss how steroids alter neuronal phenotype in *Manduca* and how these effects relate to behavior.

Dendritic Remodeling

The most detailed understanding of how the steroid-mediated remodeling of neuronal structure alters neural circuit function has come from the proleg motor system of *Manduca*. Prolegs occur in pairs on abdominal segments three through six (identified as A3–A6 in figure 18.2) and on the terminal segment. Tactile stimulation of mechanosensory planta hairs (PHs) on the proleg tip evokes the proleg withdrawal reflex (PWR), which consists of ipsi- or bilateral retraction of the prolegs in that segment. The major features of the neural circuit for the ipsilateral PWR have been identified: the sensory neurons that innervate PHs excite proleg retractor motoneurons via monosynaptic, cholinergic connections and by polysynaptic pathways involving unidentified interneurons (reviewed in Weeks et al., 1997). The muscles that retract the proleg are innervated by motoneurons designated the principal planta retractors (PPRs) and the accessory planta retractors (APRs; see figure 18.2).

Both PPR and APR dendrites regress dramatically during the larval-pupal transformation in response to the prepupal peak of ecdysteroids (reviewed in Weeks et al., 1997). Dendritic regression, which is unaffected by muscle ablation or neural isolation of ganglia and can be blocked by protein synthesis inhibitors, may be a direct response to ecdysteroids. As the motoneurons regress, PWR behavior disappears. A series of experiments was performed to test the hypothesis that dendritic regression disconnects the motoneurons from excitatory

synaptic inputs that mediate the PWR. Intracellular recordings from PPR and APR motoneurons showed that the amplitude of the compound excitatory postsynaptic potential (cEPSP) evoked by stimulating the proleg sensory nerve decreases by more than 40% during the larval-pupal transformation (Jacobs and Weeks, 1990; Streichert and Weeks, 1995). This finding was consistent with the possibility that dendritic regression weakens the motoneurons' excitatory synaptic inputs; however, changes in sensory neurons or interneurons or both could also contribute to the diminished excitation. The contribution of changes in sensory neurons was tested by taking advantage of the ability in *Manduca* to selectively perturb subsets of neurons in a circuit by hormonal manipulations. In this case, a proleg was treated with JH during the commitment pulse to block the pupal commitment of the epidermal cells and PH sensory neurons (whose cell bodies lie in the epidermis); this treatment produced pupae that bore a larval proleg. In the heterochronic mosaic hemisegments, PH sensory neurons retained larval properties, but motoneuron regression appeared normal. Significantly, a similar reduction in cEPSP amplitude occurred during the larval-pupal transformation in both normal and mosaic pupal hemisegments. Thus, metamorphic changes in PH sensory neurons are *not necessary*, and metamorphic changes in central neurons (including motoneurons) are *sufficient*, for the developmental weakening of excitatory pathways in the PWR circuit (Jacobs and Weeks, 1990; Streichert and Weeks, 1995).

To further assess the effects of dendritic regression on synaptic inputs, we tested whether a decrease would occur in the amplitude of the *monosynaptic* EPSPs produced in proleg motoneurons by PH sensory neurons. While recording EPSPs in APR motoneurons, we stimulated individual PH sensory neurons in larvae and heterochronic mosaic pupae. EPSP amplitude decreased significantly during the larval-pupal transformation (Streichert and Weeks, 1995), suggesting that the PWR reflex disappears at pupation because dendritic regression of the motoneurons disconnects the sensory synapses and functionally disables the input pathway for the reflex.

These studies of the *Manduca* PWR are significant in establishing a direct electrophysiological link between a steroid effect on neuronal morphology and the function of a neural circuit subserving behavior. Steroid hormones produce simultaneous neuroanatomical and behavioral changes in many animals, but it is often difficult to test whether the relationship is causal or correlational. One advantage offered by the simpler nervous systems of insects is the ability to investigate steroid effects on CNS function at the level of synaptic connections between identified pre- and postsynaptic neurons.

Neuronal Respecification

One hallmark of neural plasticity during metamorphosis is the respecification of larval neurons for new functions in the pupal and adult stages. This phenomenon is illustrated by the metamorphic fates of proleg motoneurons (see figure 18.2). All of the PPRs, the APRs in segments A5 and A6, and their target muscles undergo programmed death after pupation in response to the prepupal peak of ecdysteroids. In contrast, the APRs in segments A3 and A4 grow new dendritic arbors in response to the ecdysteroid elevation during the pupal stage, are respecified for new functions, and then die after adult emergence. The new functions vary by segment. In segment A4, the APRs are respecified to innervate newly formed muscles, but in segment A3 they and their surviving target muscles participate in a new rhythmic motor pattern that circulates hemolymph in the wing of the developing adult moth (Lubischer et al., 1995). Here, we have a remarkable example of functional respecification: the APRs are transformed from proleg retractors to members of the circulatory motor system. Studies of the synaptic rearrangements that underlie respecification illustrate how steroid-regulated neuronal plasticity accommodates changing behavioral requirements throughout the life cycle.

Steroid-Regulated Programmed Cell Death

Manduca has been an ideal system in which to investigate steroid-regulated programmed cell death. Changes in ecdysteroid levels cause specific subsets of identified neurons and muscles to die during metamorphosis; various studies have elucidated the roles of ecdysteroid receptors and gene expression in these events (Schwartz, 1992; Truman et al., 1994). Unlike many vertebrate systems, cellular interactions play a lesser role in regulating cell death in *Manduca* (reviewed in Weeks and Levine, 1992). For example, the segment-specific death of APRs (see figure 18.2) is negligibly affected by perturbing the APRs' interactions with target muscles, sensory inputs, and interganglionic inputs (Weeks and Davidson, 1994; Lubischer and Weeks, 1996). The findings in these studies suggest that ecdysteroids may act directly on motoneurons to trigger death; consistent with this possibility, most *Manduca* motoneurons do exhibit ecdysteroid receptors during periods of cell death (Fahrbach 1992; Truman et al., 1994). The hypothesis that ecdysteroids

have a direct role in triggering APR death has recently been confirmed by the finding that APRs express the correct segment-specific pattern of death even after they are removed from the CNS and exposed to ecdysteroids in vitro (Streichert et al., 1997). The in vitro system should be useful for investigating steroid-mediated cell death and how segmental determinants regulate the genomic effects of steroid hormones. Interestingly, the APRs in segments A5 and A6 that die at pupation do so in response to a *rise* in ecdysteroids during the prepupal peak, whereas their homologs in segments A3 and A4 die in response to the *fall* in ecdysteroids at emergence (see figure 18.2). How these cell- and stage-specific responses to ecdysteroids are regulated at the molecular level remains to be determined.

Other Effects of Ecdysteroids

In addition to remodeling dendrites and triggering cell death, ecdysteroids also regulate neurogenesis, neuropeptide expression and sensitivity, and neuronal excitability. The postembryonic production of new neurons contributes to the increase in size and complexity of the CNS during metamorphosis, and both the proliferation and differentiation of new neurons are under endocrine control (Booker and Truman, 1987; reviewed in Levine et al., 1995). The respecification of neurons can include ecdysteroid-regulated changes in neuropeptide expression (Tublitz, 1993). Ecdysteroids also regulate the maturation of the biochemical machinery required for CNS sensitivity to the neuropeptide eclosion hormone (EH), which triggers ecdysis (cuticle-shedding) behavior at molts (Morton and Truman, 1988). Finally, Hewes and Truman (1994) have shown that the fall in ecdysteroids at the culmination of a molt increases the excitability of EH-containing neurons, thus priming them to release EH and trigger ecdysis at the appropriate time. This effect appears to operate through a genomic mechanism. In summary, steroids produce a range of phenotypic effects on insect neurons that parallel the effects seen in the vertebrate CNS.

Discussion

Value of a Multispecies Approach

For basic biological processes such as the hormonal regulation of behavior, a multispecies approach maximizes the chance that fundamental mechanisms will be identified, mainly because as yet we have no one optimal system for investigating steroid effects on neural circuits and behavior. The white rat is a favored species because of its long history as an experimental subject, and findings in this animal are likely to apply to other mammals. Insects are evolutionarily distant from vertebrates, but the commonality of steroid effects on neuronal properties in insects, rats, and other vertebrate species, in addition to the conservation of the steroid receptor gene family, suggest that some molecular mechanisms may be shared.

Although the gene and protein sequences for intracellular steroid receptors are conserved, a great deal of divergence and diversity is possible in the identity of the genes whose transcription is regulated by the receptors. Even for a given type of steroid receptor in a given animal on a given day, the specific pattern of gene expression that results from the hormone's presence will vary in a tissue- and cell-specific manner. Likewise, the gene products that are produced can be modified by a variety of mechanisms that vary from cell to cell. Nevertheless, recent studies have made rapid progress in identifying steroid-regulated neural genes in insects (reviewed by Levine et al., 1995), and probes derived from these studies may provide useful tools for identifying and cloning related genes in the vertebrate CNS (e.g., Carroll, 1995). At the present time, however, the primary basis for comparing hormone-regulated plasticity in vertebrates and invertebrates is at the cellular, not the molecular, level.

Comparison of Steroid Effects in Rats and Insects

Given the conservation of basic molecular and cellular processes among living organisms, similar mechanisms may underlie some of the forms of steroid-regulated plasticity in vertebrate and invertebrate nervous systems. In the next few paragraphs, we combine parallel findings in rats and insects and discuss the similarities and differences in what is known about underlying mechanisms as well as the value of in vitro versus in vivo approaches to answering key questions in the field.

Dendritic Remodeling

In *Manduca*, ecdysteroids regulate the regression and growth of neuronal dendrites and axon terminals in a cell- and stage-specific manner. In rats, estrogen induces excitatory spine synapses on hippocampal CA1 neurons and on VMN neurons, whereas progesterone causes these synapses to regress. Glucocorticoids cause dendritic regression in hippocampal CA3 neurons, and androgens regulate the dendritic extent of SNB motoneurons. The steroids' site of action in inducing these changes and the

underlying cytoskeletal rearrangements are currently active areas of investigation.

Two important research issues are the autonomy of the changes to the cell types in which they occur and the extent to which changes can be modeled in cell culture. Cell culture studies in *Manduca* suggest that ecdysteroids act directly on motoneurons via intracellular ecdysteroid receptors to induce dendritic growth during adult development (Prugh et al., 1992). The steroid-mediated growth results from enhanced branch formation at growth cones (Matheson et al., 1995; reviewed in Levine and Weeks, 1996). In vitro studies of dendritic regression in *Manduca* neurons have not yet been performed. Estrogen appears to have an indirect effect on hippocampal CA1 neurons in the rat; the CA1 neurons lack estrogen receptors, and the growth of dendritic spines appears to depend on input from interneurons, entorhinal input, or both via a use-dependent mechanism that involves NMDA receptors (Woolley and McEwen, 1994). Studies indicate that cultured hippocampal neurons respond to estrogens by increasing tau protein levels (Ferreira and Caceres, 1991) and that there is a several-fold NMDA receptor dependent stimulation by estradiol of synaptogenesis in culture (Collin et al., 1995). However, it is unclear how relatively unspecialized embryonic hippocampal cells in culture may model the specific synapse induction seen on dendritic spines in CA1 neurons of the mature hippocampus. The androgenic regulation of SNB motoneuron dendritic extent also appears to be mediated indirectly via the target muscle (Rand and Breedlove, 1995). Finally, glucocorticoid- and stress-induced atrophy of hippocampal neurons involves asymmetric changes in CA3 neurons that point to an important role for a transsynaptic mediation via excitatory amino acids and mossy fiber input; only the apical dendritic atrophy can be blocked by NMDA receptor antagonists (Magarinos and McEwen, 1995). It is difficult to imagine how to model this atrophy in embryonic hippocampal neurons in culture.

Although the above examples give the impression that steroids alter dendritic morphology through direct effects in *Manduca* and indirect effects in rats, counterexamples do exist. Cellular interactions influence the shape of the dendritic arbors elaborated by *Manduca* motoneurons in response to ecdysteroids in vivo (Kent and Levine, 1993), and afferent innervation is essential for the dendritic organization of olfactory glomeruli during metamorphosis (Hildebrand, 1985). In vertebrates, there are examples of direct steroid actions on neurite outgrowth in embryonic hippocampal neurons (Ferreira and Caceres, 1991; Brinton, 1994). The estrogenic induction of new synapses in the hypothalamus of adult female rats may also represent a direct action of steroids on the neurons that produce the synapses (McEwen et al., 1987).

To what extent can we link steroid-mediated changes in dendritic structure to behavioral alterations? In rats, some studies show differences in spatial learning or seizure threshold correlated with gonadal or adrenal steroid effects on the hippocampus, but the extent to which these structural changes *cause* the functional changes remains unexplored. In the female rat hypothalamus, it is highly likely that increased synaptic density contributes to the enhanced lordosis response. However, in both cases other cellular actions of estrogens undoubtedly contribute to the altered function. In *Manduca*, electrophysiological techniques do show that steroid-mediated changes in neuronal arbors alter the function of neural circuits and thereby alter behavior. Hopefully, electrophysiological and behavioral approaches will increasingly be applied to vertebrates to help us better understand the functional consequences of neuroanatomical effects of steroids.

Neuronal Death

In vitro studies suggest that the programmed cell death of proleg motoneurons in *Manduca* results from a direct action of ecdysteroids and does not require cellular interactions (Streichert et al., 1997). Studies of the death of other *Manduca* motoneurons during metamorphosis are consistent with a direct steroid action (discussed in Weeks and Levine, 1992); in at least one case, however, the ecdysteroid-regulated death of an identified motoneuron is modulated by descending neural input (Fahrbach and Truman, 1987). The death of granule neurons of the dentate gyrus may involve a mechanism similar to the one found in *Manduca* (Gould and McEwen, 1993), although more information is needed to evaluate this possibility. In contrast, the glucocorticoid-induced necrosis of hippocampal pyramidal neurons involves excitatory amino acid neurotoxicity (Sapolsky, 1992). That is, glucocorticoids do not kill hippocampal neurons outright but rather establish a state of "vulnerability" that makes the neurons more susceptible to other insults involving excitatory amino acids, which can kill neurons via NMDA receptors and free radicals. Cultured hippocampal neurons have been used successfully to model the synergism between glucocorticoids and excitatory amino acids in causing cell death (Packan and Sapolsky, 1990). Presently, no analogous mechanism has been identified in the insect CNS.

Excitability and Neuropeptide Expression

Orchinik and McEwen (1995) review many examples that show how steroids regulate neuropeptide gene expression as well as neuronal excitability in the vertebrate CNS. Parallel results have been seen in insects, although the number of examples is smaller. We still do not know, however, whether the non-genomic effects of steroids on neuronal excitability in vertebrates have parallels in insects.

Relationship between Life Cycle and Steroid-Mediated Plasticity

In insects, the steroid-regulated remodeling of the nervous system is linked primarily to the developmental transitions of metamorphosis. After metamorphosis is complete, however, steroid-regulated plasticity in adults is difficult to study because the ecdysteroid-secreting glands typically degenerate early in adult life. Thus, rats and insects share extensive steroid-mediated neural plasticity during the *postembryonic* period, but the striking effects of steroids on the *adult* rat CNS lack parallels in *Manduca*. Interestingly, however, JH often reappears as an important regulator of physiology and behavior in adult insects. Adult female honeybees, for instance, progress through a series of behavioral roles in the colony that are regulated by JH levels. The behavioral transitions are associated with JH-regulated changes in brain structure (Fahrbach and Robinson, 1995) in much the same way as ecdysteroids regulate neural circuits and behavior in the larval and pupal stages. Thus, in both rodents and insects, hormones play key roles in the construction, expression, and modulation of the neural circuits that subserve behavior.

Acknowledgments

Research in the Weeks laboratory is supported by NIH grants R01 NS23208 and K04 NS01473, and by an NSF Presidential Young Investigator Award. Research in the McEwen laboratory is supported by NS07080 and MH41256.

References

Baker FC, Tsai LW, Reuter CC, Schooley DA (1987) In vivo fluctuation of JH, JH acid, ecdysteroid titer, and JH esterase activity during the development of fifth stadium *Manduca sexta. Insect Biochem* 17:989–996.

Becker J, Breedlove SM, Crews D (1992) *Behavioral Endocrinology*. Cambridge, Mass.: MIT Press.

Booker R, Truman JW (1987) Postembryonic neurogenesis in the CNS of the tobacco hornworm, *Manduca sexta*. II. Hormonal control of imaginal nest cell degeneration and differentiation during metamorphosis. *J Neurosci* 7:4107–4114.

Breedlove SM, Arnold AP (1980) Hormone accumulation in a sexually dimorphic motor nucleus of the rat spinal cord. *Science* 210:564–566.

Brinton RD (1994) The neurosteroid 3-α-hydroxy-5α-pregnan-20-one induces cytoarchitectural regression in cultured fetal hippocampal neurons. *J Neurosci* 14:2763–2774.

Cameron HA, Gould E (1996) The control of neuronal birth and death. In: *Receptor Dynamics in Neural Development* (Shaw C, ed.), 141–157. Boca Raton, Fla.: CRC.

Cameron HA, McEwen BS, Gould E (1995) Regulation of adult neurogenesis by excitatory input and NMDA receptor activation in the dentate gyrus. *J Neurosci* 15:4687–4692.

Carroll S (1995) Homeotic genes and the evolution of arthropods and chordates. *Nature* (London) 376:479–485.

Collin C, Miyaguchi K, Segal M (1995) Dendritic spines in hippocampal neurons: Correlating structure and function. *Soc Neurosci Abstr* 21:1811.

DeLeon M, Golomb J, George AE, Convit A, Tarshish CY, McRae T, DeSanti S, Smith G, Ferris SH, Noz M, Rusinek H (1993) The radiologic prediction of Alzheimer's Disease: The atrophic hippocampal formation. *Am J Neuroradiol* 14:897–906.

DeVries GJ (1995) Studying neurotransmitter systems to understand the development and function of sex differences in the brain: The case of vasopressin. In: *Neurobiological Effects of Sex Steroid Hormones* (Micevych PE, Hammer RP Jr, eds.), 254–280. New York: Cambridge University Press.

Diamond DM, Bennett MC, Fleshner M, Rose GM (1992) Inverted-U relationship between the level of peripheral corticosterone and the magnitude of hippocampal primed burst potentiation. *Hippocampus* 2:421–430.

Fahrbach SE (1992) Developmental regulation of ecdysteroid receptors in the nervous system of *Manduca sexta*. *J Exp Zool* 261:245–253.

Fahrbach SE, Robinson GE (1995) Behavioral development in the honey bee: Toward the study of learning under natural conditions. *Learning and Memory* 2:199–224.

Fahrbach SE, Truman JW (1987) Possible interactions of a steroid hormone and neural inputs in controlling the death of an identified neuron in the moth, *Manduca sexta*. *J Neurobiol* 18:497–508.

Ferreira A, Caceres A (1991) Estrogen-enhanced neurite growth: Evidence for a selective induction of tau and stable microtubules. *J Neurosci* 11:392–400.

Flanagan LM, McEwen BS (1995) Ovarian steroid interactions with hypothalamic oxytocin circuits involved in reproductive behavior. In: *Neurobiological Effects of Sex Steroid* Hormones (Micevych P, Hammer RP, Jr, eds.), 117–142. New York: Cambridge University Press.

Forger NG, Breedlove SM (1991) Steroid influences on a mammalian neuromuscular system. *Semin Neurosci* 3:459–468.

Frankfurt M, Gould E, Woolley C, McEwen BS (1990) Gonadal steroids modify dendritic spine density in ventromedial hypothalamic neurons: A Golgi study in the adult rat. *Neuroendocrinology* 51:530–535.

Freidin M, Pfaff D (1995) Molecular actions of steroid hormones and their possible relations to reproductive behaviors. In: *Neurobiological Effects of Sex Steroid Hormones* (Micevych P, Hammer RP, Jr, eds.), 350–362. New York: Cambridge University Press.

Getting PA (1989) Emerging principles governing the operation of neural networks. *Ann Rev Neurosci* 12:185–204.

Gould E, McEwen BS (1993) Neuronal birth and death. *Curr Opin Neurobiol* 3:676–682.

Handa RJ, Burgess LH, Keer JE, O'Keefe JA (1994) Gonadal steroid hormone receptors and sex differences in the hypothalamo-pituitary-adrenal axis. *Horm Behavior* 28:464–476.

Hewes RS, Truman JW (1994) Steroid regulation of excitability in identified insect neurosecretory cells. *J Neurosci* 14:1812–1819.

Hildebrand JG (1985) Metamorphosis of the insect nervous system: Influences of the periphery on the postembryonic development of the antennal sensory pathway in the brain of the moth, *Manduca sexta*. In: *Model Neural Networks and Behavior* (Selverston AI, ed.), 129–148. New York: Plenum.

Insel TR, Wang ZX, Ferris CF (1994) Patterns of brain vasopressin receptor distribution associated with social organization in microtine rodents. *J Neurosci* 14:5381–5392.

Jacobs GA, Weeks JC (1990) Postsynaptic changes at a sensory-to-motoneuron synapse contribute to the developmental loss of a reflex behavior during insect metamorphosis. *J Neurosci* 10:1341–1356.

Kent KS, Levine RB (1993) Dendritic reorganization of an identified neuron during metamorphosis of the moth *Manduca sexta*: The influence of interactions with the periphery. *J Neurobiol* 24:1–22.

Koelle MR, Talbot WS, Segraves WA, Bender WA, Cherbas P, Hogness DS (1991) The *Drosophila EcR* gene encodes an ecdysone receptor, a new member of the steroid receptor superfamily. *Cell* 67:59–78.

Koob GF, Heinrichs SC, Menzaghi F, Pich EM, Britton KT (1994) Corticotropin releasing factor, stress, and behavior. *The Neurosciences* 6:221–229.

Kow LM, Mobbs CV, Pfaff DW (1994) Roles of second-messenger systems and neuronal activity in the regulation of lordosis by neurotransmitters, neuropeptides, and estrogen: A review. *Neurosci Biobehav Rev* 18:251–268.

Kurz EM, Sengelaub DR, Arnold AP (1986) Androgens regulate the dendritic length of mammalian motoneurons in adulthood. *Science* 232:395–398.

Levine RB, Morton DB, Restifo LL (1995) Remodeling of the insect nervous system. *Curr Opin Neurobiol* 5:28–35.

Levine RB, Weeks JC (1996) Cell culture approaches to understanding the actions of steroid hormones on the insect nervous system. *Devel Neurosci* 18:73–86.

Lewis C, McEwen BS, Frankfurt M (1995) Estrogen-induction of dendritic spines in ventromedial hypothalamus and hippocampus: Effects of neonatal aromatase blockade and adult GDX. *Devel Brain Res* 87:91–95.

Steroid Modulation of Neural Circuits

Lubischer JL, Verhegge L, Weeks JC (1995) Evidence that larval *Manduca* proleg muscles are respecified for hemolymph circulation in pupae. *Soc Neurosci Abstr* 21:426.

Lubischer JL, Weeks JC (1996) Target muscles and sensory afferents do not influence steroid-regulated, segment-specific death of identified motoneurons in *Manduca sexta*. J Neurobiol 31:449–460.

Magarinos AM, McEwen BS (1995) Stress-induced atrophy of apical dendrites of hippocampal CA3c neurons: Involvement of glucocorticoid secretion and excitatory amino acid receptors. *Neuroscience* 69:89–98.

Matheson SF, Della Croce K, Levine RB (1995) Steroid-enhanced neurite outgrowth in insect motoneurons involves higher-order branching and increased growth cone complexity. *Soc Neurosci Abstr* 21:1773.

Matsumoto A, Arai Y (1986) Male-female difference in synaptic organization of the ventromedial nucleus of the hypothalamus in the rat. *Neuroendocrinology* 42:232–236.

McCarthy MM, Masters DB, Rimvall K, Schwartz-Giblin S, Pfaff D (1994) Intracerebral administration of antisense oligodeoxynucleotides to GAD_{65} and GAD_{67} mRNAs modulate reproductive behavior in the female rat. *Brain Res* 636:209–220.

McEwen BS (1991a) Non-genomic and genomic effects of steroids on neural activity. *Trends Pharm Sci* 112:141–147.

McEwen BS (1991b) Our changing ideas about steroid effects on an ever-changing brain. *Semin Neurosci* 3:497–507.

McEwen BS, Albeck D, Cameron H, Chao HM, Gould E, Hastings N, Kuroda Y, Luine VN, Magarinos A-M, McKittrick CM, Orchinik M, Pavlides C, Vaher P, Watanabe Y, Weiland N (1995a) Stress and the brain: A paradoxical role for adrenal steroids. *Vitamins and Hormones* 51:371–402.

McEwen BS, Gould E, Orchinik M, Weiland NG, Woolley CS (1995b) Oestrogens and the structural and functional plasticity of neurons: Implications for memory, ageing and neurodegenerative processes. In: *Ciba Foundation Symposium*, no. 191: *The Non-Reproductive Actions of Sex Steroids* (Bock G, Goode J, eds.), 52–73. New York: J. Wiley.

McEwen BS, Jones K, Pfaff DW (1987) Hormonal control of sexual behavior in the female rat: Molecular, cellular, and neurochemical studies. *Biol Reprod* 36:37–45.

McEwen BS, Sapolsky RM (1995) Stress and cognitive function. *Curr Opin Neurobiol* 5:205–216.

Meaney MJ, Tannenbaum B, Francis D, Bhatnagar S, Shanks N, Viau V, O'Donnell D, Plotsky PM (1994) Early environmental programming hypothalamic-pituitary-adrenal responses to stress. *Semin Neurosci* 6:247–249.

Meyrand P, Simmers J, Moulins M (1994) Dynamic construction of a neural network from multiple pattern generators in the lobster stomatogastric nervous system. *J Neurosci* 14:630–644.

Miller MA, DeVries GJ, Al-Shamma HA, Dorsa DM (1992) Decline of vasopressin immunoreactivity and mRNA levels in the bed nucleus of the stria terminalis following castration. *J Neurosci* 12:2881–2887.

Morton DB, Truman JW (1988) The EGPs: The eclosion hormone and cyclic GMP-regulated phosphoproteins. II. Regulation of appearance by the steroid hormone 20-hydroxyecdysone in *Manduca sexta*. *J Neurosci* 8:1338–1345.

Nordeen EJ, Nordeen KW, Sengelaub DR, Arnold AP (1985) Androgens prevent normally occurring cell death in a sexually dimorphic spinal nucleus. *Science* 229:671–673.

Orchinik M, McEwen B (1995) Rapid steroid actions in the brain: A critique of genomic and nongenomic mechanisms. In: *Genomic and Nongenomic Effects of Aldosterone* (Wehling M, ed.), 77–108. Boca Raton, Fla.: CRC.

Packan DR, Sapolsky RM (1990) Glucocorticoid endangerment of the hippocampus: Tissue, steroid, and receptor specificity. *Neuroendocrinology* 51:613–618.

Parsons B, MacLusky N, Krey LC, Pfaff DW, McEwen BS (1980) The temporal relationship between estrogen-inducible progestin receptors in the female rat brain and the time course of estrogen activation of mating behavior. *Endocrinology* 107:774–779.

Pfaff DW (1980) *Estrogens and Brain Function*. New York: Springer.

Prugh J, Della Croce K, Levine RB (1992) Effects of the steroid hormone, 20-hydroxyecdysone, on the growth of neurites by identified insect motoneurons in vitro. *Devel Biol* 154:331–347.

Rand MN, Breedlove SM (1995) Androgen alters the dendritic arbors of SNB motoneurons by acting upon their target muscles. *J Neurosci* 15:4408–4416.

Riddiford LM, Truman JW (1994) Hormone receptors and the orchestration of development during insect metamorphosis. In: *Perspectives in Comparative Endocrinology* (Davey KG, Peter RE, Tobe SS, eds.), 389–394. Ottawa: National Research Council of Canada.

Sapolsky RM (1992) *Stress, the Aging Brain, and the Mechanisms of Neuron Death*. Cambridge, Mass.: MIT Press.

Schumacher M, Coirini H, Flanagan L, Frankfurt M, Pfaff D, McEwen BS (1992) Ovarian steroid modulation of oxytocin receptor binding in the ventromedial hypothalamus. In: *Oxytocin in Maternal, Sexual, and Social Behaviors*. (Pedersen C, Caldwell J, Jirikowski G, Insel T, eds.) *Ann New York Acad Science* 652:374–386.

Schumacher M, Coirini H, McEwen BS (1989) Regulation of GABAa receptors in specific brain regions by ovarian hormones. *Neuroendocrinology* 50:315–320.

Schwartz LM (1992) Insect muscle as a model for programmed cell death. *J Neurobiol* 23:1312–1326.

Sherry DF, Jacobs LF, Gaulin SJC (1992) Spatial memory and adaptive specialization of the hippocampus. *Trends Neurosci* 15:298–303.

Streichert LC, Pierce JT, Nelson JA, Weeks JC (1997) Steroid hormones act directly to trigger segment-specific programmed cell death of identified motoneurons in vitro. *Devel Biol* 183:95–107.

Streichert LC, Weeks JC (1995) Decreased monosynaptic input to an identified motoneuron is associated with steroid-mediated dendritic regression during metamorphosis in *Manduca sexta*. *J Neurosci* 15:1484–1495.

Terasawa E, Timiras P (1968) Electrical activity during the estrous cycle of the rat: Cyclic changes in limbic structures. *Endocrinology* 83:207–216.

Truman JW, Schwartz LM (1984) Steroid regulation of neuronal death in the moth nervous system. *J Neurosci* 4:274–280.

Truman JW, Talbot WS, Fahrbach SE, Hogness DS (1994) Ecdysone receptor expression in the CNS correlates with stage-specific responses to ecdysteroids during *Drosophila* and *Manduca* development. *Development* 120:219–234.

Tublitz NJ (1993) Steroid-induced neurotransmitter plasticity in insect peptidergic neurons. *Comp Biochem Physiol* 105C:147–154.

Weeks JC, Davidson SK (1994) Influence of interganglionic interactions on steroid-mediated dendritic reorganization and death of proleg motor neurons during metamorphosis in *Manduca sexta*. *J Neurobiol* 25:535–554.

Weeks JC, Jacobs GA, Pierce JT, Sandstrom DJ, Streichert LC, Trimmer BA, Wiel DE, Wood ER (1997) Neural mechanisms of behavioral plasticity: Metamorphosis and learning in *Manduca sexta*. *Brain Behav Evolution*, in press.

Weeks JC, Levine RB (1992) Endocrine influences on the postembryonic fates of identified neurons during insect metamorphosis. In: *Determinants of Neuronal Identity* (Shankland M, Macagno E, eds.), 293–322. San Diego: Academic.

Weeks JC, Levine RB (1995) Steroid hormone effects on neurons subserving behavior. *Curr Opin Neurobiol* 5:809–815.

Winslow JT, Hastings N, Carter CS, Harbaugh CR, Insel TR (1993) A role for central vasopressin in pair bonding in monogamous prairie voles. *Nature* 365:545–548.

Woolley C, McEwen BS (1994) Estradiol regulates hippocampal dendritic spine density via an N-methyl-D-aspartate receptor dependent mechanism. *J Neurosci* 14:7680–7687.

19

Chemical Modulation of Crustacean Stomatogastric Pattern Generator Networks

Ronald M. Harris-Warrick,
Deborah J. Baro, Lisa M. Coniglio,
Bruce R. Johnson, Robert M.
Levini, Jack H. Peck, and
Bing Zhang

Abstract

The neural networks for simple rhythmic behaviors are targets of multiple modulatory inputs. Slow-acting neurotransmitters such as amines and peptides serve as neuromodulators to reconfigure the networks and alter the behaviors they control. A number of different cellular and ionic mechanisms control the number of active neurons, the cycle frequency, firing intensity, and phasing of neuronal activity. In addition, neuromodulators regulate the interactions between different networks. The networks in the crustacean stomatogastric ganglion are described as examples of these general principles of network reconfiguration.

A major advance in our understanding of motor pattern generation over the past decade has come from the realization that a single, anatomically defined neural network can generate a variety of related motor patterns. Neuromodulators can reconfigure a neural network to generate different functional circuits, each of which controls a variant of the basic behavior (Getting, 1989). In this chapter, we discuss how network reconfiguration actually occurs—a subject extensively studied in the motor networks of the crustacean stomatogastric ganglion (STG) that generates rhythmic foregut movements during feeding; most of our examples will be taken from this system (see also Selverston et al., chapter 10; Marder et al., chapter 13; Nusbaum et al., chapter 22; this volume). Many important principles on this topic have also been generated from study of the *Aplysia* feeding system, with particular emphasis on reconfiguration at the periphery (Kupfermann et al., chapter 20, this volume).

Multiple Modulatory Inputs to Behavioral Networks

Each behaviorally relevant network receives a variety of different modulatory inputs. In the STG of different crustacea, for example, immunohistochemical and biochemical analyses have shown that at least 19 transmitters, amines, and peptides are present in inputs to the ganglion. In addition, at least 18 circulating neurohormones have access to its motor networks, acting at very low concentrations to activate or modulate network function (Harris-Warrick et al., 1992; Marder et al., 1994).

In the STG, all modulatory synapses come from neurons extrinsic to the motor networks; within the motor networks, all the synapses use rapid transmitter actions (Harris-Warrick et al., 1992). In other systems, however, neurons within the pattern-generating network can use both neuromodulators and rapid neurotransmitters, a mechanism termed *intrinsic neuromodulation*. In the *Tritonia* swim network, for example, a network neuron uses serotonin as a fast transmitter and as a neuromodulator that alters the strength of synapses within the network, thus allowing the swimming behavior to be expressed by this multifunctional network (Katz and Frost, 1996; see also Frost et al., chapter 16, this volume; Kupfermann et al., chapter 20, this volume).

Modulatory neurons almost always release multiple chemical substances, a process called *co-transmission*. Co-transmission has been examined in greatest detail in the motoneurons that innervate the *Aplysia* feeding muscles (Kupfermann et al., chapter 20, this volume). Nearly all the identified modulatory neurons innervating the STG use multiple transmitters (Katz and Harris-Warrick, 1990). Co-transmission allows increased flexibility in the activity of modulatory neurons. Most modulatory neurons release both a rapid transmitter and one or more neuromodulators; the combined activity of these co-transmitters can generate a response that may be difficult for either co-transmitter to evoke alone. For example, in the crab, the sensory/modulatory GPR neurons use both serotonin and acetylcholine to evoke plateau potentials in a gastric mill motoneuron because neither transmitter alone could typically do so (Katz and Harris-Warrick, 1989). In other neurons, the co-transmitters are not always released at a constant ratio, but can vary as a function of the spike frequency and the previous history of activity in the neuron (Kupfermann et al., chapter 20, this volume). Over the long term (e.g., during development), changes in gene expression can alter the neuron's co-transmitter complement (Beltz and Kravitz, 1987), which may allow a single neuron to subserve different roles at different times.

Modulation of Ongoing Pattern-Generating Network Activity

Many modulatory neurons or neuromodulators are capable of activating a motor pattern in the quiescent STG under the appropriate experimental conditions; most likely, however, their major role is to modify the proper-

ties of an ongoing motor pattern. Nagy and Cardi (1994) recently identified a set of neurons in the commissural ganglion that appear to drive the normal pyloric motor pattern in *H. gammarus*. Depolarization to activate these P and CP cells immediately turns on the pyloric rhythm; hyperpolarization to abolish P and CP activity turns off the pyloric rhythm. These neurons serve as modulators to evoke oscillatory properties in all the pyloric neurons. The authors suggest that P and CP activity evoke a "baseline" pyloric rhythm upon which other neuromodulators act. A cholecystokinin-like peptide, acting as a hormone, may play a similar enabling role for the gastric mill rhythm (Turrigiano and Selverston, 1990).

A number of network parameters have been shown to be the targets of modulatory action:

Control of Number of Active Neurons

Although an anatomically defined neural network has a fixed number of neurons, not all of them are active for each motor pattern variant. Neuromodulators can selectively excite or inhibit neurons to determine which subcircuit will be functional at any time. Experiments on synaptically isolated neurons in the STG have shown that, in most cases, many or all of the network neurons are direct targets of modulator action (Harris-Warrick et al., 1992).

Control of Cycle Frequency

The pyloric and gastric mill networks in the STG can oscillate over a wide range of frequencies in the presence of different neuromodulators or during stimulation of identified modulatory neurons. Several different mechanisms can cause changes in cycle frequency.

First, the major pacemaker neurons can be induced to oscillate at different frequencies. For example, the AB interneuron is the major pacemaker for the pyloric network; its oscillation frequency differs depending upon the particular neuromodulator (such as dopamine, serotonin, or octopamine) that is present. Each amine acts by a different ionic mechanism to induce AB bursting with different characteristics (Harris-Warrick and Flamm, 1987). As a result, the pyloric rhythm oscillates at different frequencies in the presence of these modulators.

Second, neuromodulators can change which neurons act as the major pacemakers, thus also changing the frequency of the motor pattern. For example, in the gastric mill rhythm, a subset of neurons becomes the pacemaker "kernel" in the presence of muscarinic agonists (Elson and Selverston, 1992). Similarly, in *H. gammarus*, muscarinic agonists can excite the IC neuron so that it be-

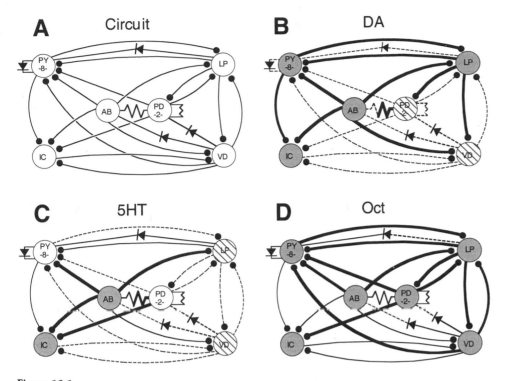

Figure 19.1

Effects of dopamine, serotonin and octopamine on synaptic efficacy within the pyloric network. (A) Wiring diagram of the known pyloric synapses without indication of the relative strengths of the synapses. Filled circles: chemical inhibitory synapses. Resistors: non-rectifying electrical synapses. Diode symbols: rectifying electrical synapses, with preferred direction of positive current indicated. Effects of (B) dopamine (DA), (C) serotonin (5-HT), and (D) octopamine (Oct) on graded synaptic strength. Thickened and dashed connections: enhancement and weakening of synaptic strength, respectively. Shaded cells: excited by the amine. Lined cells: inhibited by the amine. (Modified from Johnson et al., 1995.)

comes a major component of the pyloric pacemaker; under normal conditions, it is not (Bal et al., 1994).

Third, rhythmically active modulatory inputs can constrain the STG networks to fire with them. In *H. gammarus*, the "enabling" P and CP neurons usually fire with constant frequency. In some situations, however, they fire in bursts, causing the excited pyloric motor pattern to cycle with various fixed harmonics of the P/CP frequency (e.g., 1:1, 1:2, etc.). Under these conditions, the pyloric rhythm cannot oscillate at smoothly graded frequencies but jumps between fixed harmonics of the P/CP frequency (Nagy and Cardi, 1994).

Finally, non-pacemaker neurons can play important roles in determining the network cycle frequency. For example, the pacemaker AB neuron is electrically coupled to the PD neurons in the pyloric network. Dopamine excites the isolated AB neuron and increases its cycle frequency (Flamm and Harris-Warrick, 1986). However, in intact preparations, dopamine slightly decreases the pyloric cycle frequency (Harris-Warrick et al., 1995a) because it also inhibits and hyperpolarizes the electrically coupled PD neurons, which act as an electrical sink to reduce the AB oscillation frequency (Marder et al., 1992).

Control of Firing Intensity

A number of neuromodulators simply depolarize isolated STG neurons, increasing their spike frequency as a result. Other, more subtle changes in neurons can alter their firing frequency, however. For example, a number of neuromodulators evoke bistable plateau potentials in gastric mill neurons (Nagy et al., 1988; Elson and Selverston, 1992; Kiehn and Harris-Warrick, 1992a, 1992b). The spike frequency of the neuron is much higher when firing is due to plateau properties than when it is synaptically driven (Nagy et al., 1988). Some neuromodulators also enhance postinhibitory rebound, which can result in increased firing frequency after inhibition (Harris-Warrick et al., 1995a, 1995b).

Control of Phasing

The phase during which a neuron fires in a rhythmic motor pattern is critical for shaping the behavior. A number of mechanisms for neuromodulatory control of phasing have been demonstrated in STG motor networks.

First, changes in the synaptic interactions between network neurons can alter their phasing. Johnson and colleagues (1990, 1993a, 1993b, 1995) have determined what effects the amines dopamine, serotonin, and octop-amine have on the strength of all of the synapses in the pyloric network (figure 19.1). These amines quanti-tatively reconfigure the pyloric wiring diagram by strengthening or weakening selected synapses, silencing previously active synapses, activating previously silent synapses, and even reversing the net sign of synaptic interaction at mixed electrical/chemical synapses. These changes contribute to altering the timing of neuronal activity in the rhythm.

Altering the intrinsic electrophysiological responses of the network neurons to synaptic input can also control phasing. In the gastric mill network, the LG motoneuron normally fires in a composite discharge with an initial endogenous plateau potential followed by delayed syn-aptic drive from another neuron. A modulatory neuron, APM, radically alters the phasing of activity of the LG neuron by suppressing LG's plateau potential capability so that it fires only at a later phase upon CG synaptic drive (Nagy et al., 1988). In the pyloric network, dop-amine advances the phase of the LP and PY neurons by enhancing the rate and extent of postinhibitory rebound following synaptic inhibition (see below).

Fusion of Previously Independent Networks to Produce Novel Motor Patterns

Until recently, the various neural networks in the stoma-togastric nervous system (STNS) were studied indepen-dently of one another. However, it has now been shown that modulatory inputs can enhance the interactions be-tween these networks to generate new motor patterns. Dickinson (1995) has thoroughly reviewed this subject, so we will only briefly summarize it here. Two levels of interactions have been documented in the STNS.

First, neurons can switch their "allegiance" from one motor pattern to another. For example, when the slow cardiac sac rhythm is active in *P. vulgaris*, the pyloric network VD motoneuron fires in phase with the cardiac sac rhythm due to the loss of bursting properties and strong synaptic drive from a cardiac sac interneuron (Hooper and Moulins, 1989). Similarly, the peptide red pigment–concentrating hormone (RPCH) causes the gastric mill motoneuron AM to fire exclusively with the cardiac sac rhythm (Dickinson and Marder, 1989). In the crab, *Cancer borealis*, most neurons in the pyloric and gastric mill networks can switch to fire in rhythm with either network in the presence of peptides (Weimann et al., 1991) or after stimulation of a serotonergic sensory neuron (Katz and Harris-Warrick, 1991).

Second, two or more pattern generators can merge to produce a novel "conjoint" motor pattern. In *P. inter-ruptus*, RPCH can promote fusion of the gastric mill and cardiac sac pattern generators so that all neurons of both generators are active in a novel motor pattern whose period and phase relations are not similar to those of either parent network (Dickinson et al., 1990). An important mechanism for this fusion is a very strong enhancement of normally weak synaptic interactions between the pattern generators. Stimulation of a single neuron, PS, evokes a wholesale abolition of the oeso-phageal, pyloric, and gastric mill networks and a re-configuration of their neurons to generate a new motor pattern that may underlie rhythmic swallowing. PS acti-vation evokes modulatory actions that alter plateau or bursting properties as well as sustained depolarizations; in addition, it evokes rapid excitatory postsynaptic potentials (EPSPs) that drive follower neurons to fire in phase with it (Meyrand et al., 1991, 1994).

Ionic Mechanisms of Neuromodulation in the STG

For several cases, the ionic mechanisms underlying modulation of the intrinsic properties of STG neurons have been elucidated, possibly offering general solutions to problems that are also faced in other systems.

Dopamine Modulation of Phasing and Post-inhibitory Rebound in the Pyloric Motor Pattern

In the pyloric rhythm, the LP and PY neurons are rhyth-mically inhibited by the pacemaker AB/PD neurons; they then undergo marked postinhibitory rebound to resume firing. Dopamine excites these neurons and causes them to rebound more rapidly and to fire at an earlier phase in the rhythm. Part of this effect is due to loss of synaptic inhibition from the pacemaker PD neurons, which are hyperpolarized by dopamine (Eisen and Marder, 1984; Flamm and Harris-Warrick, 1986) and their synaptic out-put completely eliminated (Johnson and Harris-Warrick, 1990). In addition, dopamine acts directly on isolated LP and PY neurons to enhance their rate of repolarization following inhibition (Harris-Warrick et al., 1995a, 1995b). In both neurons, dopamine reduces the transient potas-sium current, I_A, which is responsible for a transient delaying current during the repolarization following synaptic inhibition: dopamine reduces I_A's maximal con-ductance and shifts its voltage dependence for activation and inactivation to more depolarized values. In the LP, dopamine also enhances the slow hyperpolarization–

activated inward current, I_h, by shifting its voltage dependence into the physiologically relevant voltage range and by increasing its rate of activation. We used the dynamic clamp method developed by Sharp and colleagues (1993) to simulate I_h in the LP cell. Our experiments showed that modulation of I_h alone accounted for about only 20% of the effect of dopamine, whereas reducing I_A accounted for more than 70% of dopamine's effect (Harris-Warrick et al., 1995b). Dopamine also markedly increases spike frequency in the LP and PY neurons. Experimental and modeling studies show that this effect also appears to be due to I_A reduction and I_h enhancement. Thus, modulation of small subthreshold ionic currents can lead to marked changes in phasing of activity in a cyclic motor pattern.

Serotonergic Induction of Plateau Potential Capability in the Dorsal Gastric Motoneuron

Stimulation of the serotonergic/cholinergic GPR cells, or a brief puff of serotonin, can evoke plateau potentials in a quiescent dorsal gastric (DG) neuron. Following a brief depolarization, the neuron remains depolarized for many seconds and spikes tonically at high frequency. To evoke the neuron's capability of firing a plateau, serotonin modulates a large number of different ionic currents in the DG neuron (Kiehn and Harris-Warrick, 1992b; Zhang et al., 1995a, 1995b). Following a period of inhibition, I_h is enhanced to help initiate the plateau and to maintain depolarization during the initial period. A voltage-dependent calcium current (I_{Ca}) is also enhanced to help depolarize the cell and to provide intracellular calcium that will activate other currents. As an indirect consequence of I_{Ca} enhancement, a calcium-activated neutral current, I_{CAN}, is also enhanced; I_{CAN} is a slow and noninactivating inward current that is relatively nonselective for cations and is activated purely by increases in intracellular Ca^{2+} (Partridge and Swandulla, 1988). It appears to be the major current maintaining the DG neuron plateau for most of its duration. The maximal conductance of a calcium-activated outward current is reduced, as is an additional calcium-independent K^+ current. All of these ionic mechanisms change the resting conductance to an equilibrium above threshold for spike initiation, thus sustaining the plateau. Induction of plateau potential capability is clearly a very complex, multiconductance process.

Enhancement of Tonic Spike Activity by Proctolin

Proctolin activates the pyloric motor pattern in a state-dependent fashion; its maximal effects occur when the pyloric rhythm is weak or quiescent (Nusbaum and Marder, 1989). Proctolin evokes a slow depolarization accompanied by an increase in spike frequency in the LP neuron. To do this, proctolin activates an inward current that is carried primarily by sodium, is blocked by extracellular Ca^{2+}, and shows very marked rectification; the current is maximal near the threshold for action potential generation and decreases with either depolarization or hyperpolarization (Golowasch and Marder, 1992), which may explain why proctolin has its strongest effect on quiescent pyloric networks and decreasing effects as the cells become more depolarized and spike at higher frequencies.

Conclusion

The principles of network reconfiguration by modulation of synaptic efficacy and intrinsic electrophysiological properties, which we have described using examples from the crustacean STG, have been found in many other systems (Kupfermann et al., chapter 20, this volume; Sillar et al., chapter 17, this volume) and are likely to be general. This work shows how fundamental cellular and molecular mechanisms—studied in detail in isolated neurons—are combined in interesting ways to generate changes in motor patterns that lead to altered behavior. Neuromodulators play critical roles in generating behavioral flexibility, which allows all animals, from lobsters to man, to adapt their movements to the demands of the moment.

Acknowledgments

Supported by NIH NS17323 and NS25915 and by the Human Frontiers Science Program.

References

Bal T, Nagy F, Moulins M (1994) Muscarinic modulation of a pattern-generating network: Control of neuronal properties. *J Neurosci* 14: 3019–3035.

Beltz BA, Kravitz EA (1987) Physiological identification, morphological analysis and development of identified serotonin-proctolin containing neurons in the lobster ventral nerve cord. *J Neurosci* 7:533–546.

Dickinson PS (1995) Interactions between neural networks for behavior. *Curr Opinion Neurobiol* 5:792–798.

Dickinson PS, Marder E (1989) Peptidergic modulation of a multioscillator system in the lobster. I. Activation of the cardiac sac motor pattern by the neuropeptides proctolin and red pigment concentrating hormone. *J Neurophysiol* 61:833–844.

Dickinson PS, Mecsas C, Marder E (1990) Neuropeptide fusion of two motor pattern generator circuits. *Nature* 344:155–158.

Eisen JS, Marder E (1984) A mechanism for the production of phase shifts in a pattern generator. *J Neurophysiol* 51:1375–1393.

Elson RC, Selverston AI (1992) Mechanisms of gastric rhythm generation in the isolated stomatogastric ganglion of spiny lobsters: Bursting pacemaker potentials, synaptic interactions, and muscarinic modulation. *J Neurophysiol* 68:890–907.

Flamm RE, Harris-Warrick RM (1986) Aminergic modulation in the lobster stomatogastric ganglion. II. Target neurons of dopamine, octopamine, and serotonin within the pyloric circuit. *J Neurophysiol* 55:866–881.

Getting PA (1989) Emerging principles governing the operation of neural networks. *Ann Rev Neurosci* 12:185–204.

Golowasch J, Marder E (1992) Proctolin activates an inward current whose voltage-dependence is modified by extracellular Ca^{++}. *J Neurosci* 12:810–817.

Harris-Warrick RM, Coniglio LM, Barazangi N, Guckenheimer J, Gueron S (1995a) Dopamine modulation of transient potassium current evokes phase shifts in a central pattern generator network. *J Neurosci* 15:342–358.

Harris-Warrick RM, Coniglio LM, Levini RM, Gueron S, Guckenheimer J (1995b) Dopamine modulation of two subthreshold currents produces phase shifts in activity of an identified motoneuron. *J Neurophysiol* 74:1404–1420.

Harris-Warrick RM, Flamm RE (1987) Multiple mechanisms of bursting in a conditional bursting neuron. *J Neurosci* 7:2113–2128.

Harris-Warrick RM, Marder E, Selverston AI, Moulins M, eds. (1992a) *Dynamic Biological Networks. The Stomatogastric Nervous System.* Cambridge, Mass.: MIT Press.

Harris-Warrick RM, Nagy F, Nusbaum MP (1992b) Neuromodulation of stomatogastric networks by identified neurons and transmitters. In: *Dynamic Biological Networks: The Stomatogastric Nervous System* (Harris-Warrick RM, Marder E, Selverston AI, Moulins M, eds.), 87–138. Cambridge, Mass.: Bradford Books/MIT Press.

Hooper SL, Moulins M (1989) Switching of a neuron from one network to another by sensory-induced changes in membrane properties. *Science* 244:1587–1589.

Johnson BR, Harris-Warrick RM (1990) Aminergic modulation of graded synaptic transmission in the lobster stomatogastric ganglion. *J Neurosci* 10:2066–2076.

Johnson BR, Peck JH, Harris-Warrick RM (1993a) Amine modulation of electrical coupling in the pyloric network of the lobster stomatogastric ganglion. *J Comp Physiol A* 172:715–732.

Johnson BR, Peck JH, Harris-Warrick RM (1993b) Dopamine induces sign reversal at mixed chemical-electrical synapses. *Brain Res* 625:159–164.

Johnson BR, Peck JH, Harris-Warrick RM (1995) Distributed amine modulation of graded chemical transmission in the pyloric network of the lobster stomatogastric ganglion. *J Neurophysiol* 74:437–452.

Katz PS, Frost WN (1996) Intrinsic neuromodulation: Altering circuits from within. *Trends Neurosci* 19:54–61.

Katz PS, Harris-Warrick RM (1989) Serotonergic/cholinergic muscle receptor cells in the crab stomatogastric nervous system. II. Rapid nicotinic and prolonged modulatory effects on neurons in the stomatogastric ganglion. *J Neurophysiol* 62:571–581.

Katz PS, Harris-Warrick RM (1990) Actions of identified neuromodulatory neurons in a simple motor system. *Trends Neurosci* 13:367–373.

Katz PS, Harris-Warrick RM (1991) Recruitment of crab gastric mill neurons into pyloric motor pattern by mechanosensory afferent stimulation. *J Neurophysiol* 65:1442–1451.

Kiehn O, Harris-Warrick RM (1992a) Serotonergic stretch receptors induce plateau properties in a crustacean motor neuron by a dual-conductance mechanism. *J Neurophysiol* 68:485–495.

Kiehn O, Harris-Warrick RM (1992b) 5-HT modulation of hyperpolarization-activated inward current and calcium-dependent outward current in a crustacean motor neuron. *J Neurophysiol* 68:496–508.

Marder E, Abbott LF, Kepler TB, Hooper SL (1992) Modification of oscillator function by electrical coupling to nonoscillatory neurons. In: *Induced Rhythms in the Brain* (Baar E, Bullock TH, ed.), 287–296. Boston: Birkhauser.

Marder E, Skiebe P, Christie AE (1994) Multiple modes of network modulation. *Verh Dtsch Zool Ges* 87:177–184.

Meyrand P, Simmers J, Moulins M (1991) Construction of a pattern-generating circuit with neurons of different networks. *Nature* (London) 351:60–63.

Meyrand P, Simmers J, Moulins M (1994) Dynamic construction of a neural network from multiple pattern generators in the lobster stomatogastric nervous system. *J Neurosci* 14:630–644.

Nagy F, Cardi P (1994) A rhythmic modulatory gating system in the stomatogastric nervous system of *Homarus gammarus*. II. Modulatory control of the pyloric CPG. *J Neurophysiol* 71:2490–2502.

Nagy F, Dickinson PS, Moulins M (1988) Control by an identified modulatory neuron of the sequential expression of plateau properties of, and synaptic inputs to, a neuron in a central pattern generator. *J Neurosci* 8:2875–2886.

Nusbaum MP, Marder E (1989) A modulatory proctolin-containing neuron (MPN). II. State-dependent modulation of rhythmic motor activity. *J Neurosci* 9:1600–1607.

Partridge LL, Swandulla D (1988) Calcium-activated non-specific cation channels. *Trends in Neurosci* 11:69–72.

Sharp AA, O'Neil MB, Abbott LF, Marder E (1993) The dynamic clamp: Computer-generated conductances in real neurons. *J Neurophysiol* 69:992–995.

Turrigiano GG, Selverston AI (1990) A cholecystokinin-like hormone activates a feeding-related neural circuit in lobster. *Nature* 344:866–868.

Weimann JM, Meyrand P, Marder E (1991) Neurons that form multiple pattern generators: Identification and multiple activity patterns of gastric/pyloric neurons in the crab stomatogastric system. *J Neurophysiol* 65:111–122.

Zhang B, Harris-Warrick RM (1995a) Calcium-dependent plateau potentials in a crab stomatogastric ganglion motoneuron. I. Calcium current and its modulation by serotonin. *J Neurophysiol* 74:1929–1937.

Zhang B, Wooton JF, Harris-Warrick RM (1995b) Calcium-dependent plateau potentials in a crab stomatogastric ganglion motoneuron. II. Calcium-activated slow inward current. *J Neurophysiol* 74:1938–1946.

20

Reconfiguration of the Peripheral Plant during Various Forms of Feeding Behaviors in the Mollusc *Aplysia*

Irving Kupfermann, Vladimir Brezina, Elizabeth C. Cropper, Dillip Deodhar, William C. Probst, Steven C. Rosen, Ferdinand S. Vilim, and Klaudiusz R. Weiss

Abstract

Feeding in *Aplysia* involves at least three different behaviors accomplished by a common set of muscles—termed the *physical plant*—that contract in different phases and with different strengths for the various movements. Execution of the behaviors is regulated both by intrinsic and extrinsic modulatory mechanisms that operate on central circuitry and on the peripheral plant. Peripheral modulation is accomplished by means of different neuropeptides released as co-transmitters from motoneurons. The peptides act presynaptically and postsynaptically to reconfigure the periphery so that muscle contractions are optimal for particular behaviors.

The problem of how neurons and the peripheral plant can be reconfigured so as to control a variety of behaviors has been effectively studied in several model systems—in particular, ingestive behaviors in gastropod molluscs and crustaceans. Studies of crustaceans have largely focused on central circuits (Harris-Warrick et al., chapter 19, this volume), whereas the studies of *Aplysia* described here have emphasized an analysis of peripheral plant reconfiguration. The two research focuses complement each other because behavior is the outcome of the emergent interaction of central and peripheral properties.

Feeding in *Aplysia* Consists of Various Behavioral Responses

The consummatory aspects of feeding in *Aplysia* are executed by buccal mass muscles that move the radula in and out of the mouth in at least three distinct modes: bite, swallow, and rejection (Morton and Chiel, 1993; Kupfermann, 1974). The different behaviors can occur independently or can be linked. Thus, if food enters the buccal cavity, a bite is followed by a swallow; if the food is too tough or noxious, a swallow is transformed into a rejection (Schwarz et al., 1991). Furthermore, the behaviors can occur at different rates as a function of various factors, such as the size of the animal, the mass of the food, and water temperature.

The various modes of feeding behavior in *Aplysia* can be recognized both by observation and by nerve recordings from intact animals (Cropper et al., 1990a; Morton and Chiel, 1993). The use of two approaches offers an important advantage because data obtained strictly from isolated ganglia has resulted in confusion about which motor output, if any, that occurs during actual behavior is similar to the fictive motor output recorded from isolated ganglia (e.g., McClellan, 1983).

Central Circuitry

We have only recently begun to understand the complex feeding circuitry of *Aplysia* and other gastropod molluscs. The data from current comparative studies will not be reviewed here, but crustacean stomatogastric ganglia (STG) do have some interesting similarities to *Aplysia* ganglia. For example, the neurons of the buccal ganglion of *Aplysia* were long felt to be exclusively "conventional," but now evidence shows that, as in crustacean STG (Harris-Warrick et al., chapter 19, this volume), the feeding circuitry of *Aplysia* contains neurons that have non-spiking cell bodies and that can generate plateau potentials (Susswein and Byrne, 1988; Perrins and Weiss, 1996; Plummer and Kirk, 1990).

Doing It and Doing It Well

Many studies, particularly of *Aplysia*, have been guided by the idea that motor systems need to generate not only specific patterns, but also relatively efficient output. In other words, the analysis of behavior can be divided into two conceptually distinct (but not necessarily exclusive) functions: how to do it at all and how to do it well. In some sense, the properties of the central circuitry and of the peripheral plant must be matched (which is analogous to impedance matching), a problem complicated by the facts that the same peripheral plant is often used in different behaviors and that the matching requirements are likely to be different for the various behaviors.

Molluscan Feeding is Fine-Tuned by Specialized Modulatory Neurons

Early studies of *Aplysia*'s feeding behavior were concerned with the mechanisms underlying the gradual build-up of the rate and strength of biting (food-induced arousal) that occurs when the animals start a meal (Kupfermann, 1974). Currently, we believe that food-induced arousal is only one of a number of manifesta-

tions of mechanisms that function to optimize behavior and that it is part of an optimal control system (Baev and Shimansky, 1992).

Food-induced arousal is partly due to the action of a pair of giant serotonergic neurons (MCCs). The cell body of each MCC is in the cerebral ganglion, and each MCC sends axons into the buccal ganglion as well as to the buccal muscles. The buccal ganglion contains a central pattern generator and the motoneurons for the buccal muscles. In a quiescent preparation, firing of an MCC enhances the excitability of the motoneurons. If a motor program is occurring, the MCC increases the rate of the program. The MCC has no effect, however, on the membrane potential of the muscle cells it innervates. Nevertheless, if the muscles are caused to contract by firing of a motoneuron, MCC activity enhances the force of contraction and the relaxation rate by means of a cAMP-mediated action on the muscle (Weiss et al., 1979). Serotonin produces identical effects. An MCC's rate of firing, recorded in intact animals, correlates positively with the degree of food arousal (Kupfermann and Weiss, 1982). Furthermore, selective lesions of both MCCs do not block feeding in free-moving animals, but cause dramatic modifications of the speed and strength of biting (Rosen et al., 1989).

MCCs are extrinsic modulators: they are not a part of the basic mediating circuitry that generates the movements (Cropper et al., 1987). Indeed, when the animal is first exposed to food, the MCCs fire before any firing of buccal motoneurons has occurred, therefore altering muscle properties in an anticipatory fashion.

The cerebral ganglion of *Aplysia* (Rosen et al., 1991) and of other molluscs (Gillette et al., 1982; Delaney and Gelperin, 1990; McCrohan and Kyriakides, 1989) also contains a small group of cells that send axons to the buccal ganglion and are referred to as cerebral-buccal interneurons (CBIs). CBIs produce modulatory actions that are relatively slow and, in contrast to MCCs, evoke complex rhythmic motor outputs from the buccal ganglion. The available evidence suggests that various CBIs are simultaneously activated by stimuli that evoke different modes of feeding behavior and that each CBI produces a somewhat different effect. CBIs receive feedback from buccal neurons; therefore, they participate in both gating and generation of the central motor program. They do not appear to be essential elements for pattern generation, however. The neurotransmitters employed by the CBIs are not known; by analogy to similar cells in crustaceans, we suspect that they contain a variety of peptides and other neuromodulator substances. Indeed, very recent preliminary evidence indicates that some CBIs contain the molluscan peptide myomodulin (Xin et al., 1996).

Behavior is also Modulated by Intrinsic Neuromodulators

Although lesioning of the MCCs interferes with food-induced arousal, it does not completely eradicate arousal; animals with this lesion still exhibit remnants of arousal, suggesting that other mechanisms operate to produce the arousal (Rosen et al., 1989). Indeed, it was found that the buccal motoneurons contain a large number of neuropeptides in addition to their conventional excitatory transmitter. Particular attention has been paid to the motoneurons that innervate a single pair of muscles, the accessory radula closers (ARCs, or I5). The principles uncovered by the study of the ARCs appear to apply to other buccal muscles, although a number of muscle-specific features have also been reported (Church et al., 1993). Another type of intrinsic neuromodulator has been described for the escape swim circuit in *Tritonia*, whose serotonergic modulator neuron forms an essential element of the central pattern generator (Katz et al., 1994; Frost et al., chapter 16, this volume).

The ARCs are innervated by only two motoneurons, B15 and B16. The two motoneurons appear to innervate the same muscle fibers, and their relative firing varies according to the particular ongoing behavior of the buccal mass (Cropper et al., 1990a). Each neuron uses acetylcholine as its conventional transmitter, but each also contains a unique family of peptides—the small cardioactive peptides (SCPs), present in B15, or the myomodulins (MMs), present in B16 (Weiss et al., 1993). The MMs and the SCPs have actions similar to serotonin; they enhance the force of contraction (without affecting relaxation rate) and increase the rate of muscle relaxation by means of a protein kinase (Hooper et al., 1994a, 1994b).

Remarkably, in addition to the peptides that potentiate contraction, the two ARC motoneurons contain a variety of other peptides that act to depress the force of contraction. For both motoneurons, the primary depressing peptides are members of the same family—the buccalins, which act presynaptically and decrease the force of contraction by reducing the release of acetylcholine from the motoneuron terminals.

Although it is tempting to assume that the presence of a neuropeptide indicates that it is functional, some peptides may be expressed only because of a failure of gene regulation and might not always have a function

(Bowers, 1994). We have several reasons for asserting that the peptides contained in the motoneurons of the *Aplysia* buccal muscle actually function as co-transmitters (Mahon et al., 1985; Miller et al., 1993a, 1993b; Vilim, 1993; Hooper et al., 1994b; Cropper et al., 1990b): (1) the cells express the appropriate mRNA; the peptides are synthesized in the neuronal cell bodies and are present in terminals in the muscle; (2) the peptides co-exist in dense-cored vesicles; (3) the peptides have actions at low concentrations; (4) firing of motoneurons at rates that normally occur releases physiologically significant quantities of the peptides.

Peripheral Reconfiguration by Sensory Neurons

Some modulatory peptides found in motoneurons are also found in sensory neurons that respond to pressure stimuli applied to the radula—the chitinous structure that grasps food (Miller et al., 1994). These sensory neurons may have both central and peripheral modulatory actions (C. G. Evans, S. C. Rosen, and E. C. Cropper, unpublished observations), but these actions are currently not well understood.

Many Neuromodulators Regulate Feeding

The circuitry that generates feeding in *Aplysia* is affected not only by serotonin but also by a number of cholinergic, dopaminergic, and peptidergic substances that evoke different buccal programs and different movements (Wieland and Gelperin, 1983; Morielli et al., 1986; King et al., 1987; Teyke et al., 1993; Taussig et al., 1989). The largest number of modulators, however, appear to be those present in motoneurons. For example, molecular cloning techniques combined with traditional biochemical characterization of the peptides released in the ARC muscle has revealed that the motoneurons synthesize an astonishingly large number of peptide variants. The SCPs are present in just two forms; the buccalin mRNA, however, encodes for a precursor that contains 19 different buccalins. Similarly, the myomodulin precursor peptide contains multiple variants.

The two SCPs have similar potentiating actions on the ARC muscle, the various buccalins have similar depressing effects, and the various myomodulins have somewhat different actions (Brezina et al., 1995). Each myomodulin appears to activate two sets of partially opposing actions (figure 20.1). Like the SCPs and serotonin, myomodulins potentiate contraction by means of a cAMP-mediated action that enhances a voltage-gated L-type calcium channel. The cAMP pathway also results in the phosphorylation of a myofibrillar protein (titin or twitchin)

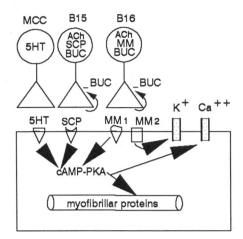

Figure 20.1
Postulated cellular mechanisms regulating the ARC muscle. The muscle is shown to be innervated by the serotonergic extrinsic modulator neuron, MCC, and by cholinergic neurons, B15 and B16 (cholinergic receptors are not shown). Three receptor types—5-HT, SCP, and MM (type 1, activated equally by all the MMs)—are linked to a cAMP–Protein kinase A cascade that acts on myofibrillar proteins (e.g., *Aplysia* twitchin) and on an L-type calcium channel. A second type of receptor (type 2, activated most effectively by MM_A) is linked to the enhancement of a potassium channel through unknown mechanisms. Activation of the other modulatory receptors may also have some effect on potassium channels, but these pathways have not been included. Each motoneuron releases buccalin (BUC), which acts on receptors on the presynaptic terminals, to produce a decrease of the release of acetylcholine and peptides. Presynaptic interactions between neurons also appear to occur but have not been illustrated here.

that may account for the enhanced relaxation (Probst et al., 1994). Another MM action results in the enhancement of a potassium current that opposes the depolarization of the muscle produced by ACh. The result is a depression of the force of contraction because the contraction of this non-spiking muscle is dependent on the level of depolarization. The various MMs differ markedly in their effectiveness in activating the K current. Consequently, their dose response signatures are not identical. Typically, they produce enhancement at the lower concentrations and depression at the higher concentrations; at intermediate concentrations, they produce an initial depression followed by an enhancement. The final effect is the result of the combined actions of the different MMs that are released. In fact, however, application of the most abundant form of MM alone produces the same effect as a mixture of the various forms. It is therefore possible, and indeed likely, that one reason for the multiple forms of peptides within a class in the ARC system is that they are redundant, thus reflecting the operation of non-adaptive or neutrally adaptive evolutionary processes (Bowers, 1994). Functional and

evolutionary explanations for multiple transmitters and co-transmitters are discussed elsewhere (Kupfermann, 1991; Brezina et al., 1996).

Reconfiguring the System

Graphical (Weiss et al., 1993) and computational (Kupfermann et al., 1993) models of the buccal neuromuscular system indicate that one important function of muscle property modulation is to reconfigure the periphery so as to produce more efficient movements when the rate and magnitude of the movements vary in different behaviors. In vertebrates, this function is partially accomplished by the use of different motoneurons that selectively innervate different muscle types whose force-velocity characteristics, metabolic efficiency, fatiguability, speed, and other properties appear to be matched to specific behavioral requirements; see Satterlie, 1993, for an example in mollusc. In *Aplysia*, as in many other invertebrates (both molluscan and non-molluscan), the same muscle can be reconfigured biochemically so as to match its properties with the required motor output. A variety of conditions increase the rate of movements or force of contraction—for example, increased firing rate of motoneurons within a burst, decreased time between motoneuron bursts, or decreased temperature. Modeling studies indicate that as contractions get larger or occur more frequently, in the absence of modulatory actions, the movements become inefficient, weak, and ineffective: the muscles contract too strongly at an inappropriate phase and do not relax quickly enough. Inefficient antagonistic co-contractions of muscles occur so that muscle contractions occur before relaxation is complete, resulting in fusion of succeeding movements instead of discrete movements.

The presynaptic actions of the buccalins, as well as the postsynaptic actions of SCPs and myomodulins, may result in a form of autoregulation that adjusts the magnitude and rate of relaxation of the muscle so as to match the requirements imposed by altered central program outputs during reconfiguration of the central circuits or by changes in the rate or intensity of motor outputs within a given configuration of the program. Neuromodulators seem to specify the values of both central and peripheral parameters that will permit the system to operate at high efficiency. Measurements of peptide release have shown that the motoneuron firing conditions that produce larger or more frequent contractions are the same conditions that result in an increase in the total amount of peptide released. Indeed, the amount of peptide released is a function not only of the total number of spikes, but also the peptide released per spike dramatically increases as a function of the overall number of spikes per unit time, independent of the exact patterns that produce the increased spike density (Vilim, 1996a, 1996b; see also Whim and Lloyd, 1994). The neurons act as if they release the peptides based on the slow accumulation of a presynaptic intracellular signal (perhaps calcium) averaged over a long period. The signal may link peptide release to the requirements of the contraction because the same type of signal acting in the muscle may affect the magnitude and duration of the contraction and may be similarly dependent on spike density.

The indication that there is parallel reconfiguration of central circuits and of the periphery emphasizes the need to consider the muscles, sensory neurons, and central circuitry as all part of a dynamic system. The behavior of such systems is an emergent property of the interacting parts, and as such it cannot be well understood by analyzing its components in isolation (Cohen, 1992; Beer, 1995). Invertebrate feeding behaviors in different species provide advantageous systems for understanding these emergent properties.

Acknowledgments

Supported in part by PHS grants MH36730, GM32099, MH35564, and MH51393. Funds provided by the Whitehall Foundation, the McKnight Endowment Fund for Neuroscience, the Irma T. Hirschl Career Scientist Award, and the Research Scientist Development Award (MH01267).

References

Baev KV, Shimansky YP (1992) Principles of organization of neural systems controlling automatic movements in animals. *Prog Neurobiol* 39:45–112.

Beer RD (1995) A dynamical systems perspective on agent-environment interaction. *Artificial Intelligence* 72:173–215.

Bowers CW (1994) Superfluous neurotransmitters. *Trends Neurosci* 17:315–320.

Brezina V, Bank B, Cropper EC, Rosen S, Vilim FS, Kupfermann I, Weiss KR (1995) Nine members of the myomodulin family of peptide cotransmitters at the B16-ARC neuromuscular junction of *Aplysia*. *J Neurophysiol* 74:54–72.

Brezina V, Orekhova IV, Weiss KR (1996) Functional uncoupling of linked neurotransmitter effects by combinatorial convergence. *Science* 273:806–810.

Church PJ, Whim MD, Lloyd PE (1993) Modulation of neuromuscular transmission by conventional and peptide transmitters released from excitatory and inhibitory motor neurons in *Aplysia*. *J Neurosci* 13:2790–2800.

Cohen AH (1992) The role of heterarchical control in the evolution of central pattern generators. *Brain Behav Evolution* 40:112–124.

Cropper EC, Kupfermann I, Weiss KR (1990a) Differential firing patterns of the peptide-containing cholinergic motor neurons B15 and B16 during feeding behavior in *Aplysia*. *Brain Res* 522:176–179.

Cropper EC, Lloyd PE, Reed W, Tenenbaum R, Kupfermann I, Weiss KR (1987) Multiple neuropeptides in cholinergic motor neurons of *Aplysia*: Evidence for modulation intrinsic to the motor circuit. *Proc Natl Acad Sci USA* 84:3486–3490.

Cropper EC, Price D, Tenenbaum R, Kupfermann I, Weiss KR (1990b) Release of peptide cotransmitters from a cholinergic motor neuron under physiological conditions. *Proc Natl Acad Sci USA* 87:933–937.

Delaney K, Gelperin A (1990) Cerebral interneurons controlling fictive feeding in *Limax maximus*. II. Initiation and modulation of fictive feeding. *J Comp Physiol (A)* 166:311–326.

Gillette R, Kovac MP, Davis WJ (1982) Control of feeding motor output by paracerebral neurons in brain of *Pleurobranchaea californica*. *J Neurophysiol* 47:885–908.

Hooper SL, Probst WC, Cropper EC, Kupfermann I, Weiss KR (1994a) Myomodulin application increases cAMP and activates cAMP-dependent protein kinase in the accessory radula closer muscle of *Aplysia*. *Neurosci Lett* 179:167–170.

Hooper SL, Probst WC, Cropper EC, Kupfermann I, Weiss KR (1994b) SCP application or B15 stimulation activates cAPK in the ARC muscle of *Aplysia*. *Brain Res* 657:337–341.

Katz PS, Getting PA, Frost WN (1994) Dynamic neuromodulation of synaptic strength intrinsic to a central pattern generator circuit. *Nature* 367:729–731.

King MS, Delaney K, Gelperin A (1987) Acetylcholine activates cerebral interneurons and feeding motor program in *Limax maximus*. *J Neurobiol* 18:509–530.

Kupfermann I (1974) Feeding behavior in *Aplysia*: A simple system for the study of motivation. *Behav Biol* 10:1–26.

Kupfermann I (1991) Functional studies of cotransmission. *Physiol Rev* 71:683–732.

Kupfermann I, Deodhar D, Rosen SR, Weiss KR (1993) The use of genetic algorithms to explore neural mechanisms that optimize rhythmic behaviors: Quasi-realistic models of feeding behavior in *Aplysia*. In: *Computation and Neural Systems* (Eeckman FH, Bower JM, eds.), 295–300. Boston: Kluwer.

Kupfermann I, Weiss KR (1982) Activity of an identified serotonergic neuron in free moving *Aplysia* correlates with behavioral arousal. *Brain Res* 241:334–337.

Mahon AC, Lloyd PE, Weiss KR, Kupfermann I, Scheller RH (1985) The small cardioactive peptides A and B of *Aplysia* are derived from a common precursor molecule. *Proc Natl Acad Sci USA* 82:3925–3929.

McClellan AD (1983) Higher order neurons in buccal ganglia of *Pleurobranchaea* elicit vomiting motor activity. *J Neurophysiol* 50:658–670.

Reconfiguration of the Peripheral Plant of *Aplysia*

McCrohan CR, Kyriakides MA (1989) Cerebral interneurones controlling feeding motor output in the snail *Lymnaea stagnalis. J Exp Biol* 147:361–374.

Miller MW, Beushausen S, Cropper EC, Eisinger K, Stamm S, Vilim FS, Vitek A, Zajc A, Kupfermann I, Brosius J, Weiss KR (1993a) The buccalin-related neuropeptides: Isolation and characterization of an *Aplysia* cDNA clone encoding a family of peptide cotransmitters. *J Neurosci* 13:3346–3357.

Miller MW, Beushausen S, Vitek A, Stamm S, Kupfermann I, Brosius J, Weiss KR (1993b) The myomodulin-related neuropeptides: Characterization of a gene encoding a family of peptide cotransmitters in *Aplysia. J Neurosci* 13:3358–3367.

Miller MW, Rosen SC, Schissel SL, Cropper EC, Kupfermann I, Weiss KR (1994) A population of SCP-containing neurons in the buccal ganglion of *Aplysia* are radula mechanoafferents and receive excitation of central origin. *J Neurosci* 14:7008–7023.

Morielli AD, Matera EM, Kovac MP, Shrum RG, McCormack KJ, Davis WJ (1986) Cholinergic suppression: A postsynaptic mechanism of long-term associative learning. *Proc Natl Acad Sci USA* 83: 4556–4560.

Morton DW, Chiel HJ (1993) In vivo buccal nerve activity that distinguishes ingestion from rejection can be used to predict behavioral transitions in *Aplysia. J Comp Physiol* (A) 172:17–32.

Perrins R, Weiss, KR (1996) Plateau generating cerebral-buccal interneurons in *Aplysia. Soc Neurosci Abstr* 22:2044.

Plummer MR, Kirk MD (1990) Premotor neurons B51 and B52 in the buccal ganglia of *Aplysia californica*: Synaptic connections, effects on ongoing motor rhythms, and peptide modulation. *J Neurophysiol* 63: 539–558.

Probst WC, Cropper EC, Heierhorst J, Hooper SL, Jaffe H, Vilim F, Beushausen S, Kupfermann I, Weiss KR (1994) cAMP-dependent phosphorylation of *Aplysia* twitchin may mediate modulation of muscle contractions by neuropeptide cotransmitters. *Proc Natl Acad Sci USA* 91:8487–8491.

Rosen SC, Teyke T, Miller MW, Weiss KR, Kupfermann I (1991) Identification and characterization of cerebral-to-buccal interneurons implicated in the control of motor programs associated with feeding in *Aplysia. J Neurosci* 11:3630–3655.

Rosen SC, Weiss KR, Goldstein RS, Kupfermann I (1989) The role of a modulatory neuron in feeding and satiation in *Aplysia*: Effects of lesioning of the serotonergic metacerebral cells. *J Neurosci* 9:1562–1578.

Satterlie RA (1993) Neuromuscular organization in the swimming system of the pteropod mollusc *Clione limacina. J Exp Biol* 181:119–140.

Schwarz M, Feldman E, Susswein AJ (1991) Vairables affecting long-term memory of learning that a food is inedible in *Aplysia. Behav Neurosci* 105:193–201.

Susswein AJ, Byrne JH (1988) Identification and characterization of neurons initiating patterned neural activity in the buccal ganglia of *Aplysia. J Neurosci* 8:2049–2061.

Taussig R, Sweet-Cordero A, Scheller RH (1989) Modulation of ionic currents in *Aplysia* motor neuron B15 by serotonin, neuropeptides, and second messengers. *J Neurosci* 9:3218–3229.

Teyke T, Rosen SC, Weiss KR, Kupfermann I (1993) Dopaminergic neuron B20 generates rhythmic neuronal activity in feeding motor circuitry of *Aplysia. Brain Res* 630:226–237.

Vilim FS, Price DA, Lesser W, Kupfermann I, Weiss KR (1996a) Co-storage and corelease of modulatory peptide cotransmitters with partially antagonistic actions on the accessory radula closer muscle of *Aplysia californica. J Neurosci* 16:8092–8104.

Vilim FS, Cropper EC, Price DA, Kupfermann I, Weiss KR (1996b) Release of peptide cotransmitters in *Aplysia*: Regulation and functional implications. *J Neurosci* 16:8105–8114.

Weiss KR, Brezina V, Cropper EC, Heierhorst J, Hooper SL, Probst WC, Rosen SC, Vilim FS, Kupfermann I (1993) Physiology and biochemistry of peptidergic cotransmission in *Aplysia. J Physiol* (Paris) 87: 141–151.

Weiss KR, Mandelbaum, DE, Schonberg M, Kupfermann I (1979) Modulation of buccal muscle contractility by the serotonergic metacerebral cells in *Aplysia*: Evidence for a role of cyclic adenosine monophosphate. *J Neurophysiol* 2:791–803.

Whim MD, Lloyd PE (1994) Differential regulation of the release of the same peptide transmitters from individual identified motor neurons in culture. *J Neurosci* 14:4244–4251.

Wieland SJ, Gelperin A (1983) Dopamine elicits feeding motor program in *Limax maximus. J Neurosci* 3:1735–1745.

Xin Y, Rosen SC, Perrins R, Hurwitz I, Weiss KR, Kupfermann I (1996) Two pairs of the cerebral to buccal interneurons that modulate buccal motor program in *Aplysia* are myomodulin peptide containing cells. *Soc Neurosci Abstr* 22:2044.

Part V

Short-Term Modulation of Pattern-Generating Circuits

21

Sensory Modulation of Pattern-Generating Circuits

Keir G. Pearson and Jan-Marino Ramirez

Abstract

Proprioceptive feedback is essential for the generation of the normal motor pattern in numerous rhythmic motor systems. Important functions of proprioceptive feedback include the regulation of frequency and the maintenance of rhythmic activity, the control of phase transitions in order to ensure that a new phase is initiated only when a certain biomechanical state has been achieved, and the shaping of motor activity within a single phase of the rhythmic movement. The influence of proprioceptive feedback is state dependent. The gain and the sign of the action of certain groups of proprioceptors can change depending on the task, or the phase of the movement, or both. Furthermore, in some systems, proprioceptive feedback reconfigures the organization and functioning of central pattern-generating networks. Neuromodulatory substances released in a state-dependent manner may contribute to this afferent-induced reconfiguration.

Two important facts regarding motor pattern generation have been established for a large number of rhythmic motor systems. The first is that a rhythmic motor pattern can be produced in the absence of any sensory feedback (Delcomyn, 1980). The neuronal network producing the rhythmic pattern is usually referred to as a central pattern generator (CPG). The second fact is that the centrally generated motor pattern can be strongly influenced by phasic signals from peripheral receptors (Rossignol et al., 1988). These sensory signals are necessary for the production of the normal motor pattern in intact behaving animals. Thus, a major problem faced by researchers has been to establish the cellular mechanisms associated with the integration of sensory information into central pattern-generating networks.

Considerable progress has been made toward solving this problem for a variety of rhythmic behaviors—mainly, flight in the locust, swimming in the lamprey (Wallen, chapter 6, this volume), respiration in mammals (Smith, chapter 9, this volume; Calabrese and Feldman, chapter 11, this volume), and walking in cats (Stein and Smith, chapter 5, this volume) and arthropods (Nusbaum et al., chapter 22, this volume). Three general principles have emerged from the investigations of these behaviors: (1) sensory feedback contributes to the generation and maintenance of rhythmic activity; (2) phasic sensory

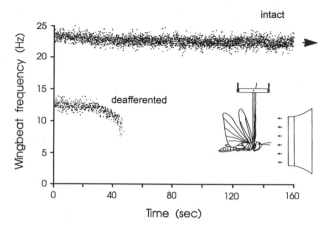

Figure 21.1
Deafferentation of the flight system of the locust reduces wingbeat frequency and shortens the period of flight activity in response to a constant wind stimulus to the head. The two sets of data (intact and deafferented) are from the same animal. Each point is the instantaneous wingbeat frequency for a single cycle. Data were recorded using EMG electrodes implanted into an animal tethered in a wind stream (inset).

signals initiate major phase transitions in intact motor systems; and (3) sensory signals regulate the magnitude of ongoing motor activity. Another important principle is that transmission in reflex pathways is extremely flexible, often depending on the motor task or the phase of the movement or both. In some systems, modification of transmission in reflex pathways depends on neuromodulatory substances that alter the cellular and synaptic properties of neurons in these pathways. The purpose of this article is to illustrate these principles with specific examples taken from a range of vertebrate and invertebrate motor systems.

Role of Sensory Feedback in the Generation and Maintenance of Rhythmic Motor Activity

The clearest example of how sensory feedback contributes to the generation and maintenance of rhythmic motor activity is found in the flight system of the locust. The importance of sensory feedback in this system is revealed by the major deficit produced by deafferentation (figure 21.1). In response to a wind stimulus to the locust's head, the normal flight rhythm occurs above 20 Hz and lasts for the duration of the stimulus. In deafferented animals, however, the frequency is initially approximately 12 Hz, declines progressively during the stimulus, and usually ceases within one minute despite the continuous presence of the wind stimulus. The change in flight behavior is associated with significant changes in the

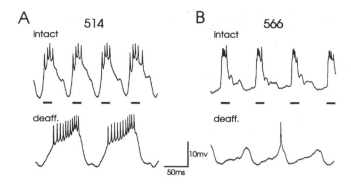

Figure 21.2
Deafferentation alters the profile of synaptic activity in flight interneurons. Intracellular recordings from interneurons 514 (A) and 566 (B) in an intact animal (intact) and deafferented animal (deaff.). Note that deafferentation abolishes the rapid initial depolarization in 514 and the burst of activity in 566. These features are triggered by phasic bursts of activity in the hindwing tegulae (see also figure 21.7). The time of tegula activity is indicated by the horizontal bars.

profile of synaptic activation in many interneurons in deafferented preparations (figure 21.2A and B) and with substantial alterations in the motor pattern itself (Pearson and Wolf, 1989). The data from this investigation demonstrate that afferent feedback does *not* contribute to the generation of the flight motor pattern by simply increasing the cycle frequency of the central pattern-generating network. Instead, as we describe below, afferent feedback reconfigures the functioning of this network and recruits additional neurons into the system that generates the motor pattern. The actions of afferent signals on central networks in the locust flight system are similar, in principle, to the action of neuromodulators on central pattern-generating networks in other systems (Harris-Warrick et al., chapter 19, this volume).

Two types of proprioceptors are involved in the generation of the flight motor pattern: stretch receptors (one for each wing) that are excited by wing elevation and tegulae (a group of about 40 receptors for each wing) that are excited by wing depression. By all the conventional criteria used for identifying neuronal elements in a rhythm-generating network, both the tegulae and the stretch receptors can be classified as elements in the neuronal system that generates the rhythm for flight: they discharge rhythmically in phase with the flight cycle, their ablation reduces the wingbeat frequency, and their stimulation can reset and entrain the flight rhythm (Wolf and Pearson, 1988; Pearson and Ramirez, 1990).

The tegulae and stretch receptors contribute to the generation of the flight rhythm in different ways. Phasic signals from the hindwing tegulae initiate the rapid depolarization of elevator motoneurons and reduce the

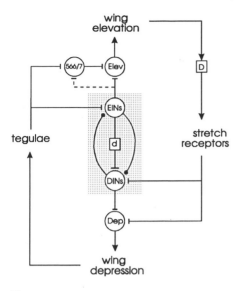

Figure 21.3
Schematic diagram illustrating how phasic afferent signals from wing proprioceptors are integrated into central networks in the flight system of the locust. Tegula input initiates wing elevation by exciting elevator interneurons (EINs) in the central pattern generator (shaded box: the central rhythm is generated by a network consisting of mutual inhibition between elevator (EINs) and depressor interneurons (DINs) and a delayed, d, excitatory connection from elevator to depressor interneurons), and interneurons (566/7) that are outside the rhythm generator. The weak subthreshold synaptic input from the CPG to interneurons 566 and 567 is indicated by the dotted line. Feedback from the forewing stretch receptors is timed to antagonize the hyperpolarization phase in DINs. This action is delayed (D) to occur on the cycle following the wing elevation that activates the stretch receptors. (Modified from Pearson and Ramirez, 1990.)

duration of elevator activity (Wolf and Pearson, 1988). The excitatory action of the hindwing tegulae on elevator motoneurons in mediated mainly via interneuronal pathways. Four interneurons have been identified that make excitatory connections to elevator motoneurons and receive monosynaptic excitatory connections from tegula afferents. Two of these interneurons, interneurons 566 and 567, usually receive only subthreshold depolarizations during flight activity in deafferented preparations (see figure 21.2B, bottom) and thus are not regarded as elements of the central pattern generator (Wolf and Pearson, 1988). However, during flight in intact animals, both interneurons are powerfully excited by phasic input from the tegulae (see figure 21.2B, top). Thus, interneurons 566 and 567 are recruited into the network that generates elevator activity by afferent signals from the tegulae. The other two interneurons in the tegula pathway, interneurons 504 and 514, are elements of the central pattern generator. Both interneurons discharge strongly during flight activity in deafferented prepara-

tions, and current injection into them resets the flight rhythm (Robertson and Pearson, 1983). Phasic signals from the forewing stretch receptors contribute to rhythm generation by antagonizing the repolarization phase in depressor neurons, thus reducing the time of their hyperpolarization phase (Pearson and Ramirez, 1990). This process allows depressor neurons to be reactivated earlier, therefore increasing the frequency of the rhythm. Figure 21.3 summarizes the organization of the afferents from tegulae and stretch receptors onto the central pattern generator.

The involvement of sensory feedback in the generation of rhythmic activity has also been demonstrated in the walking system of the stick insect, in which leg proprioceptors are integral elements of the motor pattern—generating network (Bässler, 1993). Although "locomotor-like" patterns can be induced in isolated ganglia by drug treatment (pilocarpine), they are very slow, and many features of the normal pattern are missing (Büschges et al., 1995). Some of the missing features might be established by feedback from leg proprioceptors.

Phase Switching by Sensory Signals

An important concept introduced by Sherrington early this century (1910) is that proprioceptive signals can function to regulate the transition from one phase of a rhythmic movement to another. Sherrington's own studies concentrated on analyzing the switch from the extension (stance) to the flexion (swing) phase during stepping of the hind legs in spinal cats. One important observation he made was that this transition could be initiated by extending the hips (Sherrington, 1910). He concluded that, during normal walking, proprioceptive signals arising from the hip region initiate the generation of flexor activity needed to produce swing. Additional support for this idea has come only relatively recently: initially with the demonstration that extension of the hip is necessary for initiating swing in spinal cats walking on a treadmill (Grillner and Rossignol, 1978), and then with the finding that imposed rhythmic movements at the hip can entrain and reset the fictive locomotor rhythm in spinal and decerebrate cats (Andersson and Grillner, 1983; Kriellaars et al., 1994). The proprioceptors that signal hip extension have not been positively identified, but a recent study has indicated that they may arise from muscle spindle afferents of the hip flexor muscles (Hiebert et al., 1996). Stimulation of these afferents in hip

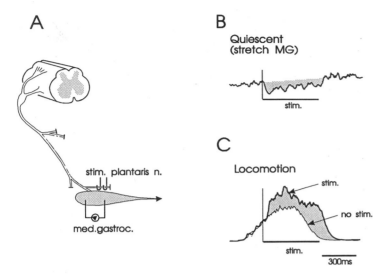

Figure 21.4

Reversal of the action of afferents from the Golgi tendon organs during locomotor activity in the cat. (A) Preparation. Acute spinal cats were treated with clonidine, and group I afferents in the plantaris nerve were stimulated in the presence and absence of locomotor activity. EMG responses were recorded in the medial gastrocnemius (MG) muscle. (B) In the quiescent state, stimulation of the plantaris nerve (horizontal line) inhibits (shaded area) tonic activity in the MG produced by muscle stretch. (C) The same stimulus train triggered during the extension phase of locomotion increases activity in MG. The average rectified and filtered bursts with (thick line) and without (thin line) stimulation have been superimposed to show this excitatory effect (shaded area). For data demonstrating that the excitatory effect during locomotion is due to activation of afferents from Golgi tendon organs, see Pearson and Collins (1993).

flexor muscles and in ankle flexor muscles during stance promotes an earlier onset of flexor burst activity.

Another sensory signal that regulates the stance-to-swing transition in the hind legs of walking cats arises from the force-sensitive Golgi tendon organs in extensor muscles (Duysens and Pearson, 1980; Conway et al., 1987). During locomotion, input from extensor group Ib afferents (arising from the tendon organs) has an excitatory action on extensor motoneurons instead of the well-known inhibition in the resting state (figure 21.4). The excitatory pathway opened during locomotion includes elements in the central pattern generator because activation of the group Ib afferents can reset and entrain the rhythm (Conway et al., 1987; Pearson et al., 1992). Furthermore, electrical stimulation of group I afferents from knee and ankle extensor muscles during the extensor phase also prolongs the stance phase in walking decerebrate cats (figure 21.5; see also Whelan et al., 1995a). The general conclusion from these recent studies is that a necessary condition for the initiation of swing during normal stepping is the unloading of extensor muscles during the latter part of stance. Unloading is signaled by a decrease in activity in the tendon organs of extensors.

The cellular mechanisms by which extensor group I afferents influence the central pattern generator have not been established. If we assume that the centrally generated rhythm is produced by mutual inhibition between flexor and extensor half-centers (Stein and Smith, chapter 5, this volume), we can identify one simple mechanism: maintained activity in extensor group I afferents excites the extensor half-center, thereby preventing burst generation in the flexor half-center. A decrease in group I afferent activity near the end of stance reduces excitatory input to the extensor half-center, but this does not necessarily terminate extensor activity to allow the flexor half-center to become active. Activation of stretch-sensitive afferents in flexor muscles takes place in association with an unloading of the limb, and it is likely that inhibitory input from these afferents normally terminates extensor activity. Figure 21.6 illustrates the pathways from the large muscle afferents known to be involved in the regulation of the transition from extension (stance) to flexion (swing; see Pearson, 1995a, for more details).

The picture emerging from the recent investigations on the walking system of the cat is similar to the one we have drawn of the mechanisms that regulate stepping in the stick insect (Bässler, 1993). In the stick insect, two groups of proprioceptors have been found to influence the timing of the onset of swing: the load-sensitive campaniform sensilla inhibit the initiation of swing (a mechanism analogous to the inhibitory effect of group Ib afferents in the cat), and stretch-sensitive afferents from

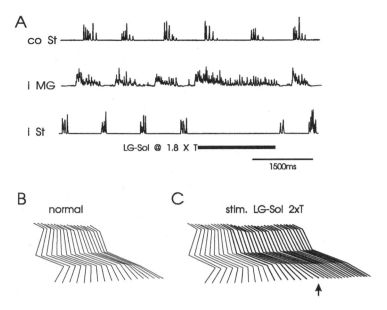

Figure 21.5

Stimulation of extensor group I afferents in walking decerebrate cats prolongs the duration of the stance phase. (A) Rectified and filtered EMGs recorded from the ipsilateral semitendinosus (i St) and medial gastrocnemius (i MG) muscles, as well as from the contralateral semitendinosus (co St) muscle, when the ipsilateral nerve supplying the lateral gastrocnemius and soleus muscle (LG-Sol) was stimulated repetitively (200 Hz, 1.8 × T) for 2 seconds (horizontal line). Note that ipsilateral extensor activity was prolonged for the duration of the stimulus train and that there was virtually no effect on the rhythm in the contralateral leg. (B and C) Stick diagrams showing the movement of the ipsilateral leg during normal steps (B) and when the LG-Sol nerve was stimulated during the extension phase (C). In C, the thick lines show the leg positions when the stimulus was being delivered, and the arrow indicates the point at which swing was normally initiated. Note that the stimulus train held the leg fully extended for the duration of the stimulus. (Modified from Whelan et al., 1995a.)

the femoral chordotonal organ promote the onset of swing (a mechanism analogous to the facilitatory action of stretch-sensitive afferents from flexor muscles in the cat). It appears, therefore, that the conditions for initiating swing in the stick insect are the same as those in the cat: namely, the leg must be unloaded, and the stance phase must have progressed beyond a critical point.

Proprioceptive signals also regulate phase transitions in rhythmic motor systems other than those that control stepping (Pearson, 1993). As we discussed in the previous section, the onset of elevator activity in the flight system of the locust is triggered by phasic signals from the hind wing tegulae (see figure 21.3). We can also observe such a mechanism in the respiratory system of mammals, where it is well established that stretch of pulmonary stretch receptors contributes to the termination of inspiration, otherwise known as the Hering-Breuer reflex (Speck et al., 1993). In addition, inspiratory inhibitory information is also provided via diaphragmatic proprioceptors. Tendon organs and muscle spindles are activated by diaphragmatic contraction, and long-lasting phrenic nerve stimulation leads to a shortening of phrenic nerve activity (Jammes et al., 1986). Furthermore, muscle spindles are also activated by diaphragmatic relaxation,

suggesting that they too may play a role in the transition from expiration to inspiration. Indeed, brief repetitive phrenic nerve stimulation early in the expiratory phase can trigger inspiration (Jammes, 1988; Marlot et al., 1987).

If it is a general rule that phase transitions are initiated by phasic signals from proprioceptors, it is reasonable to inquire into the functional advantages gained by constructing rhythmic motor systems with this feature. The most obvious possibility is that, because proprioceptors provide information about the state of the moving body parts, they function to prevent a movement that would be inappropriate for the current state of the system. The primary advantage of this regulatory mechanism is that phase transitions can be timed according to the attainment of a specific condition required for the effective functioning of the system. The importance of accurately timing phase transitions has been demonstrated in the flight system of the locust (Wolf, 1993). In this system, removal of the hindwing tegulae delays the onset of elevator activity, thus exaggerating wing depression and ultimately resulting in a severe degradation of flight performance.

Another possible advantage for relying on proprioceptive signals to initiate phase transitions is that it

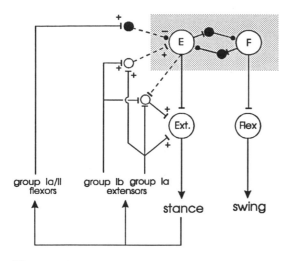

Figure 21.6
Schematic diagram illustrating the pathways from large muscle afferents from flexor and extensor muscles that influence the timing and magnitude of motor activity during stepping in the cat. Feedback from spindle and tendon organ afferents of extensors facilitates extensor activity via at least three pathways: a monosynaptic pathway from group Ia afferents, a disynaptic pathway from group Ia and Ib afferents, and a polysynaptic pathway via the extensor half-center from group Ia and Ib afferents (see Pearson, 1995a, for details). Feedback from muscle spindle afferents of flexor muscles during stance shortens the stance phase, most likely by inhibiting activity in the extensor half-center. (See Gossard et al., 1994; Pearson and Collins, 1993; Hiebert et al., 1996; and McCrea et al., 1995, for data related to this scheme.)

ensures the production of effective movements even when there are alterations in the components of the motor system, such as muscle fatigue and changes in neuronal, muscular and mechanical elements with age. This is because an ongoing phase of a rhythmic movement will proceed until a specific biomechanical state is achieved—a state being signalled by phasic signals from peripheral receptors.

Afferent Regulation of the Magnitude of Motor Activity

In virtually all motor systems, both the timing and the magnitude of the motor output has to be modifiable so that the system can adapt to external environmental conditions. The walking system of the cat offers some of the best examples of this principle because corrective responses are readily evoked by cutaneous stimulation of the skin (Forssberg, 1979) and by the loss of ground support (Gorassini et al., 1994; Hiebert et al., 1995).

A particularly interesting generalization has emerged from studies on walking systems of mammals (including man), insects, and crustaceans: namely, afferent feedback

from leg proprioceptors contributes significantly to the generation of the stance phase activity (Pearson, 1995b). Figure 21.6 illustrates the pathways that function to reinforce stance phase activity in the walking systems of the cat. The reinforcing action comes from the force-sensitive receptors in extensor muscles (the Golgi tendon organs) and from primary muscle spindle afferents in the same muscle (McCrea et al., 1995; Guertin et al., 1995; Pearson and Collins, 1993). At least three pathways are involved in reinforcing extensor activity: the well-known monosynaptic pathway from primary muscle spindle afferents; a disynaptic excitatory pathway from group Ia and Ib afferents that is opened during extension; and a polysynaptic excitatory pathway from group Ia and Ib afferents that acts via the extensor half-center of the central rhythm generator. The latter pathway is also important in regulating the transition from stance to swing. The function of the reinforcing action of proprioceptive feedback on activity in extensor muscles has not been clearly established, but it might provide a mechanism for automatically regulating the level of activity according to the load carried by the leg. For example, activity in leg extensor muscles increases substantially when animals walk up an incline, and it is conceivable that much of the increase is the result of increased feedback from extensor group Ib afferents due to elevated forces in extensor muscles.

Assuming that a substantial fraction of the extensor activity is generated by proprioceptive feedback (in man this has been estimated to be about 30%; Yang et al., 1991), then a very interesting issue arises: how is the gain of the reinforcing reflexes regulated so that it is appropriate for the current state of the animal? One possibility is that it is regulated on a moment-by-moment basis. Indeed, in the walking system of the cat, the modulation of spindle sensitivity by gamma motoneurons alters the feedback from primary spindle afferents according to the specific task (Prochazka, 1989). An additional possibility is that the gain is established slowly according both to the weight of the animal and to the tasks carried out most recently by the animal. This function is most closely analogous to the recalibration of the gain of the vestibulo-ocular reflex in response to changes in the magnification of visual images (Lisberger, 1988). If the slow establishment of gain is true, then we might expect biomechanical changes in the system to produce relatively slow changes in one or more of the excitatory reinforcing pathways. Just this type of plasticity has recently been described in the group I excitatory pathway that acts via the extensor half-center (Whelan et al.,

1995b). A few days after transection of the nerve that supplies the lateral gastrocnemius and soleus muscles (extensors of the ankle), the potency of the group I afferents from the medial gastrocnemius on the timing of the stance-to-swing transition is substantially increased. The mechanisms underlying the enhanced influence produced by the undamaged afferents from the medial gastrocnemius are unknown.

State-Dependent Modulation of Transmission in Reflex Pathways

Another important aspect of the sensory regulation of movement is that transmission in reflex pathways and hence the influence of afferent signals on motor activity are dependent on the animal's behavioral state (Sillar, 1991; Pearson, 1993), which includes both the motor task and the phase of the ongoing behavior. This dependence on task is understandable because reflexes triggered by a group of proprioceptors for one task may be completely inappropriate for another. A good example of this principle is found in the legs of crustaceans. Specialized stretch-sensitive receptors function in standing animals to stabilize posture by evoking resistance reflexes when stretched. Because none of these receptors have motor innervation, and most of them are not physically linked to muscles, their activation is similar in response to either external perturbations or active movements produced by the animal itself. If the postural resistance reflexes continued to operate when the animal is active, they would obviously impede the active movement. Not surprisingly, therefore, this does not occur. Instead, transmission in the resistance reflex pathways is reduced (Barnes et al., 1972) and, in some cases, alternative reflex pathways from the same afferents are opened to reinforce ongoing motor activity (El Manira et al., 1991)—a phenomenon known as *reflex reversal* and described in the walking systems of cats, insects, and crustaceans (see review by Pearson, 1995b).

We are just beginning to understand the range of mechanisms that modulate transmission in reflex pathways (see Sillar, 1991). Two important mechanisms include the efferent modulation of proprioceptors (Prochazka, 1989) and the presynaptic modulation of afferent pathways (Burrows, chapter 12, this volume; Nusbaum et al., chapter 22, this volume). One other mechanism depends on the state-dependent release of neuromodulatory substances. These neuromodulators may regulate phase switching, reflex reversal, and the gain of reflex pathways. Insects have provided important in-

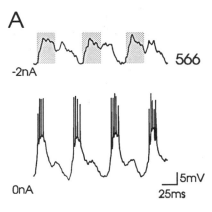

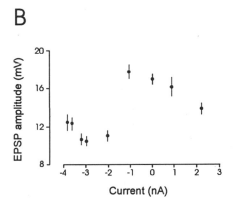

Figure 21.7

Intrinsic bursting properties of interneuron 566 in the flight system of the intact locust. (A) Intracellular recordings from 566 in an intact flying locust. When the interneuron is hyperpolarized (−2 nA, top), two peaks of depolarization can be seen for each cycle. The first peak (shaded) is generated by phasic afferent signals from the hindwing tegulae. In the absence of injected current (0 nA, bottom) the tegula input triggers a large depolarization and a burst of spikes. (B) Plot of the amplitude of the tegula-evoked EPSP against the magnitude of injected current. Note the sudden increase in amplitude when the current was reduced from −2 to −1 nA. (Modified from Ramirez and Pearson, 1993.)

sights into this type of modulation. In locusts, it has been demonstrated that the endogenous biogenic amine octopamine is released by central neurosecretory neurons at the onset of flight (Orchard et al., 1993), which probably facilitates transmission in the pathway from tegula afferents that contribute to switching from wing depression to wing elevation by inducing bursting properties in interneurons 566 and 567 (see figures 21.2 and 21.7). When stimulated in the quiescent animal, these interneurons exhibit passive membrane properties, as indicated by linear relationships between the discharge rate and the magnitude of the injected current. However, during flight activity, or in the presence of exogenously applied octopamine, the interneurons' excitability state is altered, current injection induces rhythmic bursting, and tegula-evoked EPSPs are capable of triggering regenerative bursts (Ramirez and Pearson, 1993). This state-dependent mechanism is important because phasic signals from the tegulae ensure the early activation of elevator motoneurons. This is functionally meaningful since it guarantees an all-or-none activation of elevator motoneurons in a flying animal but not in a quiescent animal.

Neuromodulators may also play an important role in mediating some reflex reversals. In most insects, octopamine is released not only during flight, but also whenever the animal is stressed or agitated. Exogenously applied to a stick insect, octopamine causes the suppression of a resistance reflex, a reflex typical for the quiescent animal, and increases the probability of inducing an "active reaction"—that is, a reflex reversal—which is typical for the agitated active animal (Büschges et al., 1993). The state-dependent release of neuromodulators may also be responsible for reflex reversal in other motor systems. In the walking system of the crayfish, for example, octopamine and proctolin are involved in regulating the reversal of leg reflexes (Skorupski et al., 1991).

Another aspect of plasticity in reflex pathways that may depend on the release of neuromodulators is the regulation of the gain of reflex pathways. Octopamine is released not only in the central nervous system, but also in the periphery, where it modulates the properties of primary afferents, including proprioceptors. For example, it increases the responsiveness of the forewing stretch receptor to wing movements (Ramirez and Orchard, 1990). A more complex modulation occurs in the multicellular femoral chordotonal organ, which plays an important role in regulating leg position in the stick insect (Ramirez et al., 1993). For this receptor organ, octopamine enhances the excitability of position-sensitive neurons without affecting the responsiveness of either velocity- or acceleration-sensitive units. Thus, octopamine alters the relative contributions of position-, velocity-, and acceleration-sensitive information to the reflex control. Modulation of primary afferents seems to be a quite general phenomenon because it has been observed in other invertebrates (Pasztor and Macmillan, 1990). Some modulatory substances are released from central neurons and affect reflex pathways that function in a cycle-by-cycle manner. Some can also be released directly from activated proprioceptors (Katz and Harris-Warrick, 1990) and can cause significant alterations in the properties of neurons in pattern-generating networks—a type of modulation that can last for minutes.

Neuromodulators also affect sensory pathways in vertebrate motor systems. This function is best illustrated by studies on the mammalian respiratory system (Smith, chapter 9, this volume; Calabrese and Feldman, chapter 11, this volume). Pulmonary reflexes are transmitted to the central respiratory network via the Nucleus Tractus Solitarius (NTS), an area that contains various neuromodulatory substances (Moss et al., 1986) known to affect respiratory control. These substances include serotonin, cholecystokinin, somatostatin, acetylcholine, endorphins, substance P, and thyrotropin-releasing hormone (TRH)—all of which are known to affect membrane properties of NTS neurons (Champagnat et al., 1993) and hence transmission of reflex pathways. For example, when released into the NTS during hypoxia, substance P contributes to the initial increased ventilatory drive by altering transmission in reflex pathways from afferents of the carotid body (Lagercrantz and Srinivasen, 1991).

Modulatory processes also directly influence the sensitivity of peripheral receptors in the respiratory system. For example, dopamine suppresses the sensitivity of chemoreceptors in the carotid body to adapt the respiratory system of the fetus to the low intrauterine O_2 levels (Hertzberg et al., 1990). A tonic modulatory influence may also be produced in central networks by afferents that arise from the carotid body because stimulation of these afferents causes an increase in the amplitude of phrenic nerve activity that outlasts the stimulus duration by several hours (Millhorn et al., 1980).

Conclusions

Many investigations have now demonstrated that feedback from proprioceptors can have a powerful influence on the timing of rhythmic motor activity. The need for proprioceptive feedback is two-fold: (1) to adjust movements to the features of the external environment and (2) to ensure that movements are executed accurately when alterations occur in the intrinsic components of the motor system. The need for the latter means that proprioceptors may be important in regulating movements that occur under fairly uniform environmental conditions—for example, in mammalian respiration, locust flight, and lamprey swimming (Wallen, chapter 6, this volume). Not unexpectedly, proprioceptors make a larger contribution to the generation of the motor pattern for movements that occur in less predictable environments. This contribution is seen most clearly in the walking systems of mammals and arthropods: motor patterns generated in the absence of proprioceptive feedback are usually unstable and often lack features of the normal pattern.

The analysis of afferent regulation of rhythmic movements has progressed rapidly over the past decade, and, generally speaking, a far greater awareness of the importance of afferent signals in controlling rhythmic movements has emerged. How has this new information advanced our general knowledge of the mechanisms for pattern generation? The concept that information from proprioceptors is integrated into central rhythm-generating networks to produce the normal motor pattern is not a new concept. In 1932, Creed and colleagues wrote, "The self-generated proprioceptive stimuli of muscles which take part in progression can regulate the act but are not essential to its rhythm." Most recent research has refined this concept with specific examples from a variety of motor systems. In two instances—locust flight and lamprey swimming—we now have a reasonable understanding of the underlying cellular mechanisms for the integration of proprioceptive signals. In many other systems, we have detailed descriptions of how central rhythms can be modified by phasic afferent signals. Thus, from one point of view, recent progress has been rapid and impressive. However, from the view of formulating new concepts, progress has been limited. Perhaps the main conceptual changes regarding afferent regulation over the past decade or so are that central pattern-generating networks are extremely flexible and—of particular relevance to this article—that transmission in reflex pathways influencing central pattern generators is task and context dependent. The influence from a specific group of proprioceptors can even be reversed from one behavioral state to another. Furthermore, we now know that afferent feedback can reconfigure the functioning of central pattern generators and thereby establish essential features of the motor pattern.

It is interesting to consider whether the present conceptual framework can sufficiently and fully account for the afferent regulation of rhythmic pattern-generating networks. For some relatively simple invertebrate behaviors it may be. Even some complex vertebrate behaviors can conceivably be explained by a flexible linking of localized neuronal networks (Grillner, 1981) that depends on afferent and central signals. It should be recognized, however, that the mechanisms for the afferent regulation of central pattern generators may be more complex than those revealed in contemporary experiments, which study the influence of only a single group of afferents or a single descending pathway. In systems where there is feedback from many different groups of sensory receptors (including visual and vestibular signals), the effects of afferent feedback may depend on some sort of weighted average of input from the different groups. The weighting need not be constant, for it may vary from animal to animal depending on its individual history and even from cycle to cycle if the overall task changes. In other words, we may have to consider afferent feedback in a more distributed manner and thus develop concepts that are analogous to those used in neural network controllers (Prochazka, 1996).

References

Andersson O, Grillner S (1983) Peripheral control of the cat's step cycle. II. Entrainment of the central pattern generators for locomotion by sinusoidal hip movements during fictive locomotion. *Acta Physiol Scand* 118:229–239.

Barnes WJP, Spirito CP, Evoy WH (1972) Nervous control of walking in the crab, *Cardisoma Guanhumi*. II. Role of resistance reflexes in walking. *Z Vergl Physiol* 76:16–31.

Bässler U (1993) The femur-tibia control system of stick insects—a model system for the study of the neural basis of joint control. *Brain Res Rev* 18:207–226.

Büschges A, Kittmann R, Ramirez JM (1993) Octopamine effects mimic state-dependent changes in a proprioceptive feedback system. *J Neurobiol* 24:598–610.

Büschges A, Schmitz J, Bässler U (1995) Rhythmic patterns in the thoracic nerve cord of the stick insect induced by pilocarpine. *J Exp Biol* 198:435–456.

Champagnat J, Barnchereau P, Denavit-Saubie M, Fortin G, Jacquin T, Schweitzer P (1993) New insights on synaptic transmission in the nucleus tractus solitarius. In: *Respiratory Control: Central and Peripheral Mechanisms* (Speck DF, Dekin MS, Revelette WR, Frazier DT, eds.), 15–20. Lexington: University Press of Kentucky.

Conway BA, Hultborn H, Kiehn O (1987) Proprioceptive input resets central locomotor rhythm in the spinal cat. *Exp Brain Res* 68:643–656.

Creed RS, Denny-Brown D, Eccles JC, Liddell EGT, Sherrington CS (1932) *Reflex Activity of the Spinal Cord.* Oxford: Clarendon.

Delcomyn F (1980) Neural basis of rhythmic behavior in animals. *Science* 210:492–498.

Duysens JD, Pearson KG (1980) Inhibition of flexor burst generation by loading ankle extensor muscles in walking cats. *Brain Res* 187:321–332.

El Manira A, DiCaprio RA, Cattaert D, Clarac F (1991) Monosynaptic interjoint reflexes and their central modulation during fictive locomotion in crayfish. *Eur J Neurosci* 3:1219–1231.

Forssberg H (1979) Stumbling corrective reaction: A phase dependent compensatory reaction during locomotion. *J Neurophysiol* 42:936–953.

Gorassini M, Prochazka A, Hiebert GW, Gauthier MJA (1994) Corrective responses to loss of ground support during walking. I. Intact cats. *J Neurophysiol* 71:603–610.

Gossard JP, Brownstone RM, Barajon I, Hultborn H (1994) Transmission in a locomotor-related group Ib pathway from hindlimb extensor muscles in the cat. *Exp Brain Res* 98:213–228.

Grillner S (1981) Control of locomotion in bipeds, tetrapods and fish. In: *Handbook of Physiology*, sec. 1, vol. 2, (Brooks VB, ed.), 1179–1236. Bethesda, Md.: American Physiological Society.

Grillner S, Rossignol S (1978) On the initiation of the swing phase of locomotion in chronic spinal cats. *Brain Res* 146:269–277.

Guertin P, Angel M, Perreault M-C, McCrea DA (1995) Ankle extensor group I afferents excite extensors throughout the hindlimb during fictive lomotion in the cat. *J Physiol (Lond)* 487:197–209.

Hertzberg T, Hellström S, Lagercrantz H, Pequignot JM (1990) Resetting of arterial chemoreceptors and carotid body catecholamines in the newborn rat. *J Physiol* 425:211–225.

Hiebert GW, Whelan PJ, Prochazka A, Pearson KG (1995) Suppression of the corrective response to loss of ground support by stimulation of extensor group I afferents. *J Neurophysiol* 73:416–420.

Hiebert GW, Whelan PJ, Prochazka A, Pearson KG (1996) Contribution of hindlimb flexor muscle afferents to the timing of phase transitions in the cat step cycle. *J Neurophysiol* 75:1126–1137.

Jammes Y (1988) Chest wall and diaphramatic afferents: Their role during external mechanical loading and respiratory muscle ischemia. In: *Respiratory Muscles in Chronic Obstructive Pulmonary Disease* (Grassino A, ed.), 49–57. London: Springer.

Jammes Y, Buchler B, Delpierre S, Rassidakeis C, Grimaud C, Roussos C (1986) Phrenic afferents and their role in inspiratory control. *J Appl Physiol* 60:854–860.

Katz PS, Harris-Warrick RM (1990) Actions of identified neuromodulatory neurons in a simple motor system. *Trends neurosci* 13:367–372.

Kriellaars DJ, Brownstone RM, Noga BR, Jordan LM (1994) Mechanical entrainment of fictive locomotion in the decerebrate cat. *J Neurophysiol* 71:2074–2086.

Lagercrantz H, Srinivasan M (1991) Development and function of neurotransmitter/neuromodulator systems in the brainstem. In: *Fetal and Neonatal Brainstem* (Hanson M, ed.), 1–19. Cambridge, UK: Cambridge University Press.

Lisberger SG (1988) The neural basis of learning of simple motor skills. *Science* 242:728–735.

Marlot D, Macron JM, Duron B (1987) Inhibitory and excitatory effects on respiration by phrenic nerve afferent stimulation in cats. *Resp Physiol* 69:321–333.

McCrea DA, Shefchyk SJ, Stephens MJ, Pearson KG (1995) Disynaptic group I excitation of synergist ankle extensor motoneurones during fictive locomotion. *J Physiol (Lond)* 487:527–539.

Millhorn DE, Eldridge FL, Waldrop TG (1980) Prolonged stimulation of respiration by endogenous central serotonin. *Resp Physiol* 42:171–181.

Moss IR, Denavit-Saubie M, Eldridge RA, Gillis M, Herkenham M, Lahiri S (1986) Neuromodulators and transmitters in respiratory control. *Fed Proc* 45:2133–2147.

Orchard I, Ramirez JM, Lange AB (1993) A multifunctional role of octopamine in locust flight. *Ann Rev Entomol* 38:227–249.

Pasztor VM, Macmillan DL (1990) The action of proctolin, octopamine on crustacean proprioceptors show species and neurone specifics. *J Exp Biol* 152:485–504.

Pearson KG (1993) Common principles of motor control in vertebrates and invertebrates. *Ann Rev Neurosci* 16:265–297.

Pearson KG (1995a) Proprioceptive regulation of locomotion. *Curr Opin Neurobiol* 5:786–791.

Pearson KG (1995b) Reflex reversal in the walking systems of mammals and arthropods. In: *Neural Control of Movement* (Ferrell WR, Proske U, eds.), 135–141. London: Plenum.

Pearson KG, Collins DF (1993) Reversal of the influence of group Ib afferents from plantaris on activity in medial gastrocnemius muscle during locomotor activity. *J Neurophysiol* 70:1009–1017.

Pearson KG, Ramirez JM (1990) Influence of input from the forewing stretch receptors on motoneurones in flying locusts. *J Exp Biol* 151:317–340.

Pearson KG, Ramirez JM, Jiang W (1992) Entrainment of the locomotor rhythm by group Ib afferents from ankle extensor muscles in spinal cats. *Exp Brain Res* 90:557–566.

Pearson KG, Wolf H (1989) Timing of forewing elevator activity during flight in the locust. *J Comp Physiol (A)* 165:217–227.

Prochazka A (1989) Sensorimotor gain control: A basic strategy of motor systems? *Prog Neurobiol* 33:281–307.

Prochazka A (1996) Proprioceptive feedback and movement regulation. In: *Handbook of Physiology*. Sec. 12, (Rowell LB, Shepherd JT, eds.), 89–127. New York: Oxford University.

Ramirez JM, Büschges A, Kittmann R (1993) Octopaminergic modulation of the femoral chordotonal organ in the stick insect. *J Comp Physiol (A)* 173:209–219.

Ramirez JM, Orchard I (1990) Octopaminergic modulation of the forewing stretch-receptor in the locust, *Locusta migratoria*. *J Exp Biol* 149:255–279.

Ramirez JM, Pearson KG (1993) Alterations of bursting properties in interneurons during locust flight. *J Neurophysiol* 70:2148–2160.

Robertson RM, Pearson KG (1983) Interneurons in the flight system of the locust: Distribution, connections, and resetting properties. *J Comp Neurol* 215:33–50.

Rossignol S, Lund JP, Drew T (1988) The role of sensory inputs in regulating pattern of rhythmical movements in higher vertebrates. In: *Neural Control of Rhythmic Movements in Vertebrates* (Cohen A, Rossignol S, Grillner S, eds.), 201–283. New York: John Wiley and Sons.

Sherrington CS (1910) Flexion-reflex of the limb, crossed extension reflex, and reflex stepping and standing. *J Physiol (Lond)* 40:28–121.

Sillar KT (1991) Spinal pattern generation and sensory gating mechanisms. *Curr Opin Neurobiol* 1:583–589.

Skorupski P, Rawat BM, Bush BMH (1991) The effect of octopamine and the neuropeptide proctolin on centrally generated and reflex activity in crayfish thoracic ganglia. In: *Locomotor Neural Mechanisms in Arthopods and Vertebrates* (Armstrong DM, Bush BMH, eds.), 173–179. Manchester: Machester University Press.

Speck DF, Karius DR, Ling L (1993) Respiratory afferents and the inhibition of inspiration. In: *Respiratory control: Central and Peripheral*

Mechanisms (Speck DF, Dekin MS, Revelette WR, Frazier DT, eds.), 100–103. Lexington: University Press of Kentucky.

Whelan PJ, Hiebert GW, Pearson KG (1995a) Stimulation of the group I extensor afferents prolongs the stance phase in walking cats. *Exp Brain Res* 103:20–30.

Whelan PJ, Hiebert GW, Pearson KG (1995b) Plasticity of the extensor group I pathway controlling the stance to swing transition in the cat. *J Neurophysiol* 74:2782–2787.

Wolf H (1993) The locust tegula: Significance for flight rhythm generation, wing movement control, and aerodynamic force production. *J Exp Biol* 182:229–253.

Wolf H, Pearson KG (1988) Proprioceptive input patterns elevator activity in the locust flight system. *J Neurophysiol* 59:1831–1853.

Yang JF, Stein RB, James KB (1991) Contribution of peripheral afferents to the activation of the soleus muscle during walking in humans. *Exp Brain Res* 87:679–687.

22

Presynaptic Mechanisms during Rhythmic Activity in Vertebrates and Invertebrates

Michael P. Nusbaum, Abdeljabbar El Manira, Jean-Pierre Gossard, and Serge Rossignol

Abstract

This chapter reviews work performed in various invertebrate and vertebrate species on presynaptic mechanisms that influence primary afferent neurons, interneurons, and projection neurons during rhythmic motor activity. The presynaptic events in sensory neurons are recorded extracellularly as dorsal root potentials (DRPs) or intracellularly from sensory neuron axons as primary afferent depolarizations (PADs) and, in some species, as antidromic discharges. During rhythmic motor activity, such as locomotion, these presynaptic events are time locked to the motor pattern, demonstrating that they can either originate from the central neural network that generates the motor pattern or arise in response to movement-related sensory activity. The rhythmic nature of PADs/DRPs during locomotion may ensure that incoming sensory information produces behavioral responses that are context appropriate for the ongoing movement. Antidromic discharges may be shunted centrally by the PAD and so not evoke transmitter release. Moreover, they may serve as a source of inhibition by colliding with orthodromic spikes or by changing the activation threshold of the receptors in the periphery. They may also invade collateral branches within the CNS that are not subject to PAD, and thereby exert postsynaptic effects on selected targets. At the level of projection neurons and interneurons, presynaptic inputs in rhythmic motor systems are facilitatory or inhibitory: they can shape pattern generation by altering the activity pattern produced by the network or, alternatively, by selectively modifying part of the output from an active network onto some of its targets. In addition, they can originate either from network components or from neurons outside the framework of the network. Thus, presynaptic mechanisms are potent influences that operate at various circuit levels to participate in regulating the input and output characteristics of rhythmically active neural networks.

Presynaptic inputs influence synaptic transmission throughout the nervous system of both vertebrates and invertebrates. Like postsynaptic inputs, presynaptic inputs operate via classical or modulatory transmission or via electrical coupling. A presynaptic input is distinct in that it is placed electrically close to transmitter release sites. Consequently, it can selectively influence transmitter release at specific sites without influencing other sites in the same neuron.

The control of afferent and central nervous system (CNS) inputs to a rhythmically active neural network, or central pattern generator (CPG), is an integral part of motor pattern generation (Rossignol et al., 1988; Rossignol, 1996). Recent evidence obtained from several species indicates that presynaptic inputs participate in this control (Nusbaum, 1994; Clarac et al., 1992; Rudomin et al., 1993), and other evidence documents presynaptic control of transmission from neural network components (Alford et al., 1991; Coleman et al., 1995; Katz and Frost, 1995). This chapter reviews the evidence for presynaptic control exerted at the level of the primary sensory neurons, interneurons, and projection neurons engaged in rhythmic motor behavior in various invertebrates and vertebrates. Our intent is to draw useful analogies that help to generalize concepts important for our understanding of sensorimotor integration.

Throughout the chapter, we use several terms that are peculiar to studies of presynaptic inhibition, particularly as it occurs in the CNS terminals of primary afferents. GABA-mediated presynaptic inhibition causes a depolarization of the presynaptic terminals of sensory neurons. With intracellular recordings of single primary afferent axons, this action is called a *primary afferent depolarization* (PAD). With extracellular dorsal root recordings, the summed depolarization of several afferent terminals transmitted electrotonically to the recording site is termed a *dorsal root potential* (DRP). With strong stimulation of an adjacent root, a PAD may be elicited strongly enough to reach spike threshold and elicit *dorsal root reflexes*, which are transmitted toward the periphery. The peripherally propagating (antidromic) spikes sometimes elicited by PADs are called *antidromic discharges*. Finally, much of our work involves recordings of *fictive motor patterns* which come from preparations in which the CNS produces the rhythmic motor activity underlying a particular rhythmic behavior, such as locomotion, but the behavior itself is not performed either because the recordings are made from an isolated nervous system or synaptic transmission at neuromuscular junctions has been blocked pharmacologically.

Presynaptic Control of Sensory Afferents during Fictive Locomotion

In the crayfish and locust thoracic locomotor systems, the CNS terminals of sensory axons from leg joint proprioceptors receive PADs. When fictive locomotion is induced in the crayfish system, PAD bursts occur at a fixed phase of the locomotor cycle and can reach an amplitude sufficient to generate antidromic discharges (see El Manira et al., 1991; Cattaert et al., 1992). The PADs result from GABAergic transmission and are mediated by an increased chloride conductance that has a reversal potential significantly more depolarized than

the resting potential (Cattaert et al., 1992, 1994). The PADs in the locust system also result from GABAergic transmission, but they do not elicit antidromic spikes, perhaps because the reversal potential is only slightly more depolarized than the resting potential (Burrows and Laurent, 1993; Burrows and Matheson, 1994; Burrows, chapter 12, this volume). The locust sensory neurons receive both tonic and rhythmic inhibitory input to their central terminals during locomotion (Wolf and Burrows, 1995). Also, rhythmic PADs coincide with the occurrence of the strongest sensory response of each sensory neuron.

During fictive locomotion, phasic depolarizations also occur in two functionally distinct axons that innervate the thoracocoxal muscle receptor organ, a crayfish leg joint receptor (Sillar and Skorupski, 1986). The sensory axons do not fire spikes but release their transmitter in a graded manner. During production of the locomotor pattern, the CNS terminals of the two axons are alternately depolarized. These locomotor-related presynaptic depolarizations are thought to enhance synaptic transmission from each axon. Because each axon is depolarized in phase with the activation of its target motoneurons, the thoracocoxal muscle receptor organ is able to reinforce the activity of leg promotor and remotor motoneurons alternately during locomotion (Skorupski and Sillar, 1986).

Cutaneous afferents in the lamprey spinal cord, known as dorsal cells and located alongside the midline in the dorsal columns (Christenson et al., 1988), are also modulated presynaptically during fictive locomotion (El Manira et al., 1997). Dual intracellular recordings from the dorsal cell soma and axon show phasic PADs that occur during the bursts of ipsilateral ventral root discharge (figure 22.1A and B). The depolarizations reach their peak amplitude at the midpoint of the burst of ventral root activity, and they are always larger in the axon than in the soma, indicating that the input synapses are located on the axons (figure 22.1B). When an increase occurs in the frequency of the locomotor motor pattern, a correlated increase in the frequency and amplitude of the PAD in the dorsal cells also takes place, suggesting that the activity level of the neurons presynaptic to the dorsal cells is dependent on that of the locomotor network. Slow potential changes recorded in the dorsal roots of the bullfrog tadpole also suggest the existence of phasic PADs in sensory axons during fictive locomotion (Stehouwer and Farel, 1981).

In cats, presynaptic inhibition of primary afferents has been studied using several different methods. By measuring the amplitude—via an intraspinal electrode (Wall,

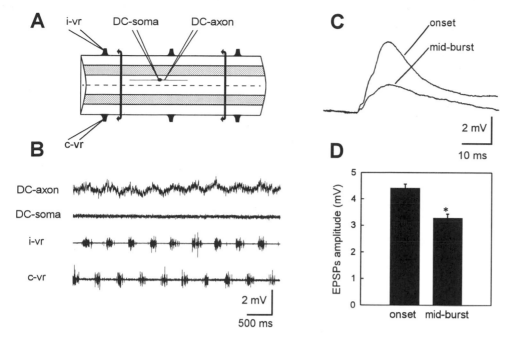

Figure 22.1

Phasic membrane potential depolarization and modulation of sensory synaptic transmission during fictive locomotion in the lamprey. (A) Experimental setup. (B) Dual intracellular recordings are made from a dorsal cell soma (DC-soma) and its axon (DC-axon) (see panel A) in the spinal cord during fictive locomotion. The DC-axon recording shows phasic membrane potential depolarizations that reach their peak amplitude at the midpoint of the ipsilateral ventral root (i-vr) discharge, whereas the membrane potential of the DC-soma shows no phasic depolarizations. (C) Monosynaptic compound EPSPs elicited in the giant interneuron after dorsal column stimulation, which activates axons of dorsal cells as well as other sensory neurons. During fictive locomotion, the EPSP amplitude is smaller when the stimulation is delivered at the midburst rather than at burst onset. (D) The EPSP amplitude in the giant interneuron decreases significantly when the stimulation is given at the midburst, which corresponds in time to the phase when the depolarization in the sensory axons reaches its peak amplitude. (From El Manira et al., 1997.)

1958)—of the antidromic compound action potential evoked by electrical stimulation of their CNS terminals, several researchers found that group Ib (innervating Golgi tendon organs) and group Ia (innervating muscle spindles) afferents of both flexor and extensor muscles were more excitable (i.e., more depolarized) during the flexor phase than during the extensor phase of the step cycle (Baev, 1980; Baev and Kostyuk, 1982; Duenas and Rudomin, 1988). DRP studies during fictive locomotion in thalamic or decerebrate cats and in spinal (L-Dopa-injected) cats showed that the dorsal roots at cervical and lumbar levels are depolarized twice per locomotor cycle (Baev, 1978; Dubuc et al., 1988). Maximum depolarization occurred during the flexor phase (figure 22.2B). A separate study indicated only one wave of depolarization, in the middle of the extensor phase, but the rhythmic activity was faster (Baev and Kostyuk, 1982).

In thalamic cats exhibiting spontaneous fictive locomotion, intra-axonal recordings have been made in the dorsal horn from large cutaneous axons that innervate the dorsal and plantar surfaces of the hindpaw (Gossard et al., 1989), as well as from muscle afferents (Gossard et

al., 1991). As Dubuc and colleagues (1988) found in their DRP studies, a large wave of depolarization generally occurred during the flexor phase (F-PAD), and a smaller wave occurred during the extensor phase (E-PAD; see figure 22.2B). There was no obvious correlation between the PAD patterns and the size of the axon, its receptive field, or the muscle group. Intra-axonal recordings from a variety of preparations during fictive locomotion have shown that most large cutaneous and muscle primary afferents exhibit comparable PAD profiles—two phasic waves synchronous with the two major phases of the step cycle. Additionally, recent work in anesthetized cats shows that different collateral arborizations of the same Ia afferent may be controlled by different last-order PAD interneurons (Eguibar et al., 1994). It remains to be seen whether a variety of PAD patterns occur in different collaterals of the same axon during locomotion.

Supraspinal systems also evoke PAD in spinal sensory neurons. In the anesthetized cat, descending supraspinal systems evoke different PAD patterns in different primary afferents (Rudomin, 1990). The effects of these pathways during locomotion, however, remain largely

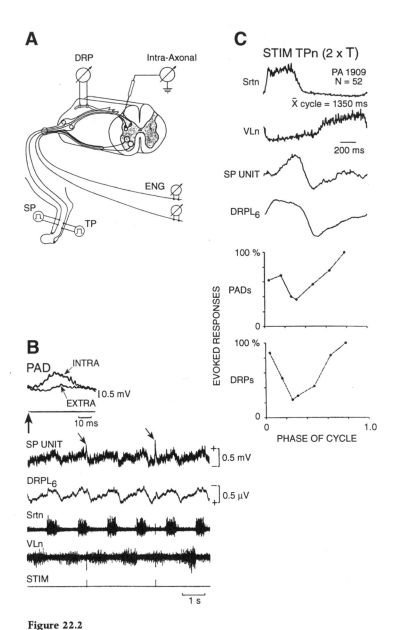

Figure 22.2
CPG-related PAD and cutaneous-evoked PAD in a cutaneous primary afferent from superficial peroneal (SP) nerve innervating hairs on the dorsal surface of the hindpaw. (A) Experimental setup. (B, Top). Averaged PAD evoked in the SP axon by tibialis posterior (TP) nerve stimulation (1 msec pulse at 2 times threshold: $2 \times T$). Intra, PAD recorded intra-axonally; Extra, PAD recorded extracellularly as DRP. (Bottom). The CPG-related PAD in the SP unit and the DRP-L6 are maximal during the flexor phase (Srtn). Superimposed on these ongoing cyclic PAD changes are brief PADs evoked by TP nerve stimulation (arrows). SP unit, intra-axonal recording; DRP, recording from an L6 dorsal rootlet; Srtn, sartorius electroneurogram (ENG); VLn, vastus lateralis ENG;

Stim, stimulus. (C) From top to bottom, first to fourth traces are the averaged activities of the raw traces shown in panel B. The averaged Srtn and VLn ENG activities represent the flexor and extensor phases of the step, respectively. "$\bar{X}$ cycle" represents the mean cycle period. Below are two phase plots of the amplitude of the PADs and DRPs evoked by stimulation of the TP nerve. During the flexor phase, the SP unit and the DRP-L6 are maximally depolarized by the CPG, but the amplitudes of the evoked PADs and DRPs are minimal. The evoked PAD and DRPs are maximal during the extensor phase (VLn). (Modified from Gossard et al., 1990, with permission.)

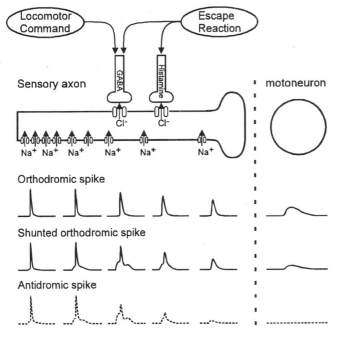

Figure 22.3
Schematic illustration of the mechanisms underlying presynaptic inhibition of the CNS terminals of sensory afferents in the crayfish and of the consequences of this presynaptic inhibition for sensory neuron elicited EPSPs in motoneurons. Presynaptic inhibition occurs during locomotion, via activation of GABA receptors, and during an escape reaction, via activation of GABA and histamine receptors (El Manira and Clarac, 1994). Orthodromic spikes propagate passively in the most central part of the sensory terminal, possibly because of decreased sodium channel density. Locomotor- and escape reaction–related PADs shunt the orthodromic spikes, thereby decreasing the amplitude of the monosynaptic EPSPs in the target motoneuron. When the PADs are large, they generate antidromic spikes in the neighboring peripheral region of the axon, where the density of sodium channels is presumably higher than in the neuropil and there is no shunting conductance change from the PAD. These spikes then propagate successfully to the periphery, but they are shunted as they propagate centrally into the neuropil, past the GABA synapse, and thus fail to induce any postsynaptic response. (Reproduced from Cattaert et al., 1994, with permission.)

unknown. Recent preliminary work (Gossard et al., 1994) has revealed that stimulation of the medullary reticular formation (MRF) evoked maximal DRPs during the extensor phase of the fictive step cycle, as did stimulation of different types of peripheral afferents.

Physiological and Pharmacological Mechanisms of PADs

Effects of PADs on Sensory Synaptic Transmission

Until recently no direct link was detected between PADs and decreased synaptic transmission, which mainly resulted from the difficulty of recording simultaneously from sensory axons and target neurons. However, analysis of the PAD influence on sensory synaptic transmission was recently undertaken in the crayfish locomotor system (Cattaert et al., 1992; Clarac et al., 1992). In these experiments, simultaneous intracellular recordings were made from a sensory axon and its postsynaptic motoneuron, revealing that the GABAergic PADs shunted the orthodromic afferent spikes and reduced their amplitude (figure 22.3). This reduced the amount of transmitter released onto the target motoneuron (Cattaert et al., 1992). Because the PADs are time locked to the locomotor rhythm, they may help to ensure that the sensory input acts only in the behaviorally appropriate phases of the locomotor cycle. For example, the same receptor mediates both a resistance reflex in quiescent preparations and an assistance reflex during fictive locomotion. Therefore, the presynaptic inhibition might be designed to eliminate the resistance reflex responses that would tend to oppose the performed movement (El Manira et al., 1991; Sillar and Skorupski, 1986). Comparable results have also been observed in the locust locomotor system (Burrows and Laurent, 1993; Burrows and Matheson, 1994; Wolf and Burrows, 1995; Burrows, chapter 12, this volume). A GABAergic-dependent reduction of group Ia-related excitatory postsynaptic potentials (EPSPs) was also recorded in cat lumbar motoneurons when PAD was evoked by sensory volleys (Stuart and Redman, 1992).

The role of phasic PADs during fictive locomotion (swimming) has also been analyzed in the lamprey spinal cord (El Manira et al., 1997). In this system, the efficacy of synaptic transmission from the dorsal column, which contains the axons of dorsal cells and other sensory neurons, onto the relay giant interneurons was measured and compared at both the onset and the midpoint of the burst of the ipsilateral ventral root discharge because these times correspond to the locomotor phases when the PAD amplitude in the dorsal cell axon is at its lowest and at its peak level, respectively (see figure 22.1B). The amplitude of the dorsal column–evoked EPSP in relay giant interneurons is smaller when the afferents are stimulated at the midpoint rather than at the onset of the burst of ventral root discharge (see figure 22.1C). The giant interneurons do not display membrane potential oscillations during fictive locomotion, nor are there any detectable changes in their input resistance between the onset and the midpoint of the ventral root bursts. Coincidentally, sensory-evoked resetting of the locomotor rhythm is more effective when delivered at burst onset. Such presynaptic locomotor-related modulation of sensory transmission may represent a mechanism for phasic gain control, which functions to depress sensory inputs activated by ongoing ipsilateral muscle contractions, such as those resulting from skin deformation.

Pharmacology of PADs

Activation of GABA receptors depolarizes sensory axons and mediates presynaptic inhibition of synaptic transmission in both vertebrates and invertebrates (Nicoll and Alger, 1979; Watson, 1992). In crayfish sensory axons, local application of GABA into the neuropil induces a chloride-mediated depolarization that has a reversal potential 20–40 mV more depolarized than the resting potential (El Manira and Clarac, 1991). This effect is activated by both $GABA_A$ and $GABA_B$ agonists, but it is insensitive to specific antagonists. It can be blocked only by picrotoxin, a relatively nonspecific antagonist (El Manira and Clarac, 1991, 1994). The PADs in locust leg sensory neurons are also GABA mediated (Burrows and Laurent, 1993).

In the bullfrog spinal cord, both $GABA_A$ and $GABA_B$ receptors produce presynaptic inhibition at synapses between muscle spindle afferents and motoneurons (Peng and Frank, 1989a, 1989b). The $GABA_A$ effect, but not the $GABA_B$ effect, is associated with a reduced afferent spike amplitude due to an increased chloride conductance. $GABA_B$ receptor activation reduces calcium current in dorsal root ganglion somata (Dunlap and Fischbach, 1981; Dolphin and Scott, 1987), suggesting a mechanism for $GABA_B$-mediated presynaptic inhibition.

In the lamprey spinal cord, synaptic transmission from the mechanosensory dorsal cells to postsynaptic targets is depressed by $GABA_B$-mediated presynaptic inhibition (Christenson and Grillner, 1991). Both GABA- and NPY-immunoreactive neurons make close appositions with dorsal cell axons in the lamprey spinal cord (Bongianni et al., 1990; Christenson et al., 1991). These neurons may be the source of the synaptic inputs that mediate the phasic depolarizations. The locomotor-related depolarizations, however, are not blocked by commonly used GABA receptor antagonists (El Manira et al., 1997).

The lamprey dorsal cells also are inhibited presynaptically by serotonin (Wikström et al., 1995). Close appositions occur between serotonin immunoreactive dorsal root axons and dorsal cell axons. The appositions may represent a substrate for sensory-sensory interactions that modulate dorsal cell output. Similarly, serotonin produces presynaptic inhibition of cutaneous synaptic transmission from the Rohon-Beard sensory neurons in the *Xenopus* tadpole (Sillar and Simmers, 1994), which reduces the ability of cutaneous stimulation to elicit

fictive locomotion. In addition to depressing cutaneous synaptic transmission, serotonin acts postsynaptically to influence the swim CPG and to increase the frequency of the swim motor pattern (Sillar et al., 1992). These actions may take place during escape behavior, when the animal should swim rapidly and ignore weak sensory inputs that would tend to interfere with the motor task (Sillar and Simmers, 1994).

Results from studies in many species thus suggest that the strength of sensory transmission is phasically modulated during fictive locomotion (see Rossignol et al., 1988; Pearson, 1993). The modulation allows the locomotor network to control the gain of sensory inputs. Such control may serve to gate reflex responses that might otherwise interfere with the ongoing network activity.

Antidromic Discharges

A Brief History of Antidromic Activity in the Cat

Despite lingering misconceptions, antidromic discharges do not result simply from the lowering of the spinal cord temperature (an experimental artifact), and they occur often enough not to be considered physiologically insignificant. Toennies (1939) systematically studied the effect of external cooling of the spinal cord and concluded that, although cooling enhanced dorsal root reflexes, these were present at normal temperature, even when no laminectomy was performed. Several subsequent studies have confirmed this point (Brooks et al., 1955; Eccles et al., 1961; Brooks and Koizumi, 1956; Habgood, 1953; Casey and Oakley, 1972). Regarding the frequency of their occurrence, Habgood (1953) stated that all dorsal rootlets in cats show antidromic discharges after the rootlets have been sectioned and after their injury discharge has died out. Recordings of antidromic discharge units in cut dorsal rootlets during both fictive and actual locomotion in the cat suggest that such discharges are not rare (Beloozerova and Rossignol, 1994, 1995).

Antidromic Discharge during Rhythmic Activity in the Cat

Using extracellular dorsal root recordings during fictive locomotion in cats, Dubuc and colleagues (1985, 1988) found that antidromic discharges of unidentified units were often superimposed on the DRPs and were generally coincident with the largest DRPs. The antidromic discharges occurred in various parts of the locomotor cycle. Whereas some units discharged more or less ton-

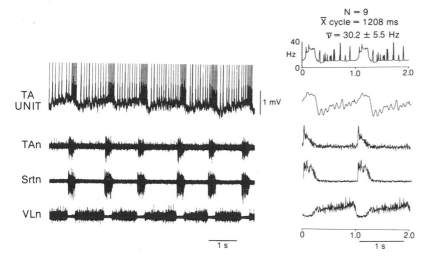

Figure 22.4
Rhythmic membrane potential and phasic firing of a provisional group Ia spindle afferent during spontaneous fictive locomotion in a decorticate cat. (Left) Intra-axonal recording from the afferent, which innervates the tibialis anterior muscle (TA unit). (Right) The firing frequency and membrane potential fluctuations of the TA axon are shown (extra-axonal potential subtracted), as are the rectified TA, Srt, and VL elec-troneurograms, which were averaged over nine cycles. The display is repeated twice to facilitate viewing the temporal relationships. Note that, even though the cycles are normalized, the time base (1 sec) is derived from the mean cycle duration and applies to all the averages. TA = tibialis anterior; Srt = sartorius; VL = vastus lateralis. (Reproduced from Gossard et al., 1991, with permission.)

ically, others exhibited brief bursts at transition phases (i.e., at stance-to-swing or swing-to-stance transitions). Units that produced well-defined bursts of antidromic discharge showed a strong correlation between burst duration and the duration of the locomotor cycle in both the decerebrate cat and the spinal cat injected with L-DOPA. Most units were also activated by stimulation of either the skin or by manipulation of the joints of the ipsi- or contralateral hindlimb or even of the forelimbs (Dubuc et al., 1987). Studies of antidromic discharge during fictive scratching in the cat (Baev and Kostyuk, 1981) and during locomotion in the rat (Pilyavskii et al., 1988, 1989) have produced similar results.

In a study done by Gossard and colleagues (1989), only 5 of 82 cutaneous axons displayed rhythmic antidromic discharges during rhythmic PADs. Surprisingly, about one-third of muscle afferents originating from flexor muscles, but none from extensors, displayed rhythmic antidromic discharges even though their locomotor PAD amplitudes were comparable (Gossard et al., 1991; figure 22.4). In some cases, it was possible to assess both the orthodromic and antidromic discharges in the same unit. The orthodromic discharge rate varied with changes in muscle length produced by passively flexing or extending the ankle. In contrast, the rhythmic antidromic bursts of highest frequency, which occurred during the flexor phase, were more or less independent of muscle length.

Although it is difficult to record DRPs during treadmill locomotion (but see Yakhnitsa et al., 1988), antidromic discharges can be easily recorded in cut or intact roots in the cat by use of spike-triggered averaging (STA). During fictive locomotion, 15–20% of rootlets had rhythmic antidromic discharges (Dubuc et al., 1988). In more recent studies that made dorsal root recordings during real locomotion, approximately 80% of the tested rootlets contained antidromically firing units (figure 22.5; see also Beloozerova and Rossignol, 1994, 1995).

In the crayfish locomotor system, as in the cat, GABAergic inputs onto the CNS terminals of sensory axons not only produce PADs, but also evoke spikes that are conveyed antidromically (El Manira et al., 1991; Cattaert et al., 1992). In contrast, sensory afferents in neither the locust nor the lamprey exhibit antidromic discharges during PAD (Wolf and Burrows, 1995; El Manira et al., 1997).

Role of Antidromic Discharges

The abundant antidromic discharges that occur in the dorsal roots of cats during real locomotion suggest they are linked to the neural mechanisms that generate the movement. Indeed, the finding that antidromic discharges are also generated in the fictive state suggests

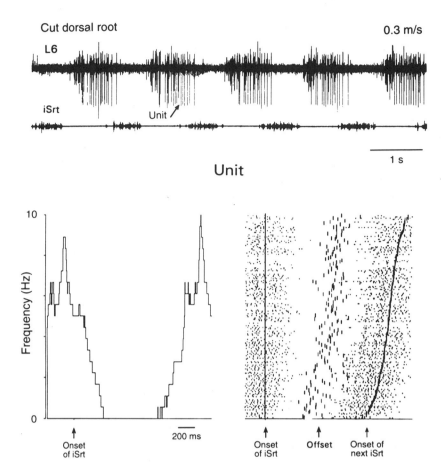

Cut dorsal root · 0.3 m/s

L6

iSrt · Unit ↗

1 s

Unit

Frequency (Hz) · 10 · 0

200 ms

Onset of iSrt

Onset of iSrt · Offset · Onset of next iSrt

Figure 22.5

Antidromic discharge recorded from dorsal root axons during controlled treadmill locomotion in the decerebrate cat. (Top) Simultaneous recordings are shown from a cut dorsal rootlet from L6 and discharge of the hip flexor sartorius on the ipsilateral side (iSrt) in a decerebrate cat walking on a treadmill at 0.3 m/s. The largest unit from the L6 recording was window discriminated, and its discharge during each locomotor cycle is represented both as a raster (bottom right) and as a firing frequency histogram (bottom left). (Bottom right) For the raster plot, the onset of the iSrt in each cycle was chosen as a trigger (vertical line labelled: Onset of iSrt) and all the step cycles (∼ 100) in the sequence were rank ordered, with the longest step cycle at the top. The second, wavy line indicates the end of each cycle (defined by the onset of the next iSrt burst). The arrow labeled "Offset" points to the end of the iSrt burst within each cycle and is represented as small vertical bars. Each row of dots represents the time of occurrence of all spikes from the window discriminated unit within one step cycle. This unit starts to discharge well before iSrt burst onset and continues its activity through approximately one-third of the iSrt burst. It is then silent until the last third of the cycle. The discharge of this unit closely follows the variation in cycle duration, as seen from the successive rows of dots. (Bottom left) In the histogram, the cycles, which are also triggered on iSrt onset, are normalized to 256 bins. The onset of iSrt defines the beginning of the cycle, and the end of the X-axis defines the end of the normalized step cycle. The mean frequency discharge of the unit (in Hz) was obtained by averaging the instantaneous firing frequency of the unit throughout each cycle. Thus, the unit discharges at a peak-averaged instantaneous frequency of approximately 8–9 Hz at the stance-swing transition. The time base applies to both the histogram and the raster plot. (From Beloozerova and Rossignol, unpublished.)

that, in addition to being elicited by sensory input, they may be part of the centrally generated locomotor program.

Periphery One of the first indications that antidromic discharges could interact with the sensory mechanisms themselves came from studies done by Toennies (1939). He found that the afferent orthodromic volley in the saphenous nerve originally produced by receptive field stimulation could be markedly reduced by a preceding stimulation to the sciatic nerve. He reasoned that the antidromic activity evoked by the sciatic nerve stimulation not only collided with the orthodromic activity (resulting in a refractoriness in the previously active axons) but also interfered with sensory transduction at the level of the receptors. Clearly, spike collision is one mechanism by which antidromic discharges can modify the orthodromic activity (Wall, 1964; Eccles et al., 1961). Such collisions, however, occur only within a narrow window of time. For instance, in a 10-cm-long axon conducting at 50 m/s, only a 2 msec window follows each antidromic spike, during which time there is the possibility for a collision with an orthodromic spike.

Antidromic discharge might interfere with the sensory transduction event by changing receptor excitability. Lindblom (1958) showed that the response of a frog cutaneous receptor decreased for several milliseconds after a spike was produced by proximally stimulating the nerve. Similarly, Catton (1961) showed that, after the period of axonal refractoriness (approximately 1 msec), there is a longer period of receptor refractoriness (approximately 10 msec), followed by an even longer period of increased threshold (several hundred milliseconds). Catton suggested that these events occurred at the first node of Ranvier in the periphery. Evidence also indicates that antidromic spikes invade the first node of Ranvier, but not the receptor membrane (Loewenstein, 1959). Similar findings have been made in frog muscle receptors (Ito, 1968).

The possibility also exists that the antidromic discharge, especially when it occurs as bursts of spikes, may evoke dendritic release of a chemical in the periphery that will affect neuronal excitability (Catton, 1961; Habgood, 1950). Dendritic release of a neurotransmitter that affects sensory neuron excitability is known to occur in vertebrate primary afferent nociceptors (Levine et al., 1993) and in a crustacean stretch receptor neuron (Pasztor and Bush, 1987; Pasztor et al., 1988).

CNS Simultaneous recordings from presynaptic sensory axons and postsynaptic motoneurons in the crayfish demonstrated that PAD-elicited spikes do not evoke EPSPs (El Manira et al., 1991; Cattaert et al., 1992). The GABAergic PADs generate these spikes in the axon upstream (i.e., toward the periphery) from the GABAergic synapses. The spikes are shunted by the increased chloride conductance as they enter the neuropil and travel past the region of the GABAergic PAD. Their amplitude thus decreases considerably, resulting in the failure to evoke transmitter release (see figure 22.3). They are particularly susceptible to shunting because, even without PAD, they are not actively propagated once they enter the neuropil (see figure 22.3; Cattaert et al., 1992, 1994).

Preliminary results in a study done by Gossard (1995) also suggest that antidromic discharges recorded in dorsal rootlets have no postsynaptic effects in lumbar motoneurons or first-order interneurons in the intermediate nucleus of the cat, within the same spinal segment. The possibility exists, however, that other sensory neuron collaterals are not directly subjected to PADs and may be invaded by the antidromic discharges, thus leading to orthodromic postsynaptic effects. For example, when the L7 dorsal root is stimulated, a reflex discharge is evoked and carried centrifugally in adjacent dorsal roots, and a similar complex wave can also be recorded in the dorsal columns up to 13 cm rostral to the stimulation site (Hursh, 1940). It is thus possible that these discharges activate the dorsal column nuclei. Duchen (1986) reported that ventral root discharges could also be correlated with evoked antidromic discharges. Similarly, Eccles and colleagues (1961) showed with intracellular recordings that antidromic discharges set up in muscle afferents could produce monosynaptic EPSPs in motoneurons as well as ventral root discharges in kittens (Eccles and Willis, 1962). Further work in the cat is thus needed to better understand the potential central role of these antidromic discharges.

Finally, dorsal root recordings of antidromic discharge may represent only a crude reflection of more sophisticated mechanisms occurring in the spinal cord. For instance, Wall (1994) showed that an apparently sophisticated control is exerted on spike conduction in various collateral branches of primary afferents. Kolta and colleagues (1995) suggest that various parts of the same afferent could have different discharge patterns, with some of these parts acting as a local interneuron. If comparable events occur during locomotion, then some of the primary afferent arborizations might also participate in the generation of the locomotor motor pattern. A similar functional compartmentalization resulting from presynaptic inhibition has also been documented in a modulatory projection neuron (Coleman and Nusbaum, 1994).

Sensory-Sensory Interactions

Presynaptic inhibition can also result from sensory-sensory synaptic interactions at their CNS terminals—as happens, for example, in locust leg joint proprioceptors (Burrows and Matheson, 1994). Paired intracellular recordings from sensory axons reveal that the presence of a PAD in one sensory neuron is elicited by the stimulation of a second, functionally equivalent sensory neuron. This presynaptic event is thought to be mediated by GABAergic interneurons. PADs elicited in this way decrease the amplitude of orthodromic spikes near the presynaptic terminals of the sensory axon, thus producing smaller EPSPs in target motoneurons. Presynaptic inhibition resulting from sensory-sensory interactions appears to act as a local gain control that prevents saturation of the postsynaptic response (Burrows and Matheson, 1994; Wolf and Burrows, 1995).

Sensory-sensory interaction can also mediate presynaptic facilitation via electrical coupling between sensory axons (El Manira et al., 1993). In the crayfish locomotor system, there is electrical coupling between the central terminals of functionally equivalent leg joint proprioceptors. Consequently, an active sensory axon depolarizes the coupled axons, sometimes to the degree that spikes are elicited in the coupled axons, which enhances the postsynaptic response in target motoneurons. The spike-mediated depolarization in the coupled axons also increases the amplitude of simultaneously occurring orthodromic spikes in the axons, thus facilitating transmitter release and producing larger amplitude EPSPs in the motoneurons (El Manira et al., 1993). In the goldfish, similar electrical coupling occurs at the axon terminals of eighth nerve afferents, where they synapse with the lateral dendrite of the Mauthner cell (Pereda et al., 1995).

Interaction between CPG-related PAD and sensory-evoked PAD has been studied during fictive locomotion in thalamic or spinal cats. The interaction was studied using DRPs from cutaneous and muscle afferents (Gossard and Rossignol, 1990) and intra-axonal recordings of cutaneous axons that innervate the dorsal and plantar surfaces of the hindpaw (see figure 22.2B and C; Gossard et al., 1990). In all axons studied, the PAD evoked in cutaneous afferents by cutaneous stimulation was maximal during the extensor phase of the step, whether or not there was a large CPG-related E-PAD in the afferent. The results showed clearly that the maximum CPG-related PAD, which occurs during flexion, was out-of-phase with the maximum cutaneous-evoked PAD (see figure 22.2C). Moreover, evoked DRPs were maximal during the ipsilateral extensor phase, whether the stimulated nerve was ipsilateral or contralateral (Gossard and Rossignol, 1990), suggesting that the state of the CPG on the side of the receptive fiber is dominant in determining the size of the sensory-evoked PAD. Yakhnitsa and colleagues (1988) obtained comparable results during real locomotion in rats, and accordingly, Duenas and colleagues (1990) found that, during treadmill locomotion of thalamic cats, dorsal root reflexes evoked by cutaneous stimulation were maximal during the extensor phase of the step. One possible explanation for such results is that, during flexion, the PAD pathways recruited by the CPG and sensory inputs are occluded; during extension, however, sensory inputs can interact maximally, so the sensory-evoked PADs and DRPs are largest.

Presynaptic Control of Network Interneurons and Projection Neurons

Only recently has documentation become available on the effects that presynaptic influences have on the local interneurons and projection neurons that contribute to the generation of rhythmic motor patterns. In some cases, presynaptic control enables a selective alteration of inputs to or output from the pattern generator network without a concomitant alteration of the activity pattern generated by that network. In other cases, presynaptic effects reconfigure the network-generated pattern.

Alteration of Network Input and Output

Network Input

In the lamprey spinal cord, synaptic output from reticulospinal neurons is inhibited presynaptically, not by GABA (Alford and Grillner, 1991), but by serotonin and metabotropic glutamate receptors (Buchanan and Grillner, 1991; Krieger et al., 1996). These projection neurons are also presynaptically excited by AMPA-type glutamate receptors (Holt and Alford, 1995). The serotonin may directly influence the transmitter release machinery, downstream from Ca^{2+} influx, because serotonin does not block Ca^{2+} entry into the presynaptic terminals of these axons (Shupliakov et al., 1995). This presynaptic mechanism might enable the segmentally iterated neuronal network to control, at the segmental level, the excitability of the descending reticulospinal neurons. Serotonin also acts postsynaptically to change the firing frequency of network neurons directly by reducing their post-spike afterhyperpolarization, which in turn decreases the locomotor burst rate (Wallén et al., 1989). Serotonin thus appears to act presynaptically to reduce the level of excitatory input from the brain stem, thereby ensuring maintenance of the decreased locomotor burst frequency that results from its postsynaptic actions.

Network Output

Presynaptic control of network output onto its motoneuron targets has been documented in the leech heartbeat system, the molluscan feeding system, and the mammalian respiratory system. The leech heartbeat system includes seven pairs of segmentally iterated heart interneurons (HN cells), each of which projects an axon to posterior ganglia to inhibit other HN cells and heart excitor motoneurons (HE cells) (Calabrese, 1979; Calabrese and Feldman, chapter 11, this volume). The HN cells form a network that generates a rhythmic activity pattern that is imposed, via rhythmic synaptic inhibition, on HE cells. Each HN cell is also electrically coupled to posterior HN cells in the ganglion of origin of the posterior cell. Via the electrical synapse, posterior HN cells influence the local terminals of anterior HN cells. For example, hyperpolarizing an HN cell in ganglion 6 selectively eliminates the synaptic effects of other anterior HN cells within ganglion 6, even though they continue to have postsynaptic effects in other ganglia (Thompson and Stent, 1976; Nicholls and Wallace, 1978; Calabrese, 1979).

Neurotransmitter-mediated presynaptic inhibition can also control the postsynaptic effects that a rhythmically active neural network has on its motoneuronal targets. In an in vitro brainstem-spinal cord preparation of the neonatal rat, Dong and Feldman (1995; see also Calabrese and Feldman, chapter 11, this volume) showed that adenosine A_1 receptors regulate phrenic motoneuron excitation by means of bulbospinal neurons that are rhythmically active during the respiratory rhythm. The presynaptic nature of the adenosine-mediated inhibition on the axon terminals of the bulbospinal neurons was confirmed using several analyses of events that occurred in the postsynaptic motoneuron. Dong and Feldman (1995) also showed that presynaptic control of transmitter release is a naturally occurring event. Thus, adenosine receptor antagonists not only blocked the inhibitory effects of the applied adenosine agonist, but they also enhanced the synaptic response of inspiratory motoneurons to ongoing bulbospinal activity in the absence of the applied agonist.

A similar presynaptic control is exerted on the axon terminals of identified projection neurons that transmit the rhythmic feeding motor pattern in the mollusc *Aplysia californica* from the buccal ganglion, where it originates, to the cerebral ganglion (Chiel et al., 1988). The projection neurons synapse with feeding-related motoneurons in the cerebral ganglion. The synaptic efficacy from the projection neurons onto the motoneurons is presynaptically reduced by activation of an identified histaminergic mechanoafferent neuron. As in Dong and Feldman's study (1995) of respiration, Chiel and colleagues identified a presynaptic locus of action in several complementary analyses that were centered primarily on intrasomatic recordings from the postsynaptic neurons. In addition, based on the soma response of the projection neurons to histamine application, they suggested that the presynaptic inhibition is likely to shunt the spikes by causing a conductance-increase hyperpolar-

ization. They also hypothesized (Chiel et al., 1990) that the presynaptic inhibition might play a behaviorally appropriate role during feeding because the histaminergic neuron is strongly activated by an increased load, such as an unexpectedly tough piece of food. The combined pre- and postsynaptic effects of this neuron on feeding-related neurons might strengthen and prolong the swallowing phase to overcome an unexpected obstacle.

Neural Network Reconfiguration

Individual rhythmically active neural networks produce a series of distinct activity patterns as a result of modulatory inputs received from the CNS and from the periphery (Harris-Warrick and Marder, 1991; Marder and Calabrese, 1996). Modulatory inputs alter network activity by changing the membrane properties and/or the synaptic effects of network components. Most studies of neural network modulation have focused on the consequences of postsynaptic modulation (Harris-Warrick et al., chapter 19, and Kiehn et al., chapter 4, this volume), but recent work has shown that focal, presynaptic influences also contribute to the reconfiguration of neural networks.

In the stomatogastric nervous system (Selverston and Moulins, 1987; Harris-Warrick et al., 1992), the amines octopamine, dopamine, and serotonin each elicit a distinct pyloric motor pattern when bath applied to the stomatogastric ganglion (STG) of the spiny lobster, *Panulirus interruptus* (Flamm and Harris-Warrick, 1986a). The modified pyloric rhythm results at least partly from alterations in the membrane properties of pyloric network neurons (Flamm and Harris-Warrick, 1986b; Johnson and Harris-Warrick, 1990; Harris-Warrick et al., chapter 19, this volume). Some of those alterations, however, do not correlate with measurable changes in the input resistance of either the pre- or postsynaptic neuron, thereby suggesting that the applied amine has a focal influence at the synapse (Johnson and Harris-Warrick, 1990).

Dickinson and colleagues (1990, 1993) obtained even stronger evidence of presynaptic control of transmitter release in the spiny lobster STG. They showed that superfusion of the neuropeptide red pigment concentrating hormone (RPCH) to the isolated stomatogastric nervous system not only excited the pyloric network in the STG, but also activated the gastric mill and cardiac sac networks. The gastric mill network occurs in the STG, whereas cardiac sac network neurons are distributed among all four ganglia of the stomatogastric nervous system, including the STG. RPCH's activation of the cardiac sac network appears to result primarily from its ability to elicit rhythmic bursting activity in the inferior ventricular nerve (IVN) neurons, a pair of cardiac sac network neurons that project to all four ganglia to influence their network targets. Interestingly, in addition to eliciting rhythmic bursts from the IVN neurons, RPCH dramatically increases the postsynaptic potentials (PSPs) produced by these neurons in their network targets. This synaptic facilitation appears to be presynaptic in nature, in part because no change was recorded in either postsynaptic input resistance or PSP reversal potential (Dickinson et al., 1990). Although RPCH application to any single ganglion elicited rhythmic bursting from the IVN neurons that extended to its branches in other ganglia, PSP facilitation was significantly greater in the ganglion to which the peptide was directly applied, suggesting a direct RPCH influence on transmitter release (Dickinson et al., 1993). RPCH's presynaptic facilitation not only contributed to strengthening the cardiac sac motor pattern, but also enabled a functional fusion of the cardiac sac and gastric mill networks (Dickinson et al., 1990). The conjoint cardiac sac–gastric mill motor pattern results largely from the RPCH-mediated presynaptic enhancement of the IVN neurons' synaptic effects on gastric mill network neurons.

Recently, studies of the functional reconfiguration of CPG activity by presynaptic influences have progressed from the use of exogenously applied transmitters to a focus on the activation of individual identified neurons. Using the well-characterized escape network of the marine mollusc *Tritonia diomedea* (Getting, 1989), Katz and colleagues showed that presynaptic facilitation of transmitter release is a critical factor in determining whether the *Tritonia* escape network produces a relatively simple reflexive withdrawal response or the more complex escape swimming behavior (Katz et al., 1994; Katz and Frost, 1995). Although they could not test directly for the presence of presynaptic facilitation, Katz and Frost (1995; Frost et al., chapter 16, this volume) used a series of complementary approaches to document the presynaptic nature of the facilitation. The facilitatory neurons are a small group of serotonergic interneurons that are integral members of the escape network. The activity of the facilitated neuron, called C2, appears to be pivotal in the decision whether to withdraw or to swim. The presynaptic facilitation of C2 enables the system to produce the escape swimming response. The effects of serotonergic neuron stimulation were also mimicked by bath application of serotonin (Katz et al., 1994). In the *Tritonia* system, the placement of the facilitatory events at the presynaptic side of the C2 synapses enables sero-

tonin to reconfigure the functional network more elaborately, thereby contributing further to swim pattern generation. Specifically, the released serotonin concomitantly decreases the synaptic strength of the serotonergic neurons themselves onto the same postsynaptic neurons that receive facilitated excitation from C2 (Katz and Frost, 1995).

Presynaptic influences on the terminals of interneurons in the lamprey spinal cord and the crab stomatogastric system have been directly documented recently. In the lamprey swimming system (Grillner et al., 1995), intra-axonal recordings from excitatory and inhibitory interneurons belonging to the locomotor network have shown that the interneurons are depolarized in phase with each burst of ipsilateral ventral root discharge during the swimming motor pattern (Alford et al., 1991). The depolarizations are mediated by the combined activation of $GABA_A$ and $GABA_B$ receptors (Alford et al., 1991). In contrast to the phasic depolarizations in the sensory dorsal cells, these depolarizations are blocked by commonly used GABA receptor antagonists.

The mechanism underlying GABA-mediated presynaptic inhibition in lamprey network interneurons has been studied by simultaneously recording from the axons of the inhibited interneurons and their postsynaptic target neurons. Exogenously applied GABA or the $GABA_B$ agonist, baclofen, reduces the amplitude of monosynaptic PSPs in the target neurons (Alford and Grillner, 1991). Baclofen's effect is mediated via a pertussis toxin-sensitive G-protein that blocks calcium channels and decreases transmitter release (Matsushima et al., 1993). Whereas baclofen affects only the duration of the presynaptic spikes, GABA reduces both the amplitude and duration of the spike. GABA activates $GABA_A$ and $GABA_B$ receptors, which act through different, but complementary, mechanisms to decrease the ability of spikes to evoke transmitter release (Alford and Grillner, 1991; Grillner et al., 1995). The GABAergic presynaptic inhibition may allow local segmental networks to modulate interneuronal synaptic output in relation to the ongoing motor pattern. Furthermore, the level of such GABAergic presynaptic inhibition can modulate the overall activity of the locomotor network, thus changing the rate and intersegmental coordination of motoneuron activity along the spinal cord (Tegnér et al., 1993).

Recent studies of the isolated crab stomatogastric system has shown that presynaptic inhibition can selectively suppress chemical transmission without affecting electrical transmission from the same presynaptic neuron (Coleman et al., 1995). In this preparation, it is possible

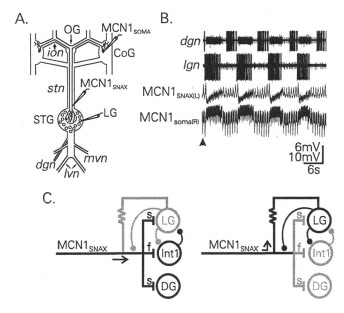

Figure 22.6

An example of presynaptic inhibition in the isolated crab stomatogastric nervous system (STNS). Presynaptic inhibition is pivotal to activation of the gastric mill rhythm by MCN1, a modulatory projection neuron in the crab STNS. (A) Schematic of the STNS, including the intrasomatic and intra-axonal recording sites of MCN1 and the LG neuron, a gastric mill network neuron. Abbreviations: CoG, commissural ganglion; *dgn*, dorsal gastric nerve; *ion*, inferior oesophageal nerve; *lvn*, lateral ventricular nerve; MCN1$_{SNAX}$, stomatogastric nerve axon of modulatory commissural neuron 1; *mvn*, medial ventricular nerve; OG, oesophageal ganglion; STG, stomatogastric ganglion; *stn*, stomatogastric nerve. (Reproduced from Coleman and Nusbaum, 1994, with permission.) B. Activation of the gastric mill rhythm by continual intracellular stimulation of MCN1$_{soma-RIGHT}$ (arrowhead). Prior to MCN1$_{soma}$ stimulation, all gastric mill neurons were inactive. During this rhythm, MCN1$_{SNAX-LEFT}$ receives rhythmic inhibition from LG (*lgn*). MCN1$_{SNAX-LEFT}$ is silent, but it undergoes pyloric rhythm–timed membrane potential oscillations between bouts of gastric mill rhythm–timed inhibition from LG. Note that MCN1$_{soma-RIGHT}$ activity persists in the CoG despite its own STG terminals also being inhibited by LG. The fast rhythmic inhibition in MCN1$_{soma}$ results from feedback it receives in the CoG (as well as in the STG) from the pyloric network. (Reproduced from Nusbaum, 1994, with permission.) C. Presynaptic inhibition switches the effective mode of MCN1 transmission and, consequently, the targets activated by MCN1. (Left) When LG is inactive (grey shading), MCN1 chemically excites the gastric mill neurons. Interneuron 1 (Int1) is activated faster than LG and its inhibitory effects delay LG burst onset. This enables DG to also burst. Eventually, the MCN1 excitation of LG enables LG to escape from (Int1) inhibition and fire spikes. (Right) When LG is active (black shading), it inhibits Int1 and presynaptically inhibits MCN1$_{SNAX}$, silencing Int1 and DG. At this time, LG also loses its chemical excitatory input, but it repolarizes slowly. During the first few seconds of this repolarization, the electrical EPSPs that it receives from MCN1 are sufficient to maintain the LG burst. Eventually, LG stops firing, and MCN1 again releases transmitter and excites Int1, thereby silencing LG. (Reproduced from Coleman et al., 1995, with permission.)

to make intra-axonal recordings, at the entrance to the STG, from modulatory projection neurons that originate in other ganglia (figure 22.6A). These intra-axonal recordings are electrotonically close to the STG terminals of these projection neurons and are distant from their ganglion of origin. Using this approach, Nusbaum and colleagues (1992) showed that the STG terminals of a modulatory projection neuron called MCN1 receives inhibitory postsynaptic potentials (IPSPs) from an STG network neuron. This presynaptic inhibition causes a fast-onset, glutamate-mediated hyperpolarization that effectively inhibits chemical synaptic transmission from MCN1 in the STG (Coleman and Nusbaum, 1994). MCN1 is a multitransmitter neuron whose activity excites and activates the pyloric and gastric mill rhythms in the STG (see figure 22.6B; Nusbaum et al., 1992; Coleman and Nusbaum, 1994; Christie et al., 1993).

The gastric mill rhythm controls chewing. When this rhythm is elicited by tonic activation of the MCN1 soma, the STG terminals of MCN1 are rhythmically inhibited by the lateral gastric (LG) neuron, a gastric mill protractor neuron (see figure 22.6B). For several reasons, this presynaptic inhibition is pivotal in enabling MCN1 to elicit the gastric mill rhythm. First, each rhythmic LG burst reduces or eliminates all of the transmitter-mediated excitatory effects of MCN1, thereby effectively terminating activity of the gastric mill retractor neurons (see figure 22.6C): the slow, transmitter-mediated excitation that LG receives from MCN1 during each retractor phase enables LG to escape from the inhibition it receives from a retractor phase neuron (labeled interneuron 1 in figure 22.6C) and to begin to fire. Second, the presynaptic inhibition contributes to the activation of LG and other protractor neurons: although the protractor neurons lose their neurotransmitter-elicited excitatory input from MCN1, they also receive electrical excitation from MCN1, and this input in not suppressed by the presynaptic inhibition (see figure 22.6C; Coleman et al., 1995; Coleman, 1995).

The rhythmic switching of MCN1 output from neurotransmitter to electrical excitation occurs only in the STG. It does not influence the MCN1 synaptic interactions in its ganglion of origin (Coleman and Nusbaum, 1994). Traditionally, projection neurons such as MCN1 have been considered only as inputs to rhythmically active networks but not as integral network components. Indeed, using only the information obtained from intrasomatic recordings, it does appear that MCN1 serves only as an input to the gastric mill network, not as a network component. However, the local synaptic interactions involving the STG terminals of MCN1 clearly indicate that it is a member of the gastric mill network itself, whose rhythmic activity it also initiates.

Conclusions and Future Directions

Presynaptic inputs clearly influence rhythmic motor systems. They rhythmically gate both the sensory input to central neural networks and the output from that network onto its motoneuronal targets. These influences seem, in part, to enable sensory input to be better coordinated with an ongoing movement. Moreover, presynaptic inputs alter centrally generated rhythmic patterns by modifying transmission to the network and between the network neurons. Presumably, such effects contribute to the selection of one particular motor pattern over others. We have yet to determine how presynaptic inputs influence rhythmic CPG systems during real, rather than fictive, performance of various motor behaviors, however.

Both the placement of presynaptic inputs near transmitter release sites and their tendency to influence the neuron only focally at these sites have made it technically daunting to learn directly about the mechanisms by which these inputs alter transmitter release. Most work to date has studied these influences indirectly—either downstream via the postsynaptic neuron, or upstream via the axon proximal to the synapse. Although these experimental approaches have been complemented by modeling studies (e.g., Segev, 1990; Zytnicki and L'Hote, 1993; Graham and Redman, 1994; Hatsopoulos et al., 1995), new approaches such as optical recording techniques (Salzberg and Obaid, 1988; Parsons et al., 1992) and patch clamp recordings (Bielefeldt and Jackson, 1993) will offer better access to the sites of presynaptic input than can be achieved by the use of intracellular recording electrodes.

One particularly intriguing feature of presynaptic input is the ability of such inputs to compartmentalize a neuron into regions with specific functions, which enables some branches of the neuron to release more or less transmitter than other branches. This feature has already been documented in a few cases, and it may occur in others. Clearly, presynaptic mechanisms considerably expand the computational power of the nervous system, but it also makes it more difficult for modelers and experimental neurobiologists to understand the neuronal basis of behavior. The growing attention being paid to presynaptic inputs will hopefully engender new insights regarding their roles in rhythmic motor control and in other aspects of signaling within the central nervous system.

Acknowledgments

Work in the lab of Michael P. Nusbaum is supported by NIH (NS-29436), NSF (IBN94-96264), and the Human Frontiers Science Program. Abdeljabbar El Manira is supported by the Swedish MRC (project # 11562) and Karolinska Institute Funds. Jean-Pierre Gossard and Serge Rossignol wish to thank the Canadian MRC and the FRSQ for their support and Dr. I. Beloozerova for figure 22.5.

References

Alford S, Christenson J, Grillner S (1991) Presynaptic GABA$_A$ and GABA$_B$ receptor-mediated phasic modulation in axons of spinal motor interneurons. *Eur J Neurosci* 3:107–117.

Alford S, Grillner S (1991) The involvement of GABA$_B$ receptors and coupled G-proteins in spinal GABAergic presynaptic inhibition. *J Neurosci* 11:3718–3726.

Baev KV (1978) Periodic changes in primary afferent depolarization during fictitious locomotion by thalamic cats. *Neurophysiology* 10:316–317.

Baev KV (1980) Polarization of primary afferent terminals in the lumbar spinal cord during fictitious locomotion. *Neurophysiology* 12:305–311.

Baev KV, Kostyuk PG (1981) Primary afferent depolarization evoked by the activity of spinal scratching generator. *Neuroscience* 6:205–215.

Baev KV, Kostyuk PG (1982) Polarization of primary afferent terminals of lumbosacral cord elicited by the activity of spinal locomotor generator. *Neuroscience* 7:1401–1409.

Beloozerova IN, Rossignol S (1994) Antidromic activity of dorsal root filaments during treadmill locomotion in thalamic cats. *Soc Neurosci Abstr* 20:1755.

Beloozerova I, Rossignol S (1995) Antidromic activity in uncut dorsal roots of the cat. *Soc Neurosci Abstr* 21:413.

Bielefeldt K, Jackson MB (1993) A calcium-activated potassium channel causes frequency-dependent action potential failures in a mammalian nerve terminal. *J Neurophysiol* 70:284–298.

Bongianni F, Christenson J, Hökfelt T, Grillner S (1990) Neuropeptide Y-immunoreactive spinal neurons make close appositions on axons of primary sensory afferents. *Brain Res* 523:337–341.

Brooks C, Koizumi K (1956) Origin of the dorsal root reflex. *J Neurophysiol* 19:61–74.

Brooks CM, Koizumi K, Malcolm JL (1955) Effects of changes in temperature on reactions of spinal cord. *J Neurophysiol* 18:205–216.

Buchanan JT, Grillner S (1991) 5-Hydroxytryptamine depresses reticulospinal excitatory postsynaptic potentials in motoneurons of the lamprey. *Neurosci Lett* 112:71–74.

Burrows M, Laurent G (1993) Synaptic potentials in the central terminals of locust proprioceptive afferents generated by other afferents from the same sense organ. *J Neurosci* 13:808–819.

Burrows M, Matheson T (1994) A presynaptic gain control mechanism among sensory neurons of a locust leg proprioceptor. *J Neurosci* 14: 272–282.

Calabrese RL (1979) The roles of endogenous membrane properties and synaptic interaction in generating the heartbeat rhythm of the leech, *Hirudo medicinalis*. *J Exp Biol* 82:163–176.

Casey KL, Oakley B (1972) Intraspinal latency, cutaneous fiber composition, and afferent control of the dorsal root reflex in cat. *Brain Res* 47: 353–369.

Cattaert D, El Manira A, Clarac F (1992) Direct evidence for presynaptic inhibitory mechanisms in crayfish sensory afferents. *J Neurophysiol* 67:610–624.

Cattaert D, El Manira A, Clarac F (1994) Chloride conductance produces both presynaptic inhibition and antidromic action potentials in primary afferents. *Brain Res* 666:109–112.

Catton WT (1961) Threshold, recovery, and fatigue of tactile receptors in frog skin. *J Physiol (Lond)* 158:333–365.

Chiel HJ, Kupfermann I, Weiss KR (1988) An identified histaminergic neuron can modulate the outputs of buccal-cerebral interneurons in *Aplysia* via presynaptic inhibition. *J Neurosci* 8:49–63.

Chiel HJ, Weiss KR, Kupfermann I (1990) Multiple roles of a histaminergic afferent neuron in the feeding behavior of *Aplysia. Trends Neurosci* 13:223–227.

Christenson J, Boman A, Lagerbäck P, Grillner S (1988) The dorsal cell, one class of primary sensory neuron in the lamprey spinal cord. I. Touch, pressure but no nociception: A physiological study. *Brain Res* 44:1–8.

Christenson J, Bongianni F, Grillner S, Hökfelt T (1991) Putative GABAergic input to axons of spinal interneurons and primary sensory neurons in the lamprey spinal cord as shown by intracellular Lucifer Yellow and GABA immunohistochemistry. *Brain Res* 538:313–318.

Christenson J, Grillner S (1991) Primary afferents evoke excitatory amino acid receptor-mediated EPSPs that are modulated by presynaptic GABA$_B$ receptors in lamprey. *J Neurophysiol* 66:2141–2149.

Christie AE, Norris BJ, Coleman MJ, Marder E, Nusbaum MP (1993) Neuropil arborization and transmitter complement of a modulatory projection neuron. *Soc Neurosci Abstr* 19:931.

Clarac F, El Manira A, Cattaert D (1992) Presynaptic control as a mechanism of sensory-motor integration. *Curr Opin Neurobiol* 2:764–769.

Coleman MJ (1995) Dynamic modulation of a rhythmically active neural network in the stomatogastric nervous system of the crab, *Cancer borealis*. Ph.D. dissertation, University of Alabama, Birmingham, Alabama.

Coleman MJ, Meyrand P, Nusbaum MP (1995) Presynaptic inhibition mediates a switch between two modes of synaptic transmission. *Nature* 378:502–505.

Coleman MJ, Nusbaum MP (1994) Functional consequences of compartmentalization of synaptic input. *J Neurosci* 14:6544–6552.

Dickinson PS, Mecsas C, Hetling J, Terio K (1993) The neuropeptide red pigment concentrating hormone affects rhythmic pattern generation at multiple sites. *J Neurophysiol* 69:1475–1483.

Dickinson PS, Mecsas C, Marder E (1990) Neuropeptide fusion of two motor-pattern generator circuits. *Nature* 344:155–158.

Dolphin AC, Scott RH (1987) Calcium channel currents and their inhibition by (-)-baclofen in rat sensory neurones: Modulation by guanosine nucleotides. *J Physiol (Lond)* 386:1–17.

Dong X-W, Feldman JL (1995) Modulation of inspiratory drive to phrenic motoneurons by presynaptic adenosine A$_1$ receptors. *J Neurosci* 15:3458–3467.

Dubuc R, Cabelguen J-M, Rossignol S (1985) Rhythmic antidromic discharges of single primary afferents recorded in cut dorsal roots filaments during locomotion in the cat. *Brain Res* 359:375–378.

Dubuc R, Cabelguen J-M, Rossignol S (1987) Antidromic discharges of primary afferents during locomotion. In: *Motor Control* (Gantchev GN, Dimitrov B, Gatev P, eds), 165–169. New York: Plenum.

Dubuc R, Cabelguen J-M, Rossignol S (1988) Rhythmic fluctuations of dorsal root potentials and antidromic discharges of single primary afferents during fictive locomotion in the cat. *J Neurophysiol* 60:2014–2036.

Duchen MR (1986) Excitation of mouse motoneurons by GABA-mediated primary afferent depolarization. *Brain Res* 379:182–187.

Duenas SH, Loeb GE, Marks WB (1990) Monosynaptic and dorsal root reflexes during locomotion in normal and thalamic cats. *J Neurophysiol* 63:1467–1476.

Duenas SH, Rudomin P (1988) Excitability changes of ankle extensor group Ia and Ib fibers during fictive locomotion in the cat. *Exp Brain Res* 70:15–25.

Dunlap K, Fischbach GD (1981) Neurotransmitters decrease the calcium conductance activated by depolarization of embryonic chick sensory neurons. *J Physiol (Lond)* 317:519–535.

Eccles JC, Kozak W, Magni F (1961) Dorsal root reflexes of muscle group I afferent fibres. *J Physiol (Lond)* 159:128–146.

Eccles RM, Willis WD (1962) Presynaptic inhibition of the monosynaptic reflex pathway in kittens. *J Physiol (Lond)* 165:403–420.

Eguibar JR, Quevedo J, Jimenez I, Rudomin P (1994) Selective cortical control of information flow through different intraspinal collaterals of the same muscle afferent fibers. *Brain Res* 643:328–333.

El Manira A, Cattaert D, Wallén P, DiCaprio RA, Clarac F (1993) Electrical coupling of mechanoreceptor afferents in the crayfish: A possible mechanism for enhancement of sensory signal transmission. *J Neurophysiol* 69:2248–2251.

El Manira A, Clarac F (1991) GABA-mediated presynaptic inhibition in crayfish primary afferents by non-A, non-B GABA receptors. *Eur J Neurosci* 3:1208–1218.

El Manira A, Clarac F (1994) Presynaptic inhibition is mediated by histamine and GABA during the crustacean escape reaction. *J Neurophysiol* 71:1088–1095.

El Manira A, DiCaprio RA, Cattaert D, Clarac F (1991) Monosynaptic interjoint reflexes and their central modulation during fictive locomotion in crayfish. *Eur J Neurosci* 3:1219–1231.

Presynaptic Mechanisms during Rhythmic Activity

El Manira A, Tegnér J, Grillner S (1997) Locomotor-related presynaptic modulation of primary afferents in the lamprey. *Eur J Neurosci* 9:696–705.

Flamm RE, Harris-Warrick RM (1986a) Aminergic modulation in lobster stomatogastric ganglion. I. Effects on the motor pattern and individual neurons within the pyloric circuit. *J Neurophysiol* 55:847–865.

Flamm RE, Harris-Warrick RM (1986b) Aminergic modulation in lobster stomatogastric ganglion. II. Target neurons of dopamine, octopamine, and serotonin within the pyloric circuit. *J Neurophysiol* 55:866–881.

Getting PA (1989) Emerging principles governing the operation of neural networks. *Annu Rev Neurosci* 12:185–204.

Gossard J-P (1995) Do antidromic discharges in primary afferents have post-synaptic effects? *Soc Neurosci Abstr* 21:414.

Gossard J-P, Cabelguen J-M, Brustein E, Rossignol S (1994) Locomotor-related modulation of dorsal root potentials evoked by the stimulation of the medullary reticular formation (MRF) during fictive locomotion in the cat. *Soc Neurosci Abstr* 20:793.

Gossard J-P, Cabelguen J-M, Rossignol S (1989) Intra-axonal recordings of cutaneous primary afferents during fictive locomotion in the cat. *J Neurophysiol* 62:1177–1188.

Gossard J-P, Cabelguen J-M, Rossignol S (1990) Phase-dependent modulation of primary afferent depolarization in single cutaneous primary afferents evoked by peripheral stimulation during fictive locomotion in the cat. *Brain Res* 537:14–23.

Gossard J-P, Cabelguen J-M, Rossignol S (1991) An intracellular study of muscle primary afferents during fictive locomotion in the cat. *J Neurophysiol* 65:914–926.

Gossard J-P, Rossignol S (1990) Phase-dependent modulation of dorsal root potentials evoked by peripheral nerve stimulation during fictive locomotion in the cat. *Brain Res* 537:1–13.

Graham B, Redman S (1994) A simulation of action potentials in synaptic boutons during presynaptic inhibition. *J Neurophysiol* 71:538–549.

Grillner S, Deliagina T, Ekeberg Ö, El Manira A, Hill RH, Lansner A, Orlovsky GN, Wallén P (1995) Neural networks that co-ordinate locomotion and body orientation in lamprey. *Trends Neurosci* 18:270–279.

Habgood JS (1950) Sensitization of sensory receptors in the frog's skin. *J Physiol (Lond)* 111:195–213.

Habgood JS (1953) Antidromic impulses in the dorsal roots. *J Physiol (Lond)* 121:264–274.

Harris-Warrick RM, Marder E (1991) Modulation of neural networks for behavior. *Ann Rev Neurosci* 14:39–57.

Harris-Warrick RM, Marder E, Selverston AI, Moulins M, eds (1992) *Dynamic Biological Networks: The Stomatogastric Nervous System.* Cambridge, Mass.: MIT Press.

Hatsopoulos NG, Burrows M, Laurent G (1995) Hysteresis reduction in proprioception using presynaptic shunting inhibition. *J Neurophysiol* 73:1031–1042.

Holt AJ, Alford S (1995) Excitatory synaptic input to axons in the spinal cord. *Soc Neurosci Abstr* 21:1092.

Hursh JB (1940) Relayed impulses in ascending branches of dorsal root fibers. *J Neurophysiol* 3:166–174.

Ito F (1968) Recovery curves of thresholds of muscle spindle, leaf-like and tendon receptors in the frog sartorius muscle after an antidromic discharge. *Jpn J Physiol* 18:731–745.

Johnson BR, Harris-Warrick RM (1990) Aminergic modulation of graded synaptic transmission in the lobster stomatogastric ganglion. *J Neurosci* 10:2066–2076.

Katz PS, Frost WN (1995) Intrinsic neuromodulation in the *Tritonia* swim CPG: The serotonergic dorsal swim interneurons act presynaptically to enhance transmitter release from interneuron C2. *J Neurosci* 15:6035–6045.

Katz PS, Getting PA, Frost WN (1994) Dynamic neuromodulation of synaptic strength intrinsic to a central pattern generator circuit. *Nature* 367:729–731.

Kolta A, Lund JP, Westberg K-G, Clavelou P (1995) Do muscle-spindle afferents act as interneurons during mastication? *Trends Neurosci* 18:441.

Krieger P, El Manira A, Grillner S (1996) Activation of pharmacologically distinct metabotropic glutamate receptors depresses reticulospinal-evoked monosynaptic EPSPs in the lamprey spinal cord. *J Neurophysiol* 76:3834–3841.

Levine JD, Fields HL, Basbaum AI (1993) Peptides and the primary afferent nociceptor. *J Neurosci* 13:2273–2286.

Lindblom UF (1958) Excitability and functional organization within a peripheral tactile unit. *Acta Physiol Scand* 44, Suppl 153:1–84.

Loewenstein WR (1959) The generation of electric activity in a nerve ending. *Ann NY Acad Sci* 81:367–387.

Marder E, Calabrese RL (1996) Principles of rhythmic motor pattern generation. *Physiol Rev* 76:687–717.

Matsushima T, Tegnèr J, Hill RH, Grillner S (1993) GABA$_B$ receptor activation causes a depression of low and high voltage-activated Ca^{2+}-currents, postinhibitory rebound, and post-spike afterhyperpolarization in lamprey neurons. *J Neurophysiol* 70:2606–2619.

Nicoll RA, Alger BE (1979) Presynaptic inhibition: Transmitter and ionic mechanisms. *Int Rev Neurobiol* 21:217–258.

Nicholls J, Wallace BG (1978) Modulation of transmission at an inhibitory synapse in the central nervous system of the leech. *J Physiol (Lond)* 281:157–170.

Nusbaum MP (1994) Presynaptic control of neurones in pattern-generating networks. *Curr Opin Neurobiol* 4:909–914.

Nusbaum MP, Weimann JM, Golowasch J, Marder E (1992) Presynaptic control of modulatory fibers by their neural network targets. *J Neurosci* 12:2706–2714.

Parsons TD, Obaid AL, Salzberg BM (1992) Aminoglycoside antibiotics block votage-dependent calcium channels in intact vertebrate nerve terminals. *J Gen Physiol* 99:491–504.

Pasztor VM, Bush BMH (1987) Peripheral modulation of mechanosensitivity in primary afferent neurons. *Nature* 326:793–795.

Pasztor VM, Lange AB, Orchard I (1988) Stretch-induced release of proctolin from the dendrites of a lobster sense organ. *Brain Res* 458:199–203.

Pearson KG (1993) Common principles of motor control in vertebrates and invertebrates. *Annu Rev Neurosci* 16:265–297.

Peng YY, Frank E (1989a) Activation of GABA$_A$ receptors causes presnaptic and postsynaptic inhibition at synapses between muscle spindle afferents and motoneurons in the spinal cord of bullfrogs. *J Neurosci* 9:1516–1522.

Peng YY, Frank E (1989b) Activation of GABA$_B$ receptors causes presynaptic inhibition at synapses between muscles spindle afferents and motoneurons in the spinal cord of bullfrogs. *J Neurosci* 9:1502–1515.

Pereda AE, Bell TD, Faber DS (1995) Retrograde synaptic communication via gap junctions coupling auditory afferents to the Mauthner cell. *J Neurosci* 15:5943–5955.

Pilyavskii AI, Yakhnitsa IA, Bulgakova NV (1988) Studies of the antidromic impulsation of dorsal roots during real locomotion of rats. *Neirofiziologiya* 20:579–585.

Pilyavskii AI, Yakhnitsa IA, Bulgakova NV (1989) Antidromic dorsal root impulses during naturally occurring locomotion in rats. *Neurophysiology* 20:417–422.

Rossignol S (1996) Neural control of stereotypic limb movements. In: *Handbook of Physiology*, sec. 12 (Rowell LB, Shepherd JT, eds), 173–216. New York: Oxford University.

Rossignol S, Lund JP, Drew T (1988) The role of sensory inputs in regulating patterns of rhythmical movements in higher vertebrates: A comparison between locomotion, respiration, and mastication. In: *Neural Control of Rhythmic Movements in Vertebrates* (Cohen A, Rossignol S, Grillner S, eds), 201–283. New York: Wiley and Sons.

Rudomin P (1990) Presynaptic inhibition of muscle spindle and tendon organ afferents in the mammalian spinal cord. *Trends Neurosci* 13:499–505.

Rudomin P, Quevedo J, Eguibar JR (1993) Presynaptic modulation of spinal reflexes. *Curr Opin Neurobiol* 3:997–1004.

Salzberg BM, Obaid AL (1988) Optical studies of the secretory event at vertebrate never terminals. *J Exp Biol* 139:195–231.

Segev I (1990) Computer study of presynaptic inhibition controlling the spread of action potentials into axon terminals. *J Neurophysiol* 63:987–998.

Selverston AI, Moulins M, eds (1987) *The Crustacean Stomatogastric System*. Berlin: Springer.

Shupliakov O, Pieriborne VA, Gad H, Brodin L (1995) Synaptic vesicle depletion in reticulospinal axons is reduced by 5-hydroxytryptamine: Direct evidence for presynaptic modulation of glutamatergic transmission. *Eur J Neurosci* 7:1111–1116.

Sillar KT, Simmers AJ (1994) Presynaptic inhibition of primary afferent transmitter release by 5-hydroxytryptamine at a mechanosensory synapse in the vertebrate spinal cord. *J Neurosci* 14:2636–2647.

Sillar KT, Skorupski P (1986) Central input to primary afferent neurons in crayfish, *Pacifastacus leniusculus*, is correlated with rhythmic motor output of thoracic ganglia. *J Neurophysiol* 55:678–688.

Sillar KT, Wedderburn JFS, Simmers AJ (1992) Modulation of swimming rhythmicity by 5-hydroxytryptamine during post-embryonic development in *Xenopus laevis*. *Proc R Soc Lond (Biol)* 250:107–114.

Skorupski P, Sillar KT (1986) Phase-dependent reversal of reflexes mediated by the thoracocoxal muscle receptor organ in the crayfish, *Pacifastacus leniusculus*. *J Neurophysiol* 55:689–695.

Stehouwer DJ, Farel PB (1981) Sensory interactions with a central motor program in anuran larvae. *Brain Res* 218:131–140.

Stuart GJ, Redman SJ (1992) The role of GABAa and GABAb receptors in presynaptic inhibition of Ia EPSPs in cat spinal motoneurones. *J Physiol (Lond)* 447:675–692.

Tegnér J, Matsushima T, El Manira A, Grillner S (1993) The spinal GABA system modulates burst frequency and intersegmental coordination in the lamprey: Differential effects of GABA$_A$ and GABA$_B$ receptors. *J Neurophysiol* 69:647–657.

Thompson WJ, Stent GS (1976) Neuronal control of heartbeat in the medicinal leech. III. Synaptic relations of heart interneurons. *J Comp Physiol* 111:309–333.

Toennies JF (1939) Conditioning of afferent impulses by reflex discharges over the dorsal roots. *J Neurophysiol* 2:515–525.

Wall PD (1958) Excitability changes in afferent fibre terminations and their relation to slow potentials. *J Physiol (Lond)* 142:1–21.

Wall PD (1964) Presynaptic control of impulses at the first central synapse in the cutaneous pathway. *Prog Brain Res* 12:92–115.

Wall PD (1994) Control of impulse conduction in long range branches of afferents by increases and decreases of primary afferent depolarization in the rat. *Eur J Neurosci* 6:1136–1142.

Wallén P, Christenson J, Brodin L, Hill R, Lansner A, Grillner S (1989) Mechanisms underlying the serotonergic modulation of the spinal circuitry for locomotion in lamprey. *Prog Brain Res* 80:321–327.

Watson AH (1992) Presynaptic modulation of sensory afferents in the invertebrate and vertebrate nervous system. *Comp Biochem Physiol* 103:227–239.

Wikström M, El Manira A, Zhang W, Grillner S (1995) Dopamine and 5-HT modulation of synaptic transmission in the lamprey spinal cord. *Soc Neurosci Abstr* 21:1145.

Wolf H, Burrows M (1995) Proprioceptive sensory neurons of a locust leg receive rhythmic presynaptic inhibition during walking. *J Neurosci* 15:5623–5636.

Yakhnitsa IA, Pilyavskii AI, Bulgakova NV (1988) Phase-dependent changes in dorsal root potential during actual locomotion in rats. *Neurophysiology* 20:241–246.

Zytnicki D, L'Hote G (1993) Neuromimetric model of neuronal filter. *Biol Cybern* 70:115–121.

Part VI

Sensory Modification of Motor Output to Control Whole-Body Orientation

23

Control of Body Orientation and Equilibrium in Vertebrates

Jane M. Macpherson,
Tatiana G. Deliagina, and
Grigori N. Orlovsky

Abstract

Postural behaviors encompass two components, postural orientation and postural equilibrium. Orientation refers to the relative positioning of the body segments with respect to each other and with respect to the environment. Orienting behaviors are observed in both terrestrial and aquatic animals; for example, the body is often aligned with respect to such environmental cues as the gravito-inertial force. Postural equilibrium requires the control of the position and velocity of the body's center of mass in space. In order to maintain equilibrium, forces are applied at the interface between the body and the environment—for example, by the feet against the ground or by the fins against water. These forces must counteract all external forces including that due to gravity. Postural orientation and equilibrium are achieved through complex sensorimotor processes that involve the integration of information from proprioceptive, cutaneous, visual, and vestibular inputs. The various inputs are weighted differently depending on many factors such as task conditions and prior experience. Terrestrial vertebrates such as the cat depend heavily on proprioceptive inputs, particularly during stance behavior. Aquatic vertebrates such as the lamprey depend more heavily on vestibular inputs for postural orientation and equilibrium. In the lamprey, the brainstem reticular formation plays an important role in integrating sensory inputs and in organizing motor behaviors for posture. Brainstem and cerebellar structures may be equally important for postural control in higher vertebrates as well.

Adequate control of body posture is vital for the coordinated control of almost all motor behaviors in vertebrates (reviewed in Horak and Macpherson, 1996). An optimal postural orientation can facilitate the performance of a goal-directed task. Control of postural equilibrium is required for even simple behaviors, such as standing and walking. Postural behaviors are both reactive and predictive: the neuromusculoskeletal system of vertebrates is adapted for making rapid and automatic responses to disturbances of postural equilibrium. Such disturbances may arise not only from external events, such as the sudden acceleration of a bus in which one is standing, but also from self-generated movements. Voluntary movements are accompanied and even preceded by postural adjustments that are evoked in a feedforward manner as part of the central program for the movement. The adjustments stabilize the body and minimize the disturbance to balance.

This chapter focuses on two general problems related to the control of posture in vertebrates. First, the musculoskeletal system of vertebrates has many degrees of freedom to control because it is made up of hundreds of muscles and joints. One strategy the nervous system may use to reduce the number of degrees of freedom is to select a few, global variables to control (Bernstein, 1967; Horak and Macpherson, 1996). The first part of this chapter reviews some neural strategies in cats observed during postural responses to sudden movements of the support surface.

A second problem related to the control of posture concerns the organization and operation of the basic neuronal mechanisms (i.e., the networks) responsible for postural control. Little is known about where and how postural behaviors are organized in higher vertebrates. Studies of patients have suggested the involvement of the cerebellum, basal ganglia, and the cerebral cortex (reviewed in Horak and Macpherson, 1996), but the role of each region in postural control remains unclear. In contrast, lower vertebrates—such as the lamprey, *Cyclostome*—present a rich opportunity for analytical studies of the organization and operation of the neural circuits for postural control. Not only is the basic structure of the lamprey nervous system similar to that of higher vertebrates (Kappers et al., 1936), but one can directly study the neural activity of the isolated lamprey brain and spinal cord during fictive motor behaviors (i.e., patterned neural activity in the absence of movement; Grillner et al., 1995). In the second part of this chapter, we consider the neuronal mechanisms for the control of body orientation and equilibrium in the lamprey.

Postural Control in the Cat

Postural Orientation

Most vertebrates adopt habitual postures that give rise to a characteristic silhouette. Such postures are related not only to the particular morphology of a species, but also to behavioral and biomechanical factors. For example, appropriate trunk and appendage orientation to the relevant features of a task can optimize task performance. Similarly, maintaining a vertical alignment of the body segments allows humans to reduce the moments of force due to gravity and to minimize the energy required to maintain stance. Another feature of habitual postures may be the simplification or optimization of required responses to unexpected disturbances of posture. Finally, postural orientation may be used to *control* sensory inputs

in order to optimize motor performance. For example, by stabilizing the head with respect to earth vertical, the task of interpreting inputs from the head-based vestibular and visual sensors may be simplified. The cervical column in both quadrupeds and bipeds is oriented near earth vertical during quiet standing or sitting (Vidal et al., 1986), and the head and eyes are often oriented in such a way that gaze is parallel to the horizon (Pozzo et al., 1990), particularly during motor behaviors that are more challenging to the balance system. With such a postural orientation, vestibular and visual information may be more easily integrated into a coherent signal that represents the position and velocity of head-in-space.

Recent studies in cats have demonstrated certain invariant features in postural orientation. Fung and Macpherson (1995) defined an optimal stance posture in the cat characterized by a vertical forelimb axis and an inwardly inclined hindlimb axis. The trunk axis, defined as the line joining hip and shoulder joints, was aligned with the support surface. For both forelimb and hindlimb, the ground reaction forces were angled inward, resulting in a compressive force along the long axis of the trunk, which helps keep the trunk from sagging and reduces the requirement for tonic trunk muscle activity. A characteristic feature of cat stance is trunk axis invariance: regardless of whether the support surface is tilted (Lacquaniti et al., 1990) or the distance between fore- and hindlimbs is changed (Fung and Macpherson, 1995), the trunk maintains a constant orientation parallel to the support surface—a remarkable feature because in the cat the hindlimb is significantly longer than the forelimb and must be maintained in a semiflexed posture for the trunk to remain level.

We postulate that the constraints that characterize the postural orientation system may help to simplify the dynamic responses required to maintain postural equilibrium following unexpected disturbances of stance from various postures (Macpherson, 1994a).

Postural Equilibrium

Two variables must be controlled to maintain postural equilibrium: (1) the position of the center of mass (CoM) of the body and (2) the angular momentum of the body about the center of mass. This part of the chapter focuses on the first aspect of equilibrium control. During stance in a terrestrial environment, the horizontal position of the body's CoM must remain within the base of support for the body to be in equilibrium. The base of support in the standing quadruped is a quadrangle whose corners are the paws' points of contact with the ground. The

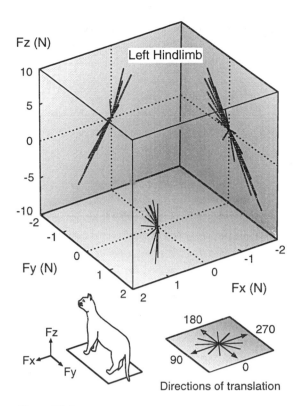

Figure 23.1
The force constraint strategy is used by the standing cat in response to unexpected movements of the supporting platform. Vectors show the mean change in force from quiet stance levels under the left hindlimb during the response evoked by linear translation of the platform in each of 16 directions in the horizontal plane. The force vectors are drawn as projections in each of three planes. Note the clustering of the vectors along two main directions and the predominance of the vertical component for both unloading (+Fz) and loading (−Fz) responses. Inset at bottom left shows the coordinate system for the ground reaction force components. Inset at bottom right shows the coordinate system for horizontal plane translation.

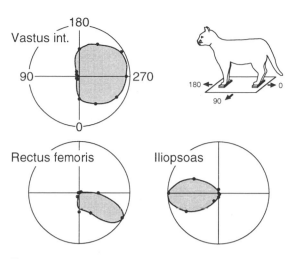

Figure 23.2
Each muscle in the cat shows a characteristic tuning curve in its response to horizontal plane translations of the platform. The polar plots show the mean EMG response of left hindlimb muscles evoked by linear translation of support surface. The radius represents the amplitude of EMG response, and the angle represents the direction of translation (see cat figurine for coordinate reference frame). Responses are normalized to the maximum mean response evoked by translation.

only way that the body can move its CoM or change its velocity is to apply force against the environment.

In experiments designed to analyze equilibrium control, stance is perturbed by the sudden movement of the support surface under the subject. When the surface under a cat is translated linearly in the horizontal plane, the paws are carried along with the support, and the trunk remains behind due to inertia. The cat must apply the appropriate force between paws and ground in order to counteract the displacement of its CoM. Regardless of the direction of surface translation, the cat responds by applying force with each limb in a constrained range of directions (Macpherson, 1988a), as illustrated in figure 23.1 for the left hindlimb. In this study, the platform was translated in each of 16 directions in the horizontal plane, yet the *change* in the force vector exerted by the limb remained primarily within one plane. Although for

any one limb the force changes were constrained to one plane, the *resultant* of the force exerted by all four paws opposed the perturbation.

The limb muscle activation patterns that give rise to the applied forces are complex (Macpherson, 1988b). Each muscle was activated for a broad range of translation directions; the amplitude of the muscle activation increased to a maximum and then decreased as a function of translation direction (figure 23.2). When the relationship of the evoked EMG activity to the forces and net joint torques was examined, it could be seen that the thigh muscles segregate into two functional groups (Jacobs and Macpherson, 1996). The first muscle group consists of the monoarticular flexors and extensors as well as some biarticular thigh muscles, including anterior sartorius, posterior biceps femoris, and semitendinosus. The activity of these muscles was correlated with the vertical force under the paw (figure 23.3A). The second group consists of the biarticular muscles rectus femoris, caudal semimembranosus, and the middle region of biceps femoris. The activity of this group was correlated with the difference in torque at knee and hip (figure 23.3B), and the torque difference was related to the direction of the force under the limb. It is tempting to speculate that the functional subdivision of the hindlimb muscles into just two groups forms the basis for a simplified control scheme for the musculoskeletal system during postural adjustments.

A. Group I: Vertical force

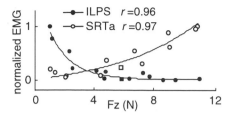

B. Group II: Torque difference

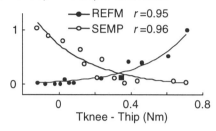

Figure 23.3
Hindlimb muscles of the cat subdivide into two functional groups in terms of their relationship to forces and torques evoked during platform translation. (A) Group I muscles were correlated with vertical force, F_z. The mean response to each of twelve directions of translation is plotted as a function of F_z. The squares indicate quiet stance EMG levels. Extensors increased activity with F_z, and flexors decreased activity. (B) Group II muscles were correlated with the difference of knee and hip torque ($T_{knee} - T_{hip}$). $T_{knee} - T_{hip}$ is a linear combination of F_z and F_y and is related to the direction of force under the limb. ILPS, iliopsoas; SRTa, anterior sartorius; REFM, rectus femoris; SEMP, caudal semimembranosus.

Sensory Control of Posture

Feedback for the control of postural equilibrium likely occurs at several levels and through multiple sensory systems (reviewed in Horak and Macpherson, 1996). Somatosensory, vestibular, and visual information together influence postural orientation and equilibrium and are thought to contribute to an internal representation, or map, of the body and its orientation with respect to environmental variables (Gurfinkel and Levick, 1991). Current models suggest that multiple channels of sensory information are integrated to generate a coherent interpretation (non-cognitive) of the current state of the body posture. This state is then compared to the internal model, and the difference is treated as an error signal that generates motor responses to correct posture (e.g., Kuo, 1995; Merfeld et al., 1993). The various sensory channels—somatosensory, vestibular, and visual—are weighted differently in their contribution to the body map, depending on the current task, central set, previous experience, and so on.

Even with the concept of an internal body map, we still do not know how the nervous system assesses and controls the body's stability for maintaining postural equilibrium. There is some debate as to whether the nervous system actually controls the position of the CoM per se (Massion, 1992). In order for the CoM to be controlled by the nervous system, its position and velocity must be encoded centrally. Because the body can assume many different postural configurations, the CoM is not fixed relative to the body segments and can actually lie outside the physical borders of the body. Because no single "CoM receptor" exists, the central representation of this variable must be derived. Inglis and Macpherson (1995) have suggested that the position and velocity of the trunk can give a good approximation of the CoM because the trunk contains the largest portion of body mass.

Information concerning the position of trunk-in-space can be derived through several sensory channels, such as proprioceptive inputs from the feet and legs, vestibular afferents, and neck proprioceptors (Mergner et al., 1993). Unidentified receptors in the trunk itself may also contribute to this computation through their apparent sensitivity to the direction of the gravito-inertial force (Mittelstaedt, 1992). Somatosensory information appears to have the highest weighting, in general, for triggering and shaping postural responses to unexpected disturbances of stance equilibrium. Evidence for the importance of proprioceptive and cutaneous inputs comes from experiments in which the vestibular end organs have been removed or deactivated by surgical intervention or drugs. In the cat, bilateral labyrinthectomy does not affect the latency and spatial pattern of EMG responses evoked by translation of the support surface, even in the absence of vision (Inglis and Macpherson, 1995). Similarly, human subjects who lack vestibular function bilaterally show a normal response to translation (Horak et al., 1994). Both the direction and velocity of the platform disturbance, which are encoded by somatosensory inputs, are reflected in the spatial pattern and amplitude of the initial burst of EMG activity (Macpherson, 1994b; Diener et al., 1988).

Vestibular information is weighted more heavily than somatosensory information in shaping postural responses under other task conditions. For example, the early response to sudden free fall is mediated by otolithic inputs (Watt, 1976), and it disappears following a bilateral labyrinthectomy. When the support surface is compliant rather than firm, subjects without vestibular inputs are not able to maintain postural equilibrium

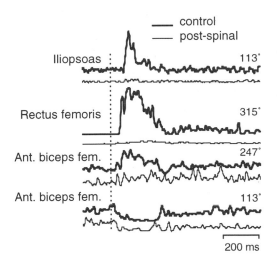

Figure 23.4
The chronic spinal cat has no lateral stability because it fails to produce postural reactions for maintaining postural equilibrium. Traces represent time series of mean EMGs recorded during translations before (control) and after (post-spinal) complete transection of the spinal cord at the T6 level. Direction of translation is indicated in degrees (coordinate reference frame as in figure 23.2). Vertical dotted line indicates onset of platform acceleration. Note the lack of response in iliopsoas and rectus femoris following lesion. Following spinalization, anterior biceps is tonically active during quiet stance; there is a small activation when the limb is loaded (247°) and inhibition when unloaded (113°).

(Black et al., 1988). In general, when the support surface is unstable or even absent (such as during leaping or rapid locomotion), proprioceptive input from the legs and feet may not be sufficient for an accurate computation of trunk-in-space. Mergner's model predicts that, under these conditions, trunk-in-space may be computed by the combination of vestibular and neck proprioceptive inputs (Mergner et al., 1991). Information from the head and neck may be most heavily weighted for determining postural equilibrium under conditions where leg proprioceptive input gives unreliable information regarding the relation between body and support surface. The current challenge is to determine what neural structures are involved in the weighting and interpretation of sensory information, the storage of the internal map, and the control of trunk position and reaction forces.

Preliminary studies of the chronic spinalized cat suggest that posture is a function not of spinal circuits, but rather of higher neural centers. The spinalized adult cat is not able to generate EMG responses appropriate for maintaining postural equilibrium. Such animals are able, through adequate training, to regain sufficient extensor muscle tonus for weight support during stance (Lovely et al., 1986; Rossignol et al., 1986; Carter and Smith, 1986). Moreover, they can maintain a relatively normal postural orientation with the trunk axis parallel to the support surface (Macpherson et al., 1997). However, they are not able to generate the appropriate pattern of EMG response to platform translation, as is shown in figure 23.4 (Macpherson et al., 1997). The only muscles that appear to respond to perturbations are those extensors that are tonically active during weight support. It is worth noting that weight support and equilibrium control are *not* equivalent and thus may be controlled independently. Even though postural response to translation is primarily driven by somatosensory inputs from the limbs, the isolated lumbar spinal circuitry cannot generate the appropriate balance responses. Therefore, the control of postural equilibrium must lie in higher neural centers, above the level of the spinal cord.

Structures in the brainstem and the cerebellum may integrate multisensory inputs for postural control and generate the appropriate descending commands to the lower spinal circuits. The vestibular nuclei and reticular formation receive inputs not only from the vestibular end organs but also from visual and somatosensory systems (reviewed in Wilson and Melvill Jones, 1979). These regions interact strongly with the cerebellar fastigial nuclei and vermal cortex. Damage to midline cerebellar regions is associated with severe balance problems. In addition, various brainstem reticular nuclei have been associated with effects on postural tonus (Luccarini et al., 1990; Mori, 1989).

More detailed insight into the identity of neural circuits responsible for posture control is gained from studies of lower vertebrates such as the lamprey. The next section of this chapter reviews evidence for the hypothesis that the reticulospinal system is a central component of the postural control mechanism.

Postural Control in the Lamprey

Functional Characteristics of the Control System

Postural control in the lamprey involves the control of both orientation and equilibrium, just as it does in terrestrial vertebrates. During swimming, lampreys control the position and velocity of the CoM and the angular momentum of the body about the CoM in order to maintain the postural orientation required for its natural behaviors. The lamprey swims by exerting force against the surrounding water using body undulations that propagate in a wave from head to tail. Its habitual orientation is dorsal side up with the long axis of the body parallel to the horizon (figure 23.5A and C), but it can

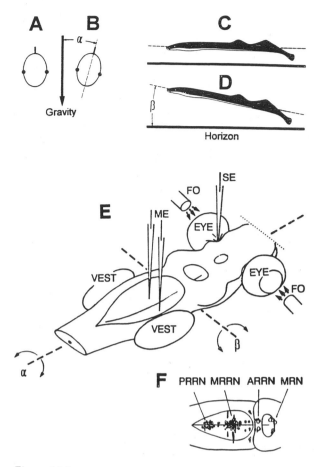

Figure 23.5
The lamprey postural control system. (A–D) Two angles characterize orientation of the lamprey in the gravity field: roll (α) and pitch (β). The lamprey habitually orients with its dorsal side up (A and B, frontal view; C and D, side view). A displacement such as that shown in B is counteracted by the roll control system. The pitch control system can stabilize various pitch angles (C, D). (E) In vitro preparation for studying the roll and pitch control systems. The brain stem with intact vestibular organs (Vest) and eyes could be rotated around its longitudinal axis (α, ±180°) or transverse axis (β, ±180°). The eyes could be illuminated by fiber optic light source (FO), or the optic nerve could be stimulated by an electrode (SE). The activity of reticulospinal neurons from different nuclei was recorded by microelectrodes (ME). (F) Location of reticular nuclei in the brain stem: PRRN, MRRN, and ARRN represent the posterior, middle, and anterior rhombencephalic reticular nuclei, MRN, the mesencephalic reticular nucleus.

also swim at any angle to the horizon (figure 23.5D). It has two control systems for postural orientation: one for roll tilt (figure 23.5B) and one for pitch (figure 23.5D). Roll angle is adjusted by a combination of sagittal and horizontal plane flexion, whereas pitch angle is altered only by sagittal plane flexion of the body (Ullén et al., 1995a).

The aquatic environment places quite different constraints on the postural control system than does the terrestrial one. The surrounding water exerts force (pressure) on the body from all directions so that cutaneous and proprioceptive information does not give a good indication of the body-in-space orientation. Instead, vestibular and visual inputs are more likely to dominate in determining posture control in the aquatic environment for both aquatic *and* terrestrial animals.

Vestibular inputs are both necessary and sufficient for posture control in the lamprey. Both blinded animals and intact animals in darkness orient themselves perfectly well with the help of the vestibular apparatus. Following bilateral labyrinthectomy, lampreys are unable to maintain any specific orientation in space (Ullén et al., 1995b). Visual input exerts only a modulatory effect on the postural control system. Illumination of one eye evokes roll tilt toward the source of light (Ullén et al., 1995b), a phenomenon initially described for bony fish and termed the *dorsal light response* (von Holst, 1935).

Neuronal Mechanisms for Gravistatic Postural Control

In the lamprey, as in terrestrial vertebrates, vestibular afferents terminate on neurons of the vestibular nuclei. The vestibulospinal tract is poorly developed in the lamprey and reaches only the rostral segments of the spinal cord. However, the vestibular nuclei also project to the reticular formation, which gives rise to the main pathways that mediate influences of the brain upon spinal mechanisms, including vestibular influences (figure 23.5F). Reticulospinal pathways reach even the caudal segments of the spinal cord (Brodin et al., 1988).

Considerable information about how the brainstem reticulospinal system processes vestibular and visual inputs has come from an in vitro lamprey preparation. In these experiments, the lamprey brain stem was isolated in a bath, along with the attached vestibular organs and eyes (figure 23.5E). The vestibular organs were stimulated by rotating the entire preparation around either the longitudinal or the transverse axis; the visual system was activated by homogeneous illumination of one eye or by electrical stimulation of the optic nerve.

Vestibular input to the postural control system in the brain stem consists mainly of otolith afferents, most of which are activated by ipsilateral roll tilt. The otolith afferents project via the vestibular nuclei to contralateral reticulospinal neurons (Deliagina et al., 1992b). Thus, reticulospinal neurons are activated by contralateral roll tilt as illustrated in figure 23.6A (Deliagina et al., 1992a). In the in vitro preparation experiments, each reticular nucleus had a characteristic angle of tilt to which it responded maximally: 45° for the mesencephalic reticular

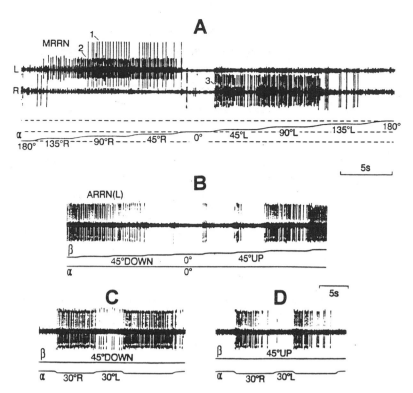

Figure 23.6

Reticulospinal neurons of the lamprey are activated by roll and pitch tilts. (A) The response to roll tilt of neurons recorded extracellularly from symmetrical sites in the two middle rhombencephalic reticular nuclei (MRRN). Units 1 and 2, recorded from the left (L) MRRN, and unit 3 from the right MRRN were activated with contralateral roll tilt.

(B–D) Anterior rhombencephalic reticular nucleus (ARRN) neuron responded to pitch tilt (B) and to roll tilt at different pitch angles (C–D). The main characteristic of the response to roll (activation with contralateral tilt) persisted at different pitch angles.

nucleus, 90° for the middle and posterior rhombencephalic reticular nuclei, and 135° for the anterior rhombencephalic reticular nucleus. Similarly, a subset of reticulospinal neurons was activated with nose-down tilt, and another with nose-up tilt.

Most reticulospinal neurons responded to both roll and pitch deflections from the normal (i.e., horizontal, dorsal-side-up) position (figure 23.6B–D). Therefore, the two control systems that stabilize roll and pitch angles share the same efferent command neurons in the brain stem, implying that information about roll and pitch tilt is not transmitted to the spinal cord by two independent sets of reticulospinal neurons, but rather through the same path. Further processing of this information and the generation of motor commands for changing the roll and pitch angles occur in the spinal cord.

From these data we have inferred a basic organizing principle whereby a given group of reticulospinal neurons, when activated by the relevant deviation of body orientation, will evoke a motor response aimed at restoring the initial position, as shown in figure 23.7A (Deliagina et al., 1993a; Grillner et al., 1995). For example, left-side-down roll tilt will activate reticulospinal neurons on the

right side of the brain (RS[R] in figure 23.7A), which will then evoke a correcting motor response to rotate the body to the right, opposite to the initial roll, and vice versa (Deliagina et al., 1993b). At the normal orientation, the activities of the two "antagonistic" groups of reticulospinal neurons are equal, so no corrective response is evoked (figure 23.7B: 0°, dorsal-side-up). This model stems from the more general idea proposed by von Holst (1935) and Mittelstaed (1975) that the system responsible for maintaining the dorsal-side-up orientation in fish continuously compares the signals from left and right otolith organs and uses the difference to generate compensatory movements for restoring balance. Data obtained in the lamprey strongly suggest that inputs from the two otolith organs are reflected in the activity of left and right groups of reticulospinal neurons. Furthermore, both the comparison of the activities of the two groups and the generation of the motor response occur at the level of the spinal cord.

The same principle applies to the control of pitch angle: reticulospinal neurons activated by nose-up and nose-down tilt will evoke nose-down and nose-up correcting responses, respectively. The pitch angle at which

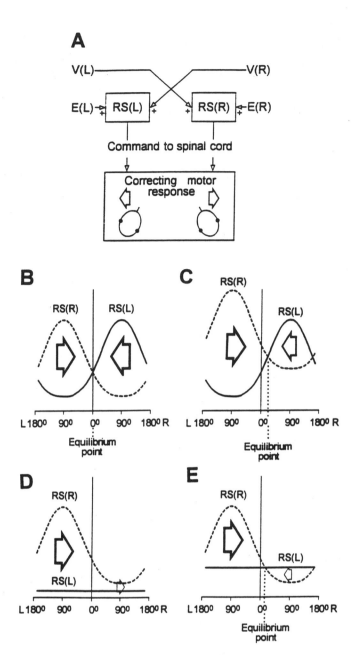

Figure 23.7
Model of the roll control system of the lamprey (A) and its operation under different conditions (B–E). (A) Vestibular inputs, V(L) and V(R), excite contralateral groups of reticulospinal neurons, RS(R) and RS(L). Inputs from the eyes, E(R) and E(L), excite ipsilateral neurons. The two groups produce reciprocal effects in the spinal cord, resulting in rotation of the animal in opposite directions. (B) Operation of the model driven by vestibular inputs only (no illumination of eyes). The curves represent activity in the two groups of RS neurons (*ordinate*) for various orientations of roll tilt (*abscissa*). Corrective motor response evoked by the group with the highest activity is indicated by the arrow. The system has an equilibrium point at 0° (dorsal-side-up) (C) Illumination of the right eye results in an upward offset of the RS(R) curve and a shift of the equilibrium point to the right. (D) Loss of input from the right labyrinth reduces activity in RS(L). The model has no equilibrium point, and activity in RS(R) evokes roll at all orientations in space (indicated by arrows). (E) The equilibrium control, impaired by removal of the labyrinth, can be restored by tonic activation of the deafferented group, RS(L), through electrical stimulation of the optic nerve or the vestibular nerve.

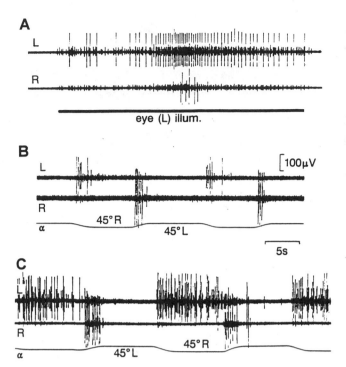

Figure 23.8
Effect of visual input on lamprey neurons of the middle rhombencephalic reticular nuclei, MRRN. (A) Homogeneous illumination of the left eye resulted in a predominant activation of the ipsilateral MRRN neurons (recordings from symmetrical sites). (B) Roll tilts of 45° to right (R) and left (L) evoked responses of similar magnitude in contralateral MRRN neurons. (C) During electrical stimulation (10 Hz) of the left optic nerve, the ipsilateral MRRN response to roll tilt increased dramatically.

activities in the two neuronal groups are equal to each other represents the equilibrium point of the pitch control system.

Integration of Visual and Vestibular Inputs

In the lamprey, vestibular and visual inputs converge on reticulospinal neurons. Illumination of one eye or stimulation of the optic nerve activates ipsilateral reticulospinal neurons (figure 23.8A), predominantly in the middle rhombencephalic reticular nucleus (Deliagina et al., 1993a). The ipsilateral excitatory effects of visual input have been incorporated in the model of the roll control system (see E[L] and E[R] in figure 23.7A).

Tonic visual input to reticulospinal neurons enhances their response to vestibular stimuli. As shown in figure 23.8B, contralateral roll tilt alone evokes rather weak dynamic excitatory responses in neurons of the middle rhombencephalic reticular nucleus. Adding a 10 Hz stimulation of the left optic nerve during roll tilt causes a significant increase in the response of ipsilateral (left) neurons, but only a modest effect on the response of contralateral neurons (figure 23.8C). As shown in the model schematic (figure 23.7C), tonic visual input on the right side will produce a positive offset of the reticulospinal activity curve on the right side. The left and right reticulospinal activity curves will intersect not at 0° but at some rightward roll tilt angle that becomes the new equilibrium point of the roll control system. Thus, the model accounts for the dorsal light response—that is, the inclination of the animal toward the more illuminated eye.

The fact that sensory inputs of different modalities are integrated in the posture control system is very important for recovery of function after damage (e.g., trauma, surgery, etc.) because it provides a mechanism for the substitution of an intact sensory input for a damaged one (Smith and Curthoys, 1989). For example, vision can partially compensate for the loss of vestibular input (Deliagina, 1995). In the lamprey, unilateral labyrinthectomy results in severe motor disorders: the animal cannot maintain equilibrium and continuously rotates around its longitudinal axis when swimming. According to the model (figure 23.7A and D), removal of the right vestibular organ, V(R), deprives reticular neurons on the left side, RS(L), of vestibular input, which leads to reduced activity in this cell group. Activity of reticular neurons on the right side, RS(R), remains high because vestibular input from the left side is intact. The reticulospinal activity curves no longer intersect, and the system thus has no equilibrium point. At any orientation in space, the dominating group—RS(R)—will evoke roll toward the lesioned side, as indicated by the arrows in figure 23.7D. To eliminate the lesion-induced rolling, the tonic activity in the deafferented reticulospinal neurons must be increased to a level at which the two curves, RS(L) and RS(R), will intersect (figure 23.7E), which will allow the roll control system to restore equilibrium control, even though it is driven by only one labyrinth. Vestibular compensation in the lamprey is rather slow, requiring about forty days. However, various means of increasing the tonic activity of deafferented reticulospinal neurons, such as a continuous 10 Hz stimulation of the optic nerve contralateral to the side of the lesion, can lead to immediate normalization of equilibrium control (i.e., "artificial" compensation; Deliagina, 1995). Plastic changes in the postural control system may contribute to the increase of tonic activity in the deafferented neurons during the process of vestibular compensation (see Dieringer, 1995; reviewed in Smith and Curthoys, 1989).

Studies on the lamprey have revealed neuronal correlates of the two aspects of postural control, orientation and equilibrium. The roll control system, based on vestibulo-reticulospinal reflexes, is responsible for the maintenance of the habitual dorsal-side-up orientation of the animal. Moreover, the system can easily be tuned to maintain any desired orientation, such as a visually evoked postural tilt or a centrally generated change in orientation. Only a simple command, such as a tonic bias in the activity of a subpopulation of reticulospinal neurons, is needed to evoke these modifications. The same control system may be used when the behavioral goal is not the stabilization of a given posture, but rather the transition from one posture to another (i.e., motor action). The concept that a movement may originate from a shift of the equilibrium point in the postural control system has been considered for a variety of movements over an extended period of time (von Holst and Mittelstaedt, 1950; Meyer et al., 1976; Feldman, 1986; Orlovsky, 1991).

Summary

Both higher and lower vertebrates exhibit highly specific motor patterns for the control of postural orientation and equilibrium. In the cat, the activation of hindlimb muscles as two functional groups, or synergies, suggests that the nervous system has devised strategies for dealing with the large number of degrees of freedom in the control of the many parts of the musculoskeletal system. Somatosensory, vestibular, and visual information is integrated—perhaps in the brain stem and/or the cerebellum—to compute the position and orientation of the body in space. The information is compared to an internal neural model of body dynamics, and the difference forms an error signal that is used to generate corrective responses. Sensory inputs are differentially weighted depending on the task; proprioceptive inputs dominate for the most common conditions of postural control in the terrestrial environment, but vestibular inputs dominate in the aquatic environment, as exemplified by experiments on the lamprey.

The reticulospinal system plays a crucial role in the control of body orientation and equilibrium in the lamprey. In the cat, the apparent inability of the lumbosacral spinal cord to generate patterned responses for postural equilibrium redirects our attention to the possible role of brainstem structures in postural control in higher vertebrates as well. One can suppose that the role of the reticulospinal system has persisted throughout the course of evolution, as suggested by the many common features of this system in both lower and higher vertebrates: the convergence of sensory inputs of different modalities on reticulospinal neurons (Pompeiano et al.,

1984); the predominance of excitatory responses to contralateral roll tilt (Bolton et al., 1992); the widespread spinal projections of reticulospinal neurons, which allow them to control the position of different body segments in a coordinated fashion (Matsuyama et al., 1988); and the dramatic effects of stimulation of the reticular formation on postural tonus (Mori, 1989).

Acknowledgments

Orlovsky is supported by the Royal Swedish Academy of Sciences (Research Grant for Swedish-Russian scientific cooperation) and by Gösta Fraenckels Fund. Deliagina is supported by Swedish Medical Research Council (grant no. 11554) and by International Research Scholars grant from the Howard Hughes Medical Institute. Macpherson is supported by grants from NINDS, NIDCD, and NASA.

References

Bernstein N (1967) *The Coordination and Modulation of Movements.* Oxford: Pergamon.

Black FO, Shupert CL, Horak FB, Nashner LM (1988) Abnormal postural control associated with peripheral vestibular disorders. *Prog Brain Res* 76:263–275.

Bolton PS, Goto T, Schor VJ, Wilson V, Yamagata Y, Yates B (1992) Response of pontomedullary reticulospinal neurons to vestibular stimuli in vertical planes: Role in vertical vestibulospinal reflexes of the decerebrate cat. *J Neurophysiol* 67:639–647.

Brodin L, Grillner S, Dubuc R, Ohta Y, Kasicki S, Hökfelt T (1988) Reticulospinal neurons in lamprey: Transmitters, synaptic interactions, and their role during locomotion. *Arch Ital Biol* 126:317–345.

Carter MC, Smith JL (1986) Simultaneous control of two rhythmical behaviors. II. Hindlimb walking with paw-shake response in spinal cat. *J Neurophysiol* 56:184–195.

Deliagina TG (1995) Vestibular compensation in the lamprey. *NeuroReport* 6:2599–2603.

Deliagina TG, Grillner S, Orlovsky GN, Ullen F (1993a) Visual input affects the response to roll in reticulospinal neurons of the lamprey. *Exp Brain Res* 95:421–428.

Deliagina TG, Orlovsky GN, Grillner S (1993b) Vestibulospinal reflexes in lamprey. *Abstr ENA Meeting* 1079:278.

Deliagina TG, Orlovsky GN, Grillner S, Wallén P (1992a) Vestibular control of swimming in lamprey. II. Characteristics of spatial sensitivity of reticulospinal neurons. *Exp Brain Res* 90:489–498.

Deliagina TG, Orlovsky GN, Grillner S, Wallén P (1992b) Vestibular control of swimming in lamprey. III. Activity of vestibular afferents: Convergence of vestibular inputs on reticulospinal neurons. *Exp Brain Res* 90:499–507.

Diener HC, Horak FB, Nashner LM (1988) Influence of stimulus parameters on human postural responses. *J Neurophysiol* 59:1888–1905.

Dieringer N (1995) "Vestibular compensation": Neural plasticity and its relations to functional recovery after labyrinthine lesions in frogs and other vertebrates. *Prog Neurobiol* 46:97–129.

Feldman AG (1986) Once more on the equilibrium-point hypothesis (lamda-model) for motor control. *J Motor Behav* 18:17–54.

Fung J, Macpherson JM (1995) Determinants of postural orientation in quadrupedal stance. *J Neurosci* 15:1121–1131.

Grillner S, Deliagina T, Ekeberg Ö, El Manira A, Hill R, Lansner A, Orlovsky G, Wallén P (1995) Neural networks controlling locomotion and body orientation in lamprey. *Trends Neurosci* 18:270–279.

Gurfinkel VS, Levick YS (1991) Perceptual and automatic aspects of the postural body scheme. In: *Brain and Space* (Paillard J, ed.), 147–162. Oxford: Oxford University Press.

Horak FB, Macpherson JM (1996) Postural orientation and equilibrium. In: *Handbook of Physiology*, section 12 (Rowell LB, Shepherd JT, eds), 255–292. New York: Oxford University Press.

Horak FB, Shupert CL, Dietz V, Horstmann G (1994) Vestibular and somatosensory contributions to responses to head and body displacements in stance. *Exp Brain Res* 100:93–106.

Inglis JT, Macpherson JM (1995) Bilateral labyrinthectomy in the cat: Effects on the postural response to translation. *J Neurophysiol* 73:1181–1191.

Jacobs R, Macpherson JM (1996) Two functional muscle groupings during postural equilibrium tasks in standing cats. *J Neurophysiol* 76:2402–2411.

Kappers ACU, Huber GC, Crosby E (1936) *The Comparative Anatomy of the Nervous System of Vertebrates, Including Man.* New York: Macmillan.

Kuo A (1995) An optimal control model for analyzing human postural balance. *IEEE Trans Biomed Eng* 42:87–101.

Lacquaniti F, le Taillanter M, Lopiano L, Maioli C (1990) The control of limb geometry in cat posture. *J Physiol (Lond)* 426:177–192.

Lovely RG, Gregor RJ, Roy RR, Edgerton VR (1986) Effects of training on the recovery of full-weight-bearing stepping in the adult spinal cat. *Exp Neurol* 92:421–435.

Luccarini P, Gahery Y, Pompeiano O (1990) Cholinoceptive pontine reticular structures modify the postural adjustments during the limb movement induced by cortical stimulation. *Arch Ital Biol* 128:19–45.

Macpherson JM (1988a) Strategies that simplify the control of quadrupedal stance. 1. Forces at the ground. *J Neurophysiol* 60:204–217.

Macpherson JM (1988b) Strategies that simplify the control of quadrupedal stance. 2. Electromyographic activity. *J Neurophysiol* 60:218–231.

Macpherson JM (1994a) Changes in a postural strategy with inter-paw distance. *J Neurophysiol* 71:931–940.

Macpherson JM (1994b) The force constraint strategy for stance is independent of prior experience. *Exp Brain Res* 101:397–405.

Macpherson JM, Fung J, Jacobs R (1997) Postural orientation, equilibrium, and the spinal cord. In: *Neuronal Regeneration, Reorganization, and Repair* (Seil F ed.), 227–232, Philadelphia: Lippincott-Raven.

Massion J (1992) Movement, posture, and equilibrium: Interaction and coordination. *Prog Neurobiol* 38:35–56.

Matsuyama K, Ohta Y, Mori S (1988) Ascending and descending projections of the nucleus reticularis gigantocellularis in the cat demonstrated by anterograde neural tracer, *Phaseolus vulgaris* leucoagglutinin (PHL-L). *Brain Res* 460:121–141.

Merfeld DM, Young LR, Oman CM, Shelhamer MJ (1993) A multidimensional model of the effect of gravity on the spatial orientation of the monkey. *J Vestib Res* 3:141–161.

Mergner T, Hlavacka F, Schweigart G (1993) Interaction of vestibular and proprioceptive inputs. *J Vestib Res* 3:41–57.

Mergner T, Siebold C, Schweigart G, Becker W (1991) Human perception of horizontal trunk and head rotation in space during vestibular and neck stimulation. *Exp Brain Res* 85:389–404.

Meyer DL, Platt C, Distel H-J (1976) Postural control mechanisms in the upside-down catfish (*Synodontis nigriventris*). *J Comp Physiol* 110:323–331.

Mittelstaedt H (1975) On the processing of postural information. *Forschb Zool* 23:128–141.

Mittelstaedt H (1992) Somatic versus vestibular gravity reception in man. In: *Sensing and Controlling Motion* (Cohen B, Tomko DL, Guedry F, eds), 124–139. New York: New York Academy of Sciences.

Mori S (1989) Contribution of postural muscle tone to full expression of posture and locomotor movements: Multi-faceted analyses of its setting brainstem-spinal cord mechanisms in the cat. *Jap J Physiol* 39:785–809.

Orlovsky G (1991) Gravistatic postural control in simpler systems. *Curr Opin Neurobiol* 1:621 627.

Pompeiano O, Manzoni D, Srivastava UC, Stampacchia G (1984) Convergence and interaction of neck and macular vestibular inputs on reticulospinal neurons. *Neuroscience* 12:111–128.

Pozzo T, Berthoz A, Lefort L (1990) Head stabilization during various locomotor tasks in humans. I. Normal subjects. *Exp Brain Res* 82:97–106.

Rossignol S, Barbeau H, Julien C (1986) Locomotion of the adult chronic spinal cat and its modification by monoaminergic agonists and antagonists. In: *Development and Plasticity of the Mammalian Spinal Cord* (Goldberger ME, Gorio A, Murray M, eds.), 323–345. Berlin: Springer.

Smith PF, Curthoys IS (1989) Mechanisms of recovery following unilateral labyrinthectomy: A review. *Brain Res Rev* 14:155–180.

Ullén F, Deliagina TG, Orlovsky GN, Grillner S (1995a) Spatial orientation in lamprey. I. Control of pitch and roll. *J Exp Biol* 198:665–673.

Ullén F, Deliagina TG, Orlovsky GN, Grillner S (1995b) Spatial orientation in lamprey. II. Visual influence on orientation during locomotion and in the attached state. *J Exp Biol* 198:675–681.

Vidal PP, Graf W, Berthoz A (1986) The orientation of the cervical vertebral column in unrestrained awake animals. *Exp Brain Res* 61:549–559.

Von Holst E (1935) Über den lichtrückenreflex bei fishen. *Pubbl Staz Zool Napoli* 15:143–158.

Von Holst E, Mittelstaedt H (1950) Das reafferenzprinzip. *Naturwissenschaften* 37:464–476.

Watt DGD (1976) Responses of cats to sudden falls: An otolith-originating reflex assisting landing. *J Neurophysiol* 39:257–265.

Wilson VJ, Melvill Jones G (1979) *Mammalian Vestibular Physiology*. New York: Plenum.

24

Centrally Patterned Behavior Generates Sensory Input for Adaptive Control

Mark A. Willis and
Edmund A. Arbas

Abstract

The successful execution and adaptation of many behaviors typically involves the blending of sensory input from the periphery with ongoing centrally patterned activity. Although it is often said that a behavior is performed in response to a particular sensory input, observations of and experimental results from many animals and robotic systems strongly suggest that behavior may often be actively expressed to acquire the sensory inputs upon which adaptations can be based. For example, the odor-guided flight of the moths that we study requires not only stabilization with respect to a fluid environment, but also strategies (perhaps active ones) to maintain contact with an elusive odor stimulus. The results of fine-scale analysis of this behavior and its underlying motor patterns suggest that the observed zigzagging flight track is organized and expressed as an active strategy to acquire the sensory information necessary to achieve source location. Sensory inputs generated by active behaviors could also aid in adapting the animal's sensorimotor processing to an ever-changing environment.

Once an animal has become active and achieved stable rhythmic locomotion (perhaps while also rhythmically processing a recently acquired meal), higher order control systems orient and direct this locomotion so that the animal can acquire critical resources, avoid stressful situations, and successfully adapt to complex environments. Our studies of the systems that control odor-guided flight in moths have led us to hypothesize that much of the behavior we observe may be organized and executed as an active strategy to acquire the sensory information that is important to successful completion of the task.

Many animals locate distant unseen resources by following trails of odor through fluid media. Certain birds and fish successfully execute this strategy to locate food and mates (see Arbas et al., 1993), but most of our knowledge of this behavior and its underlying mechanisms comes from flying insects, specifically moths (Cardé and Minks, 1997). When an animal moves, the relative movement of the world across its visual receptors creates a complex stimulus known as a *flow field* (Koenderink, 1986). All animals that follow odor trails while suspended in a fluid medium decompose the visual

Although Dr. Edmund A. Arbas died June 18, 1995, his intellect and ideas contributed significantly to the work and ideas presented here.

feedback from flow field cues into self-induced and environmentally induced (e.g., wind or current) components; they then orient their resultant movement into the direction of fluid flow—the direction that will usually "point" to the source of odor (David et al., 1982). One characteristic of odor-guided locomotion, which is remarkably consistent across many animal groups, is a movement track that describes a side-to-side zigzag (Arbas et al., 1993). In the moth *Manduca sexta*, the lateral zigzagging track has a somewhat stereotyped temporal component that is thought to be organized in the central nervous system and that is reflected in the moth's flight direction, which alternates back-and-forth across the wind approximately every 500 msec. Thus, like many complex behaviors, this one requires the integration of multiple sensory modalities—olfactory, visual, and mechanosensory—with ongoing internally generated behavior.

Functional Categories of Sensation

Although behavior is often described as being elicited by a particular stimulus or specific array of stimuli, it has become increasingly clear that discrete, internally organized behaviors may be expressed specifically to acquire sensory input. To better understand and describe the interaction of sensory input and behavior, we have divided sensation into three functional categories: passive sensation, active sensation, and dynamic sensation.

Structures responsible for transducing information about the biotic and abiotic environment into sensory information may range from the very simple (e.g., mechanosensory hairs sensitive to air currents) to the complex (e.g., the eyes of vertebrates or the compound eyes of arthropods). The neuronal networks underlying the sensory structures are adapted to extract various kinds of information from the encoded signals. For example, when an image from an object in the environment falls on one ommatidium of an insect eye, then passes on to the next ommatidium and the next, the underlying neural circuitry may extract information about the motion of the object, thus forming an elementary motion detector (Horridge, 1989; Borst and Egelhaaf, 1989; Strausfeld, chapter 25, this volume). When environmental energy impinges upon a receptor that is not moving, or whose movement has not been actively initiated, we may consider it to be a case of *passive sensation*.

A few specialized animals have evolved mechanisms for what has been termed *active sensation*. They use both specialized motor structures to emit some form of energy into the environment and specialized sensory arrays that, with their underlying neural circuitry, extract

and process information based upon the modification of the emitted signal by its interaction with the environment. Familiar examples of active sensation are echolocation in bats and electrolocation in certain fishes (e.g., Heiligenberg, 1991; Olsen and Suga, 1991a, 1991b).

In an intermediate category of sensory input and behavior, animals perform active (i.e., intrinsically organized) behaviors through which sensory information crucial for adaptive behavior may be extracted from the environment. We refer to this active exposure of sensory structures to the environment as *dynamic sensation*. The idea of generating movement to acquire sensory input (known as *active perception* in robotics literature) is not new to those who work on the design of robots and simulated agents (Bajcsy, 1993; Sandini et al., 1993), but in this field, it has been applied almost exclusively to visuomotor behaviors (Aloimonos, 1993). Those who work on robot design have argued that movement for information acquisition, with respect to vision, should be lumped in with active sensation as defined in the previous paragraph (Bajcsy, 1993). Indeed, entire volumes have been organized around this idea (e.g., Aloimonos, 1993). Because the number of examples of "moving to sense" in animals (i.e., the universality of this principle) has grown tremendously, we feel that a distinction between active sensation and dynamic sensation represents a real and fundamental difference in how behavior is organized and executed.

In the next sections, we demonstrate the ubiquity of dynamic sensation (acting to sense) in the organization of adaptive behavior and how this principle has been successfully applied to simulated agents and robots. We then extend these ideas to our interpretation of odor-guided locomotion in moths.

Acting to Sense: A Fundamental Characteristic of Sensorimotor Systems?

Behaviors that support dynamic sensation range from relatively simple movements to complex patterns of movement, such as searching behavior after the loss of some stimulus. An insect repetitively touching the ground with its antennae or a reptile flicking its tongue in a searching pattern, either to sample a chemical gradient or to discover the location of a chemical signal through sequential samples during trail following, are examples of dynamic sensation directed to the acquisition of olfactory information (Schöne, 1984; Schwenk, 1994). Lobsters actively flick their olfactory organs, the antennules, as a way of decreasing the depth of the boundary layer around the odor sensors and of driving odor molecules into close contact with the sensory receptors—in effect, "sniffing" in an aquatic environment (Schmidt and Ache, 1979).

Although historically termed *active touch*, the expression of centrally organized movements that support the acquisition of textural information through tactile stimulation should really be considered dynamic sensation. Sherrington (1900) may have been the first to note the difference between sensory information acquired during exploratory movements and information experienced passively, and since then a considerable amount of research has been directed at understanding the mechanisms at the foundation of this difference (Gordon, 1978). Recent behavioral studies on seals (Dehnhardt and Kaminski, 1995), sea lions (Dehnhardt, 1994), and rats (Carvell and Simons, 1996) have shown that the facial whiskers (mystacial vibrissae) of those animals operate much like primate hands during exploratory scanning behavior.

Animals navigating toward distant sources of auditory signals also utilize similar stereotyped scanning movements. In some species of tree frogs and crickets, the females locate males for mating by orienting and locomoting toward them in response to their species' specific auditory call (Rheinlaender et al., 1979; Rheinlaender and Blätgen, 1982). Both frog and cricket females move back and forth across a track that would take them directly to the sound source, thus producing a zigzagging track to the sound source. The performance of this active behavior appears to carry the females out of a "zone of ambiguity" directly in front of the sound source, in which their sensory capabilities are unable to determine if the sound source is to the left or right. In addition to the zigzag walking, female frogs often execute a stereotyped side-to-side head movement just prior to initiating locomotion toward the source. Jumps made after head scanning are oriented more directly toward the sound source than those made without head scanning (Rheinlaender et al., 1979).

The rocking and peering motions by which locusts obtain information on jumping distance to targets through motion parallax serve as a well-studied example of active visual scanning (Collett, 1978; Sobel, 1990). In fact, the continuous scanning movements of our own eyes, which allow the extraction of environmental features that would be unavailable otherwise, certainly qualifies as dynamic sensing (Warren and Wertheim, 1990). As flying pigeons approach a perch for landing, they initiate a precisely timed and oriented "head-bobbing" behavior (Davies and Green, 1988). This behavior is performed only during landing (i.e., the orientation and timing of head movements made during landing are unique and different from the saccadic head

bobbing commonly observed during bird walking), and it appears to enhance motion parallax cues regarding the small-scale texture and structure of the landing site (Green et al., 1994). Whether these behaviors are performed to scan the environment for cues critical for survival or to calibrate sensorimotor systems, they are examples of dynamic interactions between peripheral input and intrinsically organized motor behavior.

Recent observations of nest-building bees and wasps strongly suggest that flying insects may perform specific maneuvers to acquire information used in flight control and guidance (bees: Lehrer, 1991, 1993; solitary nesting wasps: Zeil, 1993a, 1993b; socially nesting wasps: Collett and Lehrer, 1993). In each of the species studied, an individual insect flies a stereotyped pattern upon leaving the hive or nest. It has been proposed that specific visual sampling points may be embedded in this pattern, at which information on the orientation and location of the nest and its entrance are acquired (Collett, 1992; Collett and Lehrer, 1993). In some species, visual information seems to be acquired at counterturns (at the ends of straight portions of their path, termed "straight legs" and flown at an angle to the target), during which the head and longitudinal axis of the insect are aimed at the entrance to the nest. In contrast, solitary nesting wasps studied by Zeil (1993a, 1993b) appeared to be memorizing elements of parallax fields that surround major landmarks associated with the nest and its entrance.

Inspired by flying insects, successful designs of both an autonomous simulated flying agent and an autonomous robot have utilized parallax and flow-field cues. The simulated flying agent successfully used motion parallax cues to control its airspeed and altitude as it flew over a varying topography (Mura and Franceschini, 1994). In a similar experiment, an autonomous robot was constructed with a visual control system inspired by the visual systems of flies. Using only simple movements designed to generate flow fields for the visual system, this robot was able to locomote around obstacles and to locate a target without any internal representation of the environment (Franceschini et al., 1992). In fact, the authors of the two studies noted that "the tight reciprocal interactions which are exerted between the sensory block and the motor block suggest that there is a mutual reliance between the two tasks where 'acting in order to perceive' becomes just as important as 'perceiving in order to act'" (Mura and Franceschini, 1994).

Visual flow-field feedback generated by active behavior may also be useful in tasks other than navigation. In an elegant series of experiments on the optomotor control of flight in *Drosophila melanogaster*, Heisenberg and Wolf (1984; Wolf and Heisenberg, 1990) showed that actively generated fluctuations in torque result in the continuous re-calibration of the optomotor control system. They also interpret continual minor fluctuations in torque (even during extended periods of stable flight), typically alternating in direction, as the method by which the optomotor control system actively "feels for" input. In their closed-loop tethered flight experiments, Heisenberg and Wolf (1988; Wolf and Heisenberg, 1990) discovered that the small periodic fluctuations in torque allow the flies to compute a "correlation coefficient" between some aspect of their motor performance (which they call pretorque) and the immediately subsequent visual input (i.e., the angular acceleration of the visual surround). If the correlation between the motor signal and the visual feedback indicates sufficiently coincident movement, then the control system calculates a "coupling coefficient" that allows the system to determine the direction of movement and set the internal gain that will enable the fly to compensate for any asymmetric aspect of its flight performance and thus achieve stable orientation (Wolf and Heisenberg, 1990). The optomotor control system enables the tethered fly to discriminate between self-generated movement and externally generated movement in less than 50 msec. This type of periodic sampling via self-generated movement is considered crucial to the ongoing stability of visually controlled behavior (Wolf and Heisenberg, 1990). Möhl (1988) proposed that a similar form of self-calibration underlies the visual flight stabilization system in locusts.

The work of Heisenberg and his co-workers has culminated in a proposal that the active expression of behavior to generate sensory feedback is a fundamental principle underlying any animal's successful adaptation to its environment (Wolf et al., 1992). The main thrust of this idea is that, in actively executing a behavior, an animal generates the sensory feedback necessary to enable it to distinguish an expected from an unexpected result (e.g., self-motion versus environmentally induced error). The sensory feedback (as well as the central feedback) acquired from active behavior will also assist in successful completion of a particular task or location of a specific goal. Thus, the active expression of behavior that results in an influx of sensory information is a central mechanism in the successful adaptation of any organism to its environment.

Odor-Modulated Flight in *Manduca Sexta*

Adults of *Manduca sexta* are long-lived (e.g., one to two weeks) moths and are responsive to many sensory stimuli as they fly about on summer evenings. The males and females become maximally responsive to the appropriate olfactory stimuli at specific times during the evening. Males sense and are attracted to sex attractant pheromone released by receptive females, whereas females are attracted to the odor of the larval host plant for egg laying (Willis and Arbas, 1991a). Upon encountering a wind-borne plume of attractive odor, a moth changes its behavior in an obvious and characteristic way. First, the moth turns into the wind and begins to fly upwind, controlling its altitude, ground speed, and steering movements by using feedback from visual flow fields (David, 1986). Second, it is thought that the detection of an attractive odor activates an internally generated, temporally regular pattern of counterturns (Kennedy, 1983). The simultaneous expression of these two mechanisms results in the upwind zigzagging flight track that we observe. The visual feedback control systems and the centrally generated turning appear to be modulated in a predictable way in response to changes in the intermittent structure of the odor plume as the moth approaches the odor source (Belanger and Willis, 1996; Willis and Arbas, 1997b).

It is our working hypothesis that zigzagging upwind during flight to an odor source is a behavioral strategy that is organized and expressed to acquire continuously updated information on wind speed and direction and to maintain contact with an elusive odor stimulus.

Modulation of Odor-Guided Flight Performance

As a moth flies upwind in an odor plume, it modulates its steering and velocity in a predictable fashion (Willis and Arbas, 1997a, 1997b). In studies of the upwind flight responses of male moths to female pheromone, we measured patterns of ground speed and track angle modulation that occurred predictably along the track that we observe. (The ground speed and track angles are measurements of the recorded flight track; they are thus the net result of the moth's motor behavior combined with the effects of the wind.) Most moths modulated their ground speeds so that they slowed (sometimes dropping to near zero) at the apex of most turns and then accelerated, reaching peak ground speeds during the straight legs between turns (Willis and Arbas, 1997a, 1997b). The decrease in ground speed during turns might be the result of either changing aerodynamic forces that must occur as the moth turns into the wind at the apex of the turn, or active motor outflow modulation, or a combination of both. Electromyogram recordings made from the flight muscles during flight up a pheromone plume indicate that, in at least some cases, decreases in ground speed are active maneuvers. The recordings show a decrease in wing-beat frequency, as measured by the frequency of bursts of muscle potentials in the wing depressor muscles, coincident with decreases in ground speed during some turns (Willis and Arbas, 1991b, 1994).

The angular orientation of odor-guided flight is also modulated during the performance of this behavior. The orientation of the flight track changes rapidly at or near the apices of the turns, as the moth changes its direction from one side of the wind direction to the other. Many of the straight legs between turns appear to be stabilized around a set point and to be maintained at some angle by the moths (Willis and Arbas, 1997a, 1997b). There does not seem to be any preferred angle for the straight legs, but they typically range 40°–90° either side of due upwind. It has been proposed that repeatedly flying across the wind, at an angle to the wind, exposes the moths to the effects of wind-induced drift and thus might be a strategy for acquiring information about wind direction and velocity (Kennedy, 1986). Our analyses lend support to this idea (Willis and Arbas, 1997a, 1997b).

In contrast to the visually guided parameters (i.e., velocity and steering) of odor-guided flight, the temporally regular counterturning that underlies the zigzagging flight track is modulated to a lesser extent (Willis and Arbas, 1991a). During pheromone-modulated flight, the moths execute a turn across the wind approximately every 500 msec., on average ($X = 530 \pm 20$ msec.; mean $\pm$ SD). According to our measurements, the timing of the turns is one movement parameter that remains stable in the face of the same environmental perturbations that caused the parameters controlled by visual feedback to change significantly (Willis and Arbas, 1991a). The robust nature of timing of the turns has strongly suggested the presence of a centrally generated timing cue that triggers the execution of turns (Arbas et al., 1993). However, we examined the inter-turn intervals individually, instead of on average, and observed a predictable modulation of inter-turn intervals with respect to distance from the source. This observation suggests that the inter-turn intervals may be modulated according to the fine structure of the odor plume, which is known to vary predictably with distance from the source (Belanger and Willis, 1996). Thus, if there is a central circuit underlying the regular timing of the turns, it is affected by olfactory input.

It has recently been demonstrated that tethered flying *M. sexta* males are able to execute organized, temporally regular counterturns without any olfactory stimuli or appropriate visual feedback (Baker et al., 1994). These results provide the best evidence yet for the existence of circuitry in the central nervous system of these moths that is capable of organizing and executing the temporally regular turns that we observe during odor-modulated flight. The expression of this behavior (at least in tethered moths) in the absence of odor stimuli is not necessarily problematic when considered in light of the idea that animals may perform specific maneuvers to acquire specific information. The visual flow-field feedback generated by counterturning might be critically important for orientation and stable flight performance in or out of an odor plume. Thus, we may be studying a higher-order rhythm that is centrally generated and that modulates the expression of the rhythmic locomotory pattern of wing beating.

A network of descending interneurons in the flightless domestic silkworm moth, *Bombyx mori*, are characterized by their unique state-dependent response to pheromone stimulation. They respond to pheromone stimuli by alternating between a low and high firing rate, depending on their firing rate prior to pheromone stimulation (e.g., if the neuron is at a relatively high firing rate, sensation of pheromone causes a change to a low firing rate, or vice versa; Kanzaki et al., 1994). Recent experiments with this moth have demonstrated that state changes in the descending interneurons are closely correlated with the firing of motor neurons that control the muscles underlying head turning as expressed during zigzag upwind walking toward sex pheromone (Mishima and Kanzaki, 1995). Whether similar networks exist in *M. sexta* has yet to be determined.

Conclusion

Although the strongest commonalities between vertebrate and invertebrate motor systems may be the ionic conductances that permit the unique cellular properties underlying many rhythmic motor behaviors, studies of both the higher-order organization of these cells into circuits and of the resulting behaviors have revealed common principles in the organization of motor behavior in all animals—for example, active touch in mammals and tactile scanning behaviors in insects (with possible exception of the simplest animals). It seems possible that a common property of any sensorimotor system (living or artificial) is the ability to actively organize and express behavior that results in the acquisition of information necessary to adapt subsequent behavioral outputs to the current environmental conditions and to the state of the animal (or agent).

References

Aloimonos Y, ed. (1993) *Active Perception*. Hillsdale, N.J.: Lawrence Erlbaum.

Arbas EA, Willis MA, Kanzaki R (1993) Organization of goal-oriented locomotion: Pheromone-modulated flight behavior of moths. In: *Biological Neural Networks in Invertebrate Neuroethology and Robotics* (Beer RD, Ritzmann RE, McKenna T, eds), 159–198. San Diego: Academic.

Bajcsy R (1993) Active perception and exploratory robots. In: *Robots and Biological Systems: Towards a New Bionics* (Dario P, Sandini G, Aebsicher P, eds.), 3–20. Berlin: Springer.

Baker K, Willis MA, Arbas EA (1994) Spontaneous self-generated counterturns during tethered flight of moths, *Manduca sexta*. *Soc Neurosci Abstr* 20:1025.

Belanger JH, Willis MA (1996) Adaptive control of odor-guided locomotion: Behavioral flexibility as an antidote to environmental unpredictability. *Adaptive Behavior* 4:217–253.

Borst A, Egelhaaf M (1989) Principles of visual motion detection. *Trends Neurosci* 12:297–306.

Cardé RT, Minks AK (1997) *Pheromone Research: New Directions*. London: Chapman and Hall.

Carvell GE, Simons DJ (1996) Abnormal tactile experience early in life disrupts active touch. *J Neurosci* 16:2750–2757.

Collett TS (1978) Peering: A locust behaviour pattern for obtaining motion parallax information. *J Exp Biol* 76:237–241.

Collett TS (1992) Landmark learning and guidance in insects. *Phil Trans Roy Soc B* 337:295–303.

Collett TS, Lehrer M (1993) Looking and learning: A spatial pattern in the orientation flight of the wasp, *Vespula vulgaris*. *Proc R Soc Lond B* 252:129–134.

David CT (1986) Mechanisms of directional flight in wind. In: *Mechanisms in Insect Olfaction* (Payne TL, Birch MC, Kennedy CEJ, eds), 49–57. Oxford: Clarendon.

David CT, Kennedy JS, Ludlow AR, Perry JN, Wall C (1982) A reappraisal of insect flight towards a point source of wind-borne odour. *J Chem Ecol* 8:1207–1215.

Davies MNO, Green PR (1988) Head-bobbing during walking, running, and flying: Relative motion perception in the pigeon. *J Exp Biol* 138:71–91.

Dehnhardt G (1994) Tactile size discrimination by a California sea lion (*Zalophus californianus*) using its mystacial vibrissae. *J Comp Physiol (A)* 175:791–800.

Dehnhardt G, Kaminski A (1995) Sensitivity of the mystacial vibrissae of Harbour seals (*Phoca vitulina*) for size differences of actively touched objects. *J Exp Biol* 198:2317–2323.

Franceschini N, Pichon JM, Blanes C (1992) From insect vision to robot vision. *Phil Trans R Soc Lond B* 337:283–294.

Gordon G (1978) *Active Touch: The Mechanism of Recognition of Objects by Manipulation*. Oxford: Pergamon.

Green PR, Davies MNO, Thorpe PH (1994) Head-bobbing and head orientation during landing flights of pigeons. *J Comp Physiol (A)* 174:249–256.

Heiligenberg W (1991) *Neural Nets in Electric Fish*. Cambridge, Mass.: MIT Press.

Heisenberg M, Wolf R (1984) Vision in *Drosophila*: Genetics of Microbehavior. Berlin: Springer.

Heisenberg M, Wolf R (1988) Reafferent control of optomotor yaw torque in *Drosophila melanogaster*. *J Comp Physiol (A)* 163:373–388.

Horridge GA (1989) Primitive vision based on sensing change. In: *Neurobiology of Sensory Systems* (Singh RN, Strausfeld, NJ, eds), 1–16. New York: Plenum.

Kanzaki R, Ikeda A, Shibuya T (1994) Morphological and physiological properties of pheromone-triggered flipflopping descending interneurons of the male silkworm moth, *Bombyx mori*. *J Comp Physiol (A)* 175: 1–14.

Kennedy JS (1983) Zigzagging and casting as a programmed response to windborne odour: A review. *Physiol Entomol* 8:109–120.

Kennedy JS (1986) Some current issues in orientation to odour sources. In: *Mechanisms in Insect Olfaction* (Payne TL, Birch MC, Kennedy CEJ, eds.), 11–25. Oxford: Clarendon.

Koenderink JJ (1986) Optic flow. *Vision Res* 26:161–180.

Lehrer M (1991) Bees which turn back and look. *Naturwissenschaften* 78:274–276.

Lehrer M (1993) Why do bees turn back and look? *J Comp Physiol (A)* 172:549–563.

Mishima T, Kanzaki R (1995) The function of the flipflopping neural activity in the pheromone-searching behavior of a male silkworm moth, *Bombyx mori*. In: *Nervous Systems and Behavior: Proceedings of the Fourth International Congress of Neuroethology* (Burrows M, Matheson T, Newland PL, Schuppe H, eds.), 393. Stuttgart: Georg Thieme.

Möhl B (1988) Short-term learning during flight control in *Locusta migratoria*. *J Comp Physiol (A)* 156:93–101.

Mura F, Franceschini N (1994) Visual control of altitude and speed in a flying agent. In: *From Animals to Animats 3* (Cliff D, Husbands P, Meyer J-A, Wilson SW, eds.), 91–99. Cambridge, Mass: MIT Press.

Olsen JF, Suga N (1991a) Combination-sensitive neurons in the medial geniculate body of the mustached bat: Encoding of relative velocity information. *J Neurophysiol* 65:1254–1274.

Olsen JF, Suga N (1991b) Combination-sensitive neurons in the medial geniculate body of the mustached bat: Encoding of target range information. *J Neurophysiol* 65:1275–1296.

Rheinlaender J, Blätgen G (1982) The precision of auditory lateralization in the cricket, *Gryllus bimaculatus*. *Physiol Entomol* 7:209–218.

Rheinlaender J, Gerhardt HC, Yager DD, Capranica RR (1979) Accuracy of phonotaxis by the green treefrog (*Hyla cinerea*). *J Comp Physiol (A)* 133:247–255.

Sandini G, Gandolfo F, Grosso E, Tistarelli M (1993) Vision during action. In: *Active Perception*, (Aloimonos Y, ed), 151–190. Hillsdale, N.J.: Lawrence Erlbaum.

Schmidt BC, Ache BW (1979) Olfaction: Response enhancement by flicking in a decapod crustacean. *Science* 205:204–206.

Schöne H (1984) *Spatial Orientation*. Princeton, N.J.: Princeton University Press.

Schwenk K (1994) Why snakes have forked tongues. *Science* 263:1573–1577.

Sherrington CS (1900) Cutaneous sensations. In: *Text-Book of Physiology*, vol. 2 (Schafer EA, ed.), 920–1001. Edinburgh and London: Pentland.

Sobel EC (1990) The locust's use of motion parallax to measure distance. *J Comp Physiol (A)* 167:579–588.

Warren R, Wertheim AH, eds (1990) *Perception and Control of Self-Motion*. Hillsdale: Lawrence Erlbaum.

Willis MA, Arbas EA (1991a) Odor-modulated upwind flight of the sphinx moth, *Manduca sexta. J Comp Physiol (A)* 169:427–440.

Willis MA, Arbas EA (1991b) Flight muscle activity underlying pheromone-modulated zigzagging flight in male moths, *Manduca sexta. Soc Neurosci Abstr* 17:492.15.

Willis MA, Arbas EA (1994) Motor patterns underlying pheromone-modulated flight in male moths, *Manduca sexta.* In: *Olfaction and Taste XI* (Kurihara K, Suzuki N, Ogawa H, eds), 850. Tokyo: Springer.

Willis MA, Arbas EA (1997a) Adaptive behavior and reflexive responses: Another perspective on odor-guided locomotion. In: *Pheromone Research: New Directions* (Cardé RT, Minks AK, eds.), 304–319. London: Chapman Hall.

Willis MA, Arbas EA (1997b) Locomotory performance of moths flying upwind in a pheromone plume: Individual variability in pheromone-modulated flight, *J Comp Physiol (A)* in press.

Wolf R, Heisenberg M (1990) Visual control of straight flight in *Drosophila melanogaster. J Comp Physiol (A)* 167:269–283.

Wolf R, Voss A, Hein S, Heisenberg M (1992) Can a fly ride a bicycle? *Phil Trans R Soc Lond B* 337:261–269.

Zeil J (1993a) Orientation flights of solitary wasps (*Cerceris*; Sphecidae; Hymenoptera) I. Description of flight. *J Comp Physiol (A)* 172:189–205.

Zeil J (1993b) Orientation flights of solitary wasps (*Cerceris*; Sphecidae; Hymenoptera) II. Similarities between orientation and return flights and the use of motion parallax. *J Comp Physiol (A)* 172:207–222.

25

Oculomotor Control in Insects: From Muscles to Elementary Motion Detectors

Nicholas J. Strausfeld

Abstract

Tracing the functional organization of the fly's oculomotor system from its motor output back to its visual input has provided unique insights into the cellular complexity of a motor control pathway. Control of head rotational stability during flight is rapid due to the cooperation of fast-conducting pathways from the visual system's lobula plate and organs of balance, the halteres. However, other visually evoked head movements are under the control of numerous descending premotor neurons, each carrying rather imprecise information about visual motion. To achieve precision of the motor output requires further integration of converging inputs, possibly by population coding, at the level of local interneurons in motor neuropil. Although we are virtually ignorant about how such integration is achieved, studies on single descending neurons have elucidated many principles of the functional organization of the fly's visuomotor pathways and, significantly, have led to the cellular identities of its peripheral supply. Studies on optic lobe neuropils have identified the smallest retinotopic interneurons that contribute to elementary motion-computing circuits. These interneurons provide the initial computations about motion direction and orientation that eventually lead to appropriate head movements.

Vertebrates and arthropods by and large share the same environments, so it is not surprising that they have evolved similar mechanisms to detect similar stimuli. Although very different in appearance, the nasal epithelium of the mammal and the fronded antenna of a moth or antennule of a crustacean serve equivalent roles in olfactory sampling and transduction. The brains of vertebrates and arthropods—phyla that have been evolutionarily separate for at least 560 million years—also share design principles. In olfactory and visual centers, vertebrates and insects share similar neuronal arrangements and have similar synaptic and physiological properties encoding similar parameters.

Like the olfactory organs, the eyes of insects and vertebrates appear to differ, yet they share much in common. The vertebrate eye is single lensed, recessed in a socket of the endoskeleton, and moved by a simple arrangement of a few muscles. Insect compound eyes are part of the exoskeleton. To move its eyes, an insect has to move its head. Nevertheless, visually evoked eye movements in insects can be described by the same

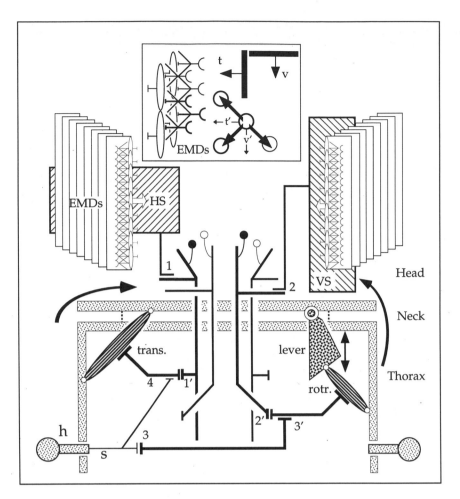

Figure 25.1

Principles of organization of the oculomotor circuit. (Inset, top right) Translational (t) or vertical (v) motion across the retina successively stimulates visual sampling units (open circles, connected by heavy arrows), arranged hexagonally in the retina, along the axes t', v.' Each sampling unit supplies a retinotopic elementary motion detector circuit arranged hexagonally in the optic lobes (left: EMDs; for details see Douglass and Strausfeld, 1995, 1996). These supply wide-field neurons in the lobula plate (HS, VS). (Main figure) Dendrites of wide-field neurons in the lobula plate (HS, VS) are arranged horizontally or vertically to receive ensembles of EMDs, here schematized as strips of elements that, in reality, comprise rectilinear networks as indicated in the left inset. Wide-field neurons respond preferentially to motion direction and orientation. Horizontal motion-sensitive neurons (HS) terminate onto intersegmental descending neurons (at 1) that branch in the prothoracic ganglion onto neck motor neurons (at 1') and then in flight motor neuropils (not shown). Neck motor neurons from HS inputs innervate direct muscles (trans) providing translatory movement of the head (arrow, left). Vertical motion–sensitive neurons (VS) terminate via electrical synapses on descending neurons (at 2) that form electrical synapses onto prothoracic motor neurons (at 2') supplying rotatory muscles (rotr). These act indirectly by moving (double arrow) the cervical sclerite (lever) that articulates with the rear of the head capsule, thus providing head rotation (arrow, right). Organs of balance (the halteres, h) provide mechanosensory axons (s) that synapse at circuits involved in translatory movement (4) and at giant interneurons (3) that project to the opposite side of the nervous system where they form electrical synapses (3') onto head rotator motor neurons, converging with the fast pathway from the lobula plate (2, 2').

criteria and essentially can perform the same functions as vertebrate eyes (Land 1992; Gilbert et al., 1995).

The compound eye's facets represent the surfaces of lenses that, in conjunction with their underlying crystalline cones, focus light onto groups of photoreceptors termed *visual sampling units* because each samples a discrete area of visual space (Franceschini, 1975). Like the vertebrate retina, sampling units relay to retinotopic interneurons that contribute to successive layers of neural filters—stratified synaptic plexi—organized concentrically in four neuropils (lamina, medulla, lobula, and lobula plate). The lobula plate contains neurons that are tuned to wide-field and local motion and that terminate on interganglionic interneurons supplying motor control centers in the thoracic ganglia (figure 25.1). In the first of these, the prothoracic ganglion, its dorsal motor neuropils provide motor neurons that innervate neck muscles.

The central representation of the insect eye is a great deal like the organization of the visual system of vertebrates. Although a detailed discussion of this issue is not possible here, there are compelling grounds for comparing the elaborate synaptic layering in the fly's lamina and medulla to the richly stratified plexiform layers of some vertebrate retinas, such as that of the pigeon (a similarity explicitly recognized much earlier by Cajal and Sanchez, 1915). In the insect lobula, the shapes and arrangements of neurons are reminiscent of pyramidal and stellate cells in mammalian visual cortex (Strausfeld, 1993), and the responses of lobula neurons suggest low-level form vision and color perception (O'Carroll, 1993; Hertel, 1980). The motion-sensitive lobula plate is an achromatic neuropil (Strausfeld and Lee, 1991), whose closest mammalian analogue is the superior colliculus, at least with regard to its visual mapping and its relevance to oculomotor patterning (see Sparks et al., chapter 2, this volume). This chapter on insect oculomotor control focuses on the relationship of uniquely identified head/neck muscles to the visual system; it extends the analysis of visuomotor control of head movements to neurons that provide the earliest computations in oculomotor control: the detection of motion and its direction (Douglass and Strausfeld, 1995, 1996).

Neck Muscle Arrangements and Motor Supply

Fly head movements are provided either by muscles that connect the rear of the head directly to the most anterior part of the prothorax ("trans" in figure 25.1), or by a pair of cervical sclerites ("levers" in figure 25.1) that articulate with the back of the head (Strausfeld et al., 1987). Although arthropod muscles are commonly multi-innervated, each muscle of the fly's head/neck system is supplied by a single motor neuron. There is no peripheral inhibition. Inactivation is central, mediated by GABAergic interneurons in prothoracic neuropil (Strausfeld et al., 1995).

As their name suggests, direct muscles (Strausfeld et al., 1987) directly link the body and the head and extend through the neck. (1) Two pairs of ventral longitudinal muscles extending beneath the gut connect the sternal prothoracic cuticle and the head. Ligaments attach the ventral muscles to the head's exoskeleton immediately beneath the opening in the head through which pass the ventral nerve cord and gut. Each of these muscles receives one motor neuron originating in the brain's suboesophageal ganglion, with a large branch that extends laterally toward the optic lobes. This branch is post-

synaptic to vertical motion detectors that respond to upward movement in the frontal visual field. (2) Pairs of oblique horizontal muscles ("trans" in figure 25.1) attach to the upper lateral prothorax and extend to the rear of the head. These muscles are supplied by motor neuron axons comprising the anterior dorsal nerve, which is supplied by descending neurons (DNs) that are postsynaptic to horizontal motion sensitive neurons (HS in figure 25.1). (3) Three pairs of short spindle-shaped horizontal oblique muscles connect the head to a reinforcement of the dorsal prothoracic exoskeleton (the pronotal apodeme) and extend to the rear of the head. All of these muscles are supplied by motor neurons that arborize in the suboesophageal ganglion.

Indirect muscles are so called because they move the head indirectly via a lever (the cervical sclerite) that articulates with the rear of the head capsule (figure 25.1). These muscles are organized into three groups. (1) Two depressor muscles, linking the lower edge of the sclerite to the sternal cuticle, pull the sclerite downward. Working against these, a levator and an adductor muscle connect the sclerite with the dorsal exoskeleton. Each of the four muscles is supplied by one motor neuron that has similar dendritic arrangements in prothoracic neck motor neuropil (Strausfeld and Seyan, 1985). (2) A quartet of muscles, anchored to the posterior face of the sclerite, extends dorsally and anteriorly to attach to the back of the head. These muscles are supplied by the motor neurons whose dendrites mingle with those supplying group 1 muscles. All the motor neurons contribute to the frontal nerve (thus, FNMNs) and have complex dendritic fields comprising many dozens of branches that divide into discrete fields of postsynaptic processes. These are visited by sensory afferents as well as by local and inter-ganglionic interneurons (Strausfeld and Seyan, 1985). (3) Other muscles abduct and retract the sclerite and are supplied by motor neurons that arise from the suboesophageal ganglion (Strausfeld et al., 1987).

The described muscular organization suggests rather straightforward biomechanics: ventral longitudinal muscles for head depression (pitch); transverse horizontal muscles for sideways head deflection (yaw); and muscles that raise and lower the pair of cervical sclerites for head roll. Cooperative action among the cervical sclerite muscles could also provide all three degrees of movement. Recordings from motor neuron axons supplying the three directional groups (Milde et al., 1987) show that they respond appropriately to the directions of panoramic visual motion (Milde and Strausfeld, 1985; Milde et al., 1987; Gronenberg et al., 1995). Motor neurons supplying head depressor muscles are activated by downward motion of horizontal gratings presented to the binocular part of the visual field. Motor neurons supplying head rotators and levators respond either to ipsilateral downward motion of horizontal gratings or to contralateral upward motion of gratings presented to the lateral (monocular) part of the visual field (Milde et al., 1987; Gilbert et al., 1995). Motor neurons supplying transverse horizontal muscles respond to front-to-back motion of vertical stripes that move around the head's vertical axis, as do motor neurons supplying the shorter oblique horizontal muscles. The three directions of response, shared among four muscle groups, suggest similarities to the functional organization of orbital muscles in primates (Land, 1992) and with the muscles that move the scanning retinas of jumping spiders (Land, 1985) or the eyes of the water flea, *Daphnia* (Consi et al., 1987).

Certain muscles—such as sclerite abductors, retractors, and rotators—are probably involved in nonvisual actions, such as stiffening. Because there is no rigid cuticle in the fly's neck, co-contraction of muscles must provide stiffening during postural control (Gronenberg et al., 1995). Evidence that the neck motor neurons mediating oculomotor responses receive a rich supply of nonvisual information from the brain (Gronenberg et al., 1995) confirms the versatility of a system that must also mediate head movements independent of visual perception (e.g., for grooming or feeding).

Sensory Supply to the Head and Neck System

Neck motor neurons have two main supplies: interganglionic DNs from the brain and primary afferents supplied by the halteres and prosternal organs (Strausfeld and Seyan, 1985).

Halteres are clublike appendages derived from the modified second wing pair. Changes in angular acceleration cause characteristic changes in the halteres' trajectory (Nalbach and Hengstenberg, 1994), which are detected by fields of strain gauges (campaniform sensilla; Gnatzy et al., 1987) on and at the base of the halteres. During flight, the detection of body yaw or roll by the halteres results in compensatory head movements (Hengstenberg, 1993). Clockwise rotation of the body around its long axis elicits counterclockwise rotation of the head. Halteres are the fly's equivalents to the human labyrinth, ensuring that the fly's eyes are in line with the horizon so as to stabilize gaze.

Compensatory head roll is mediated by one of the fastest pathways in the fly's nervous system. A pair of giant interneurons arise from haltere afferents (see figure 25.1)

on one side and terminate at neck rotator motor neurons on the other. The entire pathway is dye coupled—a phenomenon that, in the fly, indicates the presence of gap junctions and electrical coupling (Strausfeld and Bassemir, 1983; Bacon and Strausfeld, 1986).

Rotation of the body around its vertical axis elicits head yaw in the same direction, which is mediated by transverse muscles or by lateral movement of the sclerites driven by the abductor muscle (Sandeman and Markl, 1980). Although no previous comparison has been made, these movements should be slower than head roll because they must involve local interneurons that presumably are chemically postsynaptic to haltere campaniform receptor axons extending as far as the suboesophageal ganglion.

The position of the head with respect to the body is monitored by the paired prosternal organs: triangular areas on the surface of the lower front prothorax equipped with rows of mechanoreceptors. Prosternal organs are touched by a plectrum of cuticle that arises from the cervical sclerite. The position of each plectrum signals the position of the sclerites and thus the position of the head (Preuss and Hengstenberg, 1992). Axons from the prosternal organs relay information to neck motor neurons on the same side of the body (Strausfeld and Seyan, 1985).

Interganglionic Interneurons Supplying Neck Motor Neurons

Mechanosensory-driven compensatory head movements stabilize the retina for detecting motion stimuli (Hengstenberg, 1993). Insect eye movements are not restricted to compensatory actions, however, and many species employ active vision—moving their eyes to detect, fixate, and track targets (see Willis and Arbas, chapter 24, this volume, for a general discussion on active sensing). These eye actions involve fast and slow movements that are similar to the eye movements of vertebrates (Land, 1992; Gilbert et al., 1995). They include optokinetic nystagmus, smooth pursuit or tracking in the same direction as the moving target, fast saccades, rapid head movements toward a moving target in a direction opposite that of the movement, and oscillatory movements used for distance estimation by motion parallax (Collett, 1978). It is therefore important to distinguish between circuits that provide the visual equivalent of fast compensatory head movements, such as those elicited by the halteres, and circuits that underlie more subtle head movements for visual discrimination and tracking.

In general, neck motor neurons and their local inter-neuron circuits are supplied by many convergent descending interneurons (DNs), which receive a variety of visual inputs in the brain. Filling the cervical connective with fluorescent dye reveals about 350 pairs of DNs, of which more than 100 are associated with the optic lobes. DN dendrites are arranged in the brain as clusters ("optic foci" or "optic glomeruli"; Strausfeld and Gronenberg, 1990) cordoned off from each other by glial partitions (Strausfeld, 1993). Clusters are organized into two populations: anterior clusters are mainly supplied by the lobula; posterior clusters are supplied by the lobula plate. Most DNs have additional dendritic fields centrally, which are visited by mechanosensory afferents, chemosensory interneurons, and interneurons from higher cerebral centers. DNs are typically multimodal and correlate sensory information representing the same event. Matching visual and mechanical stimuli more strongly activate a DN than does either when presented by itself (Hensler, 1992).

Descending neurons send their axons down the ventral nerve cord to branch segmentally into motor neuropils (Gronenberg et al., 1995). Generally, the organization of DNs in the thorax reflects their arrangement in the brain. Posterior DN clusters send axons dorsally to neck motor neuropils and to neuropils involved in flight control; the axons branch first in neck motor neuropils (see figure 25.1) and, further posteriorly, among dendrites of motor neurons in the meso- and metathoracic ganglia (Gronenberg et al., 1995). Thus, the same DN can contribute to two motor systems—head movements and flight control—but the behavioral outputs of these systems may not necessarily be coupled.

The crucial exception to this organization is a pair of unusually large diameter DNs that terminate exclusively on motor neurons involved in head rotation (pathway VS, 2, 2', in figure 25.1). These particular descending neurons (termed DNOVS or DN-DC1; Strausfeld and Bassemir, 1985; Gronenberg et al., 1995) are the visual equivalents of giant haltere interneurons. They are dye coupled to their target motor neurons, and their dendrites in the brain are dye coupled to vertical motion-sensitive neurons in the lobula plate. The organization here again suggests an extremely rapid conduction pathway, whose function is revealed by the organization of the DNOVS's inputs. These comprise 8 of a set of 11 visual interneurons, called vertical cells (VS in figure 25.1), whose large anchor-shaped dendrites represent a corresponding array of visual sampling units in the lateral part of the retina. The eight VS cells therefore view the lateral visual field, and their dendrites collate information about visual motion from small retinotopic vertical motion-sensitive neurons called bushy T5 cells. VS cells are depolarized by downward motion of horizontal stripes, as are the motor neurons postsynaptic to DNOVS, which are themselves the postsynaptic targets of the VS neurons. Similar dye coupling can be shown between the lateral dendrites of motor neurons in the brain supplying ventral longitudinal (head depressor) muscles and the VS neurons subtending the frontal binocular field of view. Like the lateral VS cells, these elements respond to downward motion, as do their target motor neurons (Milde et al., 1987).

Segregation of Motion Information to Descending Interneurons

The organization of the VS-DNOVS pathway cannot be generalized to other DNs. The precision of visually evoked horizontal head movements (fixation, smooth pursuit, nystagmus; Land, 1975) is likely to involve cooperative activity among the multitude of other DNs that converge at motor neurons whose activity ensures fine adjustments in the horizontal plane. Any *single* DN prefers certain visual motion cues such as looming objects (Borst, 1991), small targets (Gronenberg and Strausfeld, 1992; Frye and Olberg, 1995), figure-ground stimuli (Gronenberg and Strausfeld, 1992), and visual flow fields (Gronenberg and Strausfeld, 1990). However, a *population* of DNs converging onto the same motor neuron represents a broad range of tuning, and although initially responding to one type of stimulus, some DNs can change their preference to other stimuli.

DNs that supply transverse horizontal muscle motor neurons (figure 25.1, left) approximately respond to translatory motion of wide and/or small field stimuli. Thus, the general information carried by these DNs corresponds to the contractile direction of muscles supplied by their postsynaptic motor neurons and to the directional sensitivity of tangential neurons supplying the DNs from the lobula plate. On the other hand, recordings from DNs supplying indirect muscle motor neurons demonstrate such a variety of responses that further processing by thoracic local interneurons must be necessary in order to effect a meaningful output. We are still ignorant about this part of the system, but future experiments should consider that control systems at this level may be based more on the principle of population coding (see Sparks et al., chapter 2, this volume) than on a strict correspondence between the activity of a DN and a motor neuron.

So far, evidence from premotor neurons suggests that visual information to the head and neck system is parsed into parallel pathways: (1) Rapid compensatory head roll maintains eye stability and is mediated by fast pathways from the lobula plate. The pathways show dye coupling between their constituent neurons and are congruent with an analogous mechanosensory pathway from the halteres. (2) Nystagmic head movements, involving horizontal movements, are most likely mediated by broadly tuned horizontal motion-sensitive DNs and haltere receptor axons. (3) Consensus or population coding is suggested to occur among 40–60 descending neurons, each carrying information about object or local motion, that converge to motor neurons associated with indirect muscles.

The Separation of Motion Information from Other Visual Pathways

In the fly visual system, chromatic and achromatic pathways segregate to the lobula and lobula plate, respectively. The lobula plate consists of a thin tectum-like neuropil divided into layers containing the dendrites and terminals of tangential neurons, so called because they interact with large areas of the projected retinotopic mosaic. Uptake of ^{3}H-2-deoxyglucose, an indicator of heightened metabolic activity, demonstrates direction-specific activation within four lobula plate strata (Buchner et al., 1984). Each stratum represents a different direction and orientation of visual motion and corresponds to the directional selectivities of lobula plate tangential neurons, which, in any given layer, are activated by a specific direction of motion (Hausen and Egelhaaf, 1989). Directional selectivity is also typical of wide-field afferents arriving from the contralateral lobula plate so that certain lobula plate tangential neurons respond to motion around the whole head rather than to just one side of it (Hausen and Egelhaaf, 1989).

Although all lobula plate tangentials are directionally selective, not all respond to wide-field motion. Some, such as the figure-detecting neurons (Egelhaaf, 1985), respond preferentially to the movement of small targets against a texture background. An intriguing feature of the system is that no single type of lobula plate output neuron is the sole visual input to a DN. DNs receive terminals from several lobula plate tangential neurons and from many small-field efferents arranged as palisades across the lobula plate (Strausfeld and Gilbert, 1992). These small-field neurons respond to flicker stimuli (Gilbert and Strausfeld, 1992) or to local motion (Douglass

and Strausfeld, unpublished), and it has been proposed that they may encode the position of a local stimulus in the visual field. Thus, the lobula plate may do more than simply collate information about panoramic motion; it may instead serve the more interesting role of computing where the head should move during object tracking and fixation.

The Origin of Visually Evoked Head Movements: Elementary Motion Computation

Motion detection begins by sequential changes of intensity across the retina. Although the lobula plate plays an obvious role in visuomotor control, it does not itself compute motion. A circuit for this was proposed 50 years ago from observations of beetle optomotor responses. This simple circuit, called an *autocorrelation* model (Hassenstein and Reichardt, 1956), requires the sequential activation of two parallel channels that are asymmetrically connected by a delay line. Motion is detected if the delayed signal from the channel first stimulated is combined with the signal from the second channel. The activity of only one channel is not sufficient to drive a postsynaptic neuron, and only motion in one direction will result in the two channels combining their outputs. Motion detection in the opposite direction requires symmetrical pairs of these *elementary motion detector* circuits (EMDs; figure 25.1), which can then either segregate their outputs to separate postsynaptic (summating) units or together provide an excitatory output for one direction and an inhibitory output for the other. Recordings from VS neurons, for example, demonstrate positive or negative shifts of their membrane potential, depending on motion direction (Hengstenberg, 1982). Spiking lobula plate tangentials are depolarized by one direction of movement and are inactivated or slightly hyperpolarized by movement in the opposite direction (Strausfeld et al., 1995). Recordings from spiking lobula plate tangential neurons (Franceschini et al., 1989) confirm that the smallest movement required to elicit a response is the sequential change of intensity between two neighboring visual sampling units (figure 25.1, inset).

The Cellular Basis for Elementary Motion Detection

Retinal ablation demonstrates that few synapses are interposed between lobula plate efferents and the retina (Strausfeld and Lee, 1991): rapid degeneration of an outer layer of the lobula and the entire lobula plate suggests that the transneuronal degeneration cascade is restricted to a subset of retinotopic interneurons destined for the lobula plate.

Neuroanatomical studies confirm that scotopic photoreceptors (those identified as R1–R6) supply retinotopic neurons with large axon diameters and small dendritic fields that provide relays to small bushy T-cells that supply the lobula plate, mentioned earlier in connection with the VS-DNOVS pathway. In contrast, retinotopic neurons leading to the lobula, supplied by photopic receptors (R7, R8), have larger dendritic fields and smaller axons. They terminate among columnar efferents in the lobula (Strausfeld and Gilbert, 1992).

Although bushy T-cells were once thought to contribute to an EMD, intracellular recordings demonstrate that these neurons do not themselves compute motion (Douglass and Strausfeld, 1995). Instead, only one type, the T5 cell, has directional motion-sensitive responses that are very similar, though of smaller amplitude, to those of the wide-field neurons they supply (Douglass and Strausfeld, 1995). Motion computation occurs distal to the bushy T5 cell, possibly in conjunction with its presumed presynaptic supply—the retinotopic relay neuron Tm1, which itself is supplied by a large monopolar cell (LMC) postsynaptic to the R1–R6 receptors of a visual sampling unit (Douglass and Strausfeld, 1995). Whereas LMCs do not respond to motion (Laughlin, 1984; Shaw, 1984), Tm1 is directionally sensitive. However, because Tm1's dendrites are restricted to a single retinotopic column, it must receive inputs from two neighboring columns in order for it to differentiate motion from flicker. This is problematic for the experimenter because, most peripherally, certain of the EMD's interneurons cannot be motion sensitive.

How then can one dissect this crucial circuit? Strategies currently being pursued involve phylogenetic analysis, electron microscopy, and modeling. Comparisons among taxa having widely differing flight behaviors and habitats demonstrate a phylogenetically conserved assemblage of neurons that includes the bushy T-cells, Tm1s, LMCs, and about five other types of small-field retinotopic neurons known to encode orientation, flicker, and direction (Buschbeck and Strausfeld, 1996; Douglass and Strausfeld, 1995, 1996). Elucidation of their synaptic relationships will make possible the interpretation of their intracellular responses in the context of testable models based on real neurons.

Finally, appropriate motor responses to moving stimuli do not rely exclusively on the direction of motion or on the size of the moving object on the retina. Velocity plays an important role for behaviors such as target interception, landing, and depth perception by motion parallax, where relative motion velocity, independent of direction, is essential for calculating distance (Srinivasan et al, 1993). Intracellular recordings (Douglass and Strausfeld, 1996) have now demonstrated parallel processing by both direction-dependent and direction-independent EMDs, the latter relayed by a second type of bushy T-cell (T4) that is acutely sensitive to velocity and signals motion, but not its direction.

Acknowledgments

Drs. U. K. Bassemir, Jonathan Bacon, J. J. Milde, Wulfila Gronenberg, Cole Gilbert, John K. Douglass, and the late Jong-Kyo Lee have been my valued collaborators during the last twenty years; their work is summarized in this chapter. I thank Dr. J. K. Douglass and Dr. Camilla Strausfeld for comments and improvements to the manuscript. Research is currently funded by the National Center for Research Resources (grant RR08688).

References

Bacon JP, Strausfeld NJ (1986) The dipteran "Giant Fibre " pathway: Structure and signals. *J Comp Physiol (A)* 58:529–548.

Borst A (1991) Fly visual interneurons responsive to image expansion. *Zool Jb Physiol* 95:305–313.

Buchner E, Buchner S, Bülthoff I (1984) Deoxyglucose mapping of nervous activity induced in *Drosophila* brain by visual movement. I. Wildtype. *J Comp Physiol (A)* 155:471–483.

Buschbeck EK, Strausfeld NJ (1996) Visual motion-detection circuits in flies: Small-field retintopic elements responding to motion are evolutionarily conserved across taxa. *J Neurosci* 16:4563–4578.

Cajal SR, Sanchez D (1915) Contribucion al conocimiento de los centros nerviosos de los insectos. I. Retina y centros opticos. *Trab Lab Invest Biol Univ Madrid* 13:1–168.

Collett TS (1978) Peering: A locust behaviour pattern for obtaining motion parallax information. *J Exp Biol* 76:237–241.

Consi TR, Macagno ER, Necles N (1987) Eye movements in *Daphnia magna*: The eye muscles and their motor neurons. *Cell Tissue Res* 247:515–523.

Douglass JK, Strausfeld NJ (1995) Visual motion detection circuits in flies: Peripheral motion computation by identified small field retinotopic neurons. *J Neurosci* 15:5596–5611.

Douglass JK, Strausfeld NJ (1996) Visual motion-detection circuits in flies: Parallel direction- and non-direction-sensitive pathways between the medulla and lobula plate. *J Neurosci* 16:4551–4562.

Egelhaaf M (1985) On the neuronal basis of figure-ground discrimination by relative motion in the fly. II. Figure detection cells: A new class of visual neurons. *Biol Cybern* 52:195–209.

Franceschini N (1975) Sampling of the visual environment by the compound eye of the fly: Fundamentals and applications. In: *Photoreceptor Optics* (Snyder AW, Menzel R, eds.), 98–125. Berlin, Heidelberg, New York: Springer.

Franceschini N, Riehle A, Le Nestour A (1989) Directionally selective motion detection by insect neurons. In: *Facets of Vision* (Stavenga DG, Hardie RC, eds.), 360–390. Berlin, Heidelberg: Springer.

Frye MA, Olberg RM (1995) Visual receptive field properties of feature detecting neurons in the dragonfly. *J Comp Physiol (A)* 177:569–578.

Gilbert C, Gronenberg W, Strausfeld NJ (1995) Oculomotor control in calliphorid flies: Head movements during activation and inhibition of neck motor neurons corroborate neuroanatomical predictions. *J Comp Neurol* 361:285–297.

Gilbert C, Strausfeld NJ (1992) Small-field neurons associated with oculomotor and optomotor control in muscoid flies: Functional organization. *J Comp Neurol* 316:72–86.

Gnatzy W, Grünert U, Bender M (1987) Campaniform sensilla of *Calliphora vicina* (Insecta, Diptera). I. Topography. *Zoomorphology* 106:312–319.

Gronenberg W, Milde JJ, Strausfeld NJ (1995) Oculomotor control in calliphorids flies: Multimodal descending neurons converging at frontal neck motor neuropil. *J Comp Neurol* 361:267–284.

Gronenberg W, Strausfeld NJ (1990) Descending neurons supplying the neck and flight motor of Diptera: Physiological and anatomical characteristics. *J Comp Neurol* 302:973–991.

Gronenberg W, Strausfeld NJ (1992) Premotor descending neurons responding selectively to local visual stimuli in flies. *J Comp Neurol* 316:87–103.

Hassenstein B, Reichardt W (1956) Systemtheoretische Analyse der Zeit-, Reihenfolgen-, und Vorzeichenauswertung bei der Bewegungsperzeption des Rüsselkäfers *Chlorophanus*. *Z Naturforschung* 11b:513–524.

Hausen K, Egelhaaf M (1989) Neural mechanisms of visual course control in insects. In: *Facets of Vision* (Stavenga DG, Hardie RC, eds.), 391–424. Berlin, Heidelberg, New York: Springer.

Hengstenberg R (1982) Common visual response properties of giant vertical cells in the lobula plate of the blowfly *Calliphora erythrocephala*. *J Comp Physiol (A)* 149:179–193.

Hengstenberg R (1993) Multisensory control in insect oculomotor systems. In: *Visual Motion and Its Role in the Stabilization of Gaze* (Wallman J, Miles FA, eds). *Revs Oculomotor Res* 5:285–298.

Hensler K (1992) Neuronal co-processing of course deviations and head movements in locusts. I. Descending deviation detectors. *J Comp Physiol (A)* 171:257–272.

Hertel H (1980) Chromatic properties of identified interneurons in the optic lobes of the bee. *J Comp Physiolhave (A)* 137:215–232.

Land MF (1975) Head movements and fly vision. In: *The Compound Eye and Vision in Insects* (Horridge GA, ed), 469–489. Oxford: Clarendon.

Land MF (1985) The morphology and optics of spider eyes. In: *Neurobiology of Arachnids* (Barth FG, ed), 53–78. Berlin, New York: Springer.

Land MF (1992) Visual tracking and pursuit: Humans and arthropods compared. *J Insect Physiol* 38:939–951.

Laughlin SB (1984) The roles of parallel channels in early visual processing by the arthropod compound eye. In: *Photoreception and Vision in Invertebrates* (Ali MA, ed), 457–481. New York: Plenum.

Milde JJ, Seyan HS, Strausfeld NJ (1987) The neck motor system of the fly *Calliphora erythrocephala*. II. Sensory organization. *J Comp Physiol (A)* 160:225–238.

Milde JJ, Strausfeld NJ (1986) Visuo-motor pathways in arthropods: Giant motion-sensitive neurons connect compound eyes directly to neck muscles in blow flies (*Calliphora erythrocephala*). *Naturwissenschaften* 74:151–154.

Nalbach G, Hengstenberg R (1994) The halteres of the blowfly *Calliphora*. II. Three-dimensional organization of compensatory reactions to real and simulated rotations. *J Comp Physiol (A)* 175:695–708.

O'Carroll D (1993) Feature-detecting neurons in dragonflies. *Nature (Lond)* 362:541–542.

Preuss T, Hengstenberg R (1992) Structure and kinematics of the prosternal organs and their influence on head position in the blowfly *Calliphora erythrocephala* Meig. *J Comp Physiol (A)* 17:483–493.

Sandeman DC, Markl H (1980) Head movements in flies (*Calliphora*) produced by deflexion of the halteres. *J Exp Biol* 85:43–60.

Shaw SR (1984) Early visual processing in insects. *J Exp Biol* 112:225–251.

Srinivasan MV, Zhang SW, Chandrashekra K (1993) Evidence for two distinct movement-detecting mechanisms in insect vision. *Naturwiss enshaften* 80:38–41.

Strausfeld NJ (1993) Cortex-like neural arrangements characterize an insect visual neuropil. *Soc Neurosci Abstr* 19:337.

Strausfeld NJ, Bassemir UK (1985) Lobula plate and ocellar interneurons converge onto a cluster of descending neurons leading to neck and leg motor neuropil in *Calliphora*. *Cell Tissue Res* 240:16–40.

Strausfeld NJ, Gilbert C (1992) Small-field neurons associated with oculomotor and optomotor control in muscoid flies: Cellular organization. *J Comp Neurol* 316:56–71.

Strausfeld NJ, Gronenberg W (1990) Descending neurons supplying the neck and flight motor of Diptera: Organization and neuroanatomical relationships with visual pathways. *J Comp Neurol* 302:954–972.

Strausfeld NJ, Kong B, Milde JJ, Gilbert C, Ramaiah C (1995) Oculomotor control in calliphorid flies: Neural organization in heterolateral inhibitory pathways. *J Comp Neurol* 361:298–320.

Strausfeld NJ, Lee JK (1991) Neuronal basis for parallel visual processing in the fly. *Vis Neurosci* 7:13–33.

Strausfeld NJ, Seyan HS (1985) Convergence of visual, haltere, and prosternal inputs at neck motor neurons of *Calliphora*. *Cell Tissue Res* 240:1–16.

Strausfeld NJ, Seyan HS, Milde JJ (1987) The neck motor system of the fly *Calliphora erythrocephala*. I. Muscles and motor neurons. *J Comp Physiol (A)* 160:205–224.

Contributors

Edmund A. Arbas (Deceased, June 18, 1995)
Arizona Research Laboratories
Division of Neurobiology
University of Arizona
Tucson, Arizona

Yuri I. Arshavsky
Department of Biology
University of California, San Diego
La Jolla, California
and Institute of Information Transmission Problems
Moscow, Russia

Deborah J. Baro
Section of Neurobiology and Behavior
Cornell University
Ithaca, New York

Vladimir Brezina
Department of Physiology and Biophysics
Mt. Sinai Medical Center
New York, New York

Malcolm Burrows
Department of Zoology
University of Cambridge
Cambridge, United Kingdom

Ronald L. Calabrese
Department of Biology
Emory University
Atlanta, Georgia

Lisa M. Coniglio
Section of Neurobiology and Behavior
Cornell University
Ithaca, New York

Elizabeth C. Cropper
Department of Physiology and Biophysics
Mt. Sinai Medical Center
New York, New York

Nicholas Dale
School of Biological and Medical Sciences
University of St. Andrews
St. Andrews, Scotland

Tatiana G. Deliagina
Department of Neuroscience
Nobel Institute of Neurophysiology
Karolinska Institute
Stockholm, Sweden
and A. N. Belozersky Institute of Physico-Chemical
Biology
Moscow State University
Moscow, Russia

Dillip Deodhar
Center for Neurobiology and Behavior
College of Physicians and Surgeons
Columbia University
New York, New York

Robert C. Eaton
Center for Neuroscience
and Department of Biology (EPO)
University of Colorado
Boulder, Colorado

Örjan Ekeberg
Department of Numerical Analysis and Computing
Science
Royal Institute of Technology
Stockholm, Sweden

Abdeljabbar El Manira
Department of Neuroscience
Nobel Institute of Neurophysiology
Karolinska Institute
Stockholm, Sweden

Jack L. Feldman
Departments of Physiological Science and
Neurobiology
University of California, Los Angeles
Los Angeles, California

William N. Frost
Department of Neurobiology and Anatomy
University of Texas Medical School at Houston
Houston, Texas

Apostolos P. Georgopoulos
Brain Sciences Center
Department of Veterans Affairs Medical Center
Minneapolis, Minnesota

Jean-Pierre Gossard
Center for Research in Neurological Sciences
Department of Physiology
University of Montreal
Montreal, Quebec, Canada

Sten Grillner
Nobel Institute for Neurophysiology
Department of Neuroscience
Karolinska Institute
Stockholm, Sweden

John Guckenheimer
Mathematics Department
Cornell University
Ithaca, New York

Ronald M. Harris-Warrick
Section of Neurobiology and Behavior
Cornell University
Ithaca, New York

Jørn Hounsgaard
Section of Neurophysiology
Department of Medical Physiology
University of Copenhagen
Copenhagen, Denmark

Bruce R. Johnson
Section of Neurobiology and Behavior
Cornell University
Ithaca, New York

Larry M. Jordan
Department of Physiology
University of Manitoba
Winnipeg, Manitoba, Canada

Paul S. Katz
Department of Neurobiology and Anatomy
University of Texas Medical School at Houston
Houston, Texas

Ole Kiehn
Section of Neurophysiology
Department of Medical Physiology
University of Copenhagen
Copenhagen, Denmark

Nancy Kopell
Department of Mathematics
Boston University
Boston, Massachusetts

William B. Kristan, Jr.
Department of Biology
University of California, San Diego
La Jolla, California

Norio Kudo
Department of Physiology
Institute of Basic Medical Sciences
University of Tsukuba
Tsukuba, Ibaraki, Japan

Irving Kupfermann
Center for Neurobiology and Behavior
College of Physicians and Surgeons
Columbia University
New York, New York

Anders Lansner
Department of Numerical Analysis and Computing
Science
Royal Institute of Technology
Stockholm, Sweden

Robert M. Levini
Section of Neurobiology and Behavior
Cornell University
Ithaca, New York

James R. Lieb, Jr.
Department of Neurobiology and Anatomy
University of Texas Medical School at Houston
Houston, Texas

Jane M. Macpherson
R. S. Dow Neurological Sciences Institute
Portland, Oregon

Eve Marder
Volen Center
Brandeis University
Waltham, Massachusetts

Bruce S. McEwen
Laboratory of Neuroendocrinology
The Rockefeller University
New York, New York

Brett D. Mensh
Department of Neurobiology and Anatomy
University of Texas Medical School at Houston
Houston, Texas

Michael P. Nusbaum
Department of Neuroscience
University of Pennsylvania School of Medicine
Philadelphia, Pennsylvania

Grigori N. Orlovsky
A.N. Belozersky Institute of Physico-Chemical Biology
Moscow State University
Moscow, Russia
and Nobel Institute for Neurophysiology
Department of Neuroscience
Karolinska Institute
Stockholm, Sweden

Yuri V. Panchin
Institute of Information Transmission Problems
and Moscow State University
Moscow, Russia

Keir G. Pearson
Department of Physiology
University of Alberta
Edmonton, Canada

Jack H. Peck
Section of Neurobiology and Behavior
Cornell University
Ithaca, New York

Ray Perrins
Department of Physiology and Biophysics
The Mount Sinai Medical Center
New York, New York

William C. Probst
Department of Physiology and Biophysics
Mt. Sinai Medical Center
New York, New York

Jan-Marino Ramirez
Department of Organismal Biology and Anatomy
University of Chicago
Chicago, Illinois

Roy E. Ritzmann
Department of Biology
Case Western Reserve University
Cleveland, Ohio

Alan Roberts
School of Biological Sciences
University of Bristol
Bristol, United Kingdom

Stephen C. Rosen
Center for Neurobiology and Behavior
College of Physicians and Surgeons
Columbia University
New York, New York

Serge Rossignol
Center for Research in Neurological Sciences
Department of Physiology
University of Montreal
Montreal, Quebec, Canada

Peter Rowat
Biology Department
University of California, San Diego
La Jolla, California

Allen I. Selverston
Department of Biology
University of California, San Diego
La Jolla, California

Brian K. Shaw
Department of Biology
University of California, San Diego
La Jolla, California

Keith T. Sillar
Gatty Marine Laboratory
School of Biological and Medical Sciences
University of St. Andrews
St. Andrews, Fife, Scotland

Karen Sigvardt
Department of Neurology
University of California, Davis
Davis, California

Jeffrey C. Smith
Laboratory of Neural Control
National Institute of Neurological Disorders and Stroke
Bethesda, Maryland

Judith L. Smith
Department of Physiological Science
University of California, Los Angeles
Los Angeles, California

Steve R. Soffe
School of Biological Sciences
University of Bristol
Bristol, United Kingdom

David L. Sparks
Department of Psychology
University of Pennsylvania
Philadelphia, Pennsylvania

Douglas G. Stuart
Department of Physiology
University of Arizona
Tucson, Arizona

Paul S. G. Stein
Department of Biology
Washington University
St. Louis, Missouri

Nicholas J. Strausfeld
Division of Neurobiology
Arizona Research Laboratories
University of Arizona
Tucson, Arizona

Mark J. Tunstall
Department of Neurobiology and Anatomy
University of Texas Medical School at Houston
Houston, Texas

Ferdinand S. Vilim
Department of Physiology and Biophysics
Mt. Sinai Medical Center
New York, New York

Peter Wallén
Nobel Institute for Neurophysiology
Department of Neuroscience
Karolinska Institute
Stockholm, Sweden

Janis C. Weeks
Institute of Neuroscience
University of Oregon
Eugene, Oregon

Klaudiusz R. Weiss
Department of Physiology and Biophysics
Mt. Sinai Medical Center
New York, New York

Mark A. Willis
Arizona Research Laboratories
Division of Neurobiology
University of Arizona
Tucson, Arizona

Bing Zhang
Section of Neurobiology and Behavior
Cornell University
Ithaca, New York

Author Index

Subject Index

Modulation. *See* Chemical modulation; also Neuromodulation

Modulatory neurons, 111, 212, 218–219

Module, 70

Mollusks. *See specific species*

Monkeys, 10, 12, 25, 49–50

Monoamines, 49–50

Monosynaptic EPSPs, 8, 80, 201

Monosynaptic reflex loop, 80

Monosynaptic stretch reflex, 78

Morris-Lecar model, 141–142, 153

Motion detection, 282–283

Motoneuron conductances, 52–54

Motoneurons, 50, 62, 84, 125–126, 201, 204, 219–220, 280

Motor cortex, 11, 22, 25

Mouse, 49

Movement field of cell, 22

Movement sequences, 13

Moving to sense, 270

MRF, 241

Mud puppy, 48–49

Multicomponent synaptic potentials, 111. *See also* Dual component potentials

Multiplexing, 28–29. *See also* Shared

Multispecies approach, 202–203

Muscarine, 54, 132

Myomodulins (MMs), 219

Na^+ currents, 92, 109, 121, 140

Na^+-dependent K^+ current, 92–93, 95

Negative feedback, 140

Neostriatum, 5

Neurogenesis, 200

Neuro-mechanical model, 169

Neuromodulation, 37, 111, 212, 218–219, 247

Neuromodulators, 184, 209–211, 231–232

Neuromodulatory neurons, 133

Neuronal death, 204

Neuronal respecification, 202

Neuropeptide neuromodulators, 198

Neurotensin, 187

NMA, 188. *See also* NMDA

NMDA, 50, 102

　atrophy of dendrites and, 203

　calcium influx and, 76–78

　excitatory postsynaptic potentials and, 51, 86, 128

　oscillations and, 53–55, 94, 166, 185–186

　remodeling of dendrites and, 203

　rhythm generation and, 47, 49, 86–87

　transmitter identification and, 126

N-methyl-D-aspartate. *See* NMDA

Non-genomic hormonal effects, 196, 198

Non-NMDA, 128. *See also* AMPA; Kainate

Nonspiking local interneurons, 132–135, 218

Nucleus accumbens, 4–5, 7

Nucleus cuneiformis, 3, 5–7, 14

Nucleus pedunculopontine, 5–7

　c-*fos*, 6, 7

　2-deoxyglucose, 6

Nucleus Tractus Solitarius (NTS), 232

Obstinate progression, 4

Octopamine, 38, 133, 210, 211, 232, 247

Oculomotor control in insects, 277–283

Olfaction, 269–273, 277

Optomotor control system, 272

Orienting behaviors. *See* Body orientation and equilibrium in vertebrates

Oscillations

　half-center, 159–160

　5-HT and, 87, 94

　interaction between oscillators and, 144–145

　multiple models of, 101–102

　muscarine and, 54

　NMDA and, 53–55, 94, 166, 185–186

　Xenopus embryos and, 185

Out-of-phase coordination, 63

Oxytocin, 198–199

P. vulgaris, 212

Pacemaker-driven oscillator, 100

Pacemaker-network model, 99–102

Pacemaker neurons, 97, 100, 119–120, 210

Pacemaker potentials, 107–109

PADs, 237–242

Panulirus interruptus, 152, 212, 247, 270–271

Passive Hyperpolarizing Potential (PHP) neurons, 38–39

Passive sensation, 270

Pattern generation

　adaptive control and, 269–273

　cellular properties in, 103

　central pattern generators and, 48, 237

　crustacean stomatogastric, 209–213

　network, 98, 102–103

　postsynaptic mechanisms for, 52–55

　sensory modulation of, 225–233

　　afferent regulation, 230–231, 233

　　phase switching by sensory signals, 227–230

　　sensory feedback, 226–227

　　state-dependent modulation of transmission in reflex pathways, 231–232

Paw shaking of cats, 63, 70

Pedunculopontine locomotor regions, 3

Pedunculopontine nucleus, 5–7

Peptides, 219–221

Peripheral plant, reconfiguration of during feeding behaviors of *Aplysia*, 217–221

Periplaneta americana, 26–28, 34–38

Phase difference equations, 146

Phase lags, 145–146

Phase portraits, 151–152, 154

Phase response curve (PRC) theory, 144–145

Phase switching by sensory signals, 227–230

Phasic component, 177

Phasic inhibition, 50, 100

Phasic signals, 225, 227, 229

Phonation, 126

PHP neurons, 38–39

Phrenic motoneurons, 126

Picrotoxin, 242